Natural Polymers for Inflammatory Bowel Disease Therapy

Edited by

Meenakshi Jaiswal
Department of Pharmacy
Guru Ghasidas Vishwavidyalaya
Bilaspur 495009, Chhattisgarh
India

&

S.K. Lanjhiyana
Department of Pharmacy
Guru Ghasidas Vishwavidyalaya
Bilaspur 495009, Chhattisgarh
India

Natural Polymers for Inflammatory Bowel Disease Therapy

Editors: Meenakshi Jaiswal and S.K. Lanjhiyana

ISBN (Online): 979-8-89881-726-8

ISBN (Print): 979-8-89881-727-5

ISBN (Paperback): 979-8-89881-728-2

Published by Bentham Science Publishers Pte. Ltd. Singapore,

in collaboration with Eureka Conferences, USA.

First published in 2026.

Bentham Science Publishers Pte. Ltd.
No. 9 Raffles Place
Office No. 26-01
Singapore 048619
Singapore
Email: subscriptions@benthamscience.net

BENTHAM SCIENCE

CONTENTS

FOREWORD i

PREFACE ii

LIST OF CONTRIBUTORS iii

CHAPTER 1 INFLAMMATORY BOWEL DISEASE: OVERVIEW, VARIANTS, AND UNDERLYING MECHANISMS 1

Vaishali Bharat, Mohit Rajak, Nidhi Agrawal, S.K. Lanjhiyana, Meenakshi Jaiswal and *Sanjay Kumar Bharti*

INTRODUCTION 2
MECHANISMS IN INFLAMMATORY BOWEL DISEASE 4
Genetic Factor 4
Modern Lifestyle 5
Environmental Pollution 6
Diet 6
Microbiota 6
Smoking 6
Intestinal Barrier 7
Immunological Factors 7
NSAIDs 8
TREATMENT OF INFLAMMATORY BOWEL DISEASE 8
Biologics 10
Anti-TNF Therapy 10
Anti-IL-12/23 Therapy 10
JAK Inhibitors 11
Apheresis Therapy 11
Probiotics 11
Cell Therapy 11
Dietary and Nutrition 12
Antibiotics 12
CONCLUSION 12
REFERENCES 13

CHAPTER 2 MICROENVIRONMENT IN IBD: IMPLICATIONS FOR DRUG RELEASE AND NANO-BASED TARGETING STRATEGIES 18

Mayank Garhewal, Achal Mishra, Shekhar Verma, Naresh Sahu, Arvinder Kaur and *Yogesh Vaishnav*

INTRODUCTION 18
THE IBD MICROENVIRONMENT: PATHOLOGICAL FEATURES 20
Inflammatory and Immune Dysregulation 20
Altered Gut Microbiota (Dysbiosis) 21
Epithelial Barrier Dysfunction 21
Tissue Remodeling and Fibrosis 21
Changes in pH and Enzyme Activity 22
Vascular Changes and Angiogenesis 22
IMPLICATIONS FOR DRUG RELEASE 22
THE IBD MICROENVIRONMENT AFFECTING DRUG RELEASE 23
Altered pH Implication for Drug Delivery with Example 23
Elevated Reactive Oxygen Species (ROS) — Implications for Drug Delivery with Example 23
Enzyme Overexpression — Implication for Drug Delivery with Example 24

Immune Cell Infiltration — Implication for Drug Delivery with Example ... 24
Disrupted Mucosal Barrier — Implications for Drug Delivery with Example ... 24
Dysbiosis and Microbial Enzymes ... 25
MULTIFUNCTIONAL NANOCARRIER SYSTEMS: HARNESSING THE IBD MICROENVIRONMENT ... 25
Dual pH- and ROS-Responsive Nanoparticles ... 25
Enzyme and pH Dual-Sensitive Hydrogels ... 25
CLINICAL IMPLICATIONS AND TRANSLATIONAL CONSIDERATIONS ... 26
TARGETING STRATEGIES IN NANO-BASED DELIVERY ... 27
Passive Targeting ... 27
Enhanced Permeability and Retention (EPR) Effect ... 27
Mucosal Adhesion ... 27
Active Targeting Strategies ... 27
Targeting Immune Cells ... 27
Targeting Epithelial Cells ... 28
Adhesion Molecule Targeting ... 28
Targeting That Responds to Stimuli ... 28
Delivery that is sensitive to pH ... 29
Delivery that is Enzyme-responsive ... 29
ROS-responsive Delivery ... 29
Strategies for Dual or Multifunctional Targeting ... 29
Translational Aspects and in vivo Examples ... 30
CONCLUSION ... 31
DISCLAIMER (ARTIFICIAL INTELLIGENCE) ... 32
REFRENCES ... 33
CHAPTER 3 SOURCES AND BIOMEDICAL UTILIZATION OF NATURAL POLYMERS 40
Neha Dubey, Shilpa Sahu, Sagar Sahu, Rahul Goswami, Shiv Shankar Shukla, Ravindra Kumar Pandey and *Bina Gidwani*
INTRODUCTION ... 41
Origin of Natural Polymer ... 42
Characteristics/ Importance of Natural Polymers ... 43
Renewable Source, Biocompatible, and Non-toxic ... 43
Economic ... 43
Biodegradable ... 43
Easily Accessible ... 43
Tailored Properties with Modification in Functional Group ... 43
Low Toxicity ... 43
Good Mechanical Strength and Process Ability ... 43
Advancements in Natural polymer ... 44
Natural Polymers ... 44
Cellulose ... 44
Chitosan ... 44
Collagen ... 44
Alginate ... 44
Starch ... 44
Proteins or Polypeptides ... 44
Role of Natural Polymers in Pharmaceuticals ... 45
CLASSIFICATION OF POLYMERS BASED ON THEIR SOURCE OF ORIGIN ... 45
Proteins ... 45
Cellulose ... 45

Starch ... 45
Resins ... 46
Semi-synthetic Polymers ... 46
Cellulose ... 46
Cellulose Derivatives ... 46
Starch Derivatives ... 46
Drawbacks of Herbal Polymers ... 49
Batch-to-Batch Variation ... 49
Uncontrolled Rate of Hydration ... 49
TYPES OF NATURAL POLYMERS AND THEIR APPLICATIONS IN THE BIOMEDICAL FIELD ... 50
BIOMEDICAL APPLICATION OF NATURAL POLYMERS ... 57
Antibacterial Properties ... 57
Hydrogel Preparation and Application ... 57
Applications of Hydrogels Derived from Natural Sources ... 58
Drug Delivery System ... 58
Steam Cell Morphogenesis ... 59
Wound Healing ... 60
Skin Tissue Engineering and Regenerative Medicine ... 60
Cell Encapsulation ... 61
RECENT ADVANCES AND INNOVATIONS IN THE FIELD AND FUTURE OUTLOOK 62
Recent Preclinical/ Clinical Advancements in Natural Polymers ... 63
Chitosan (derived from crustacean shells/ fungi) ... 63
Hyaluronic Acid (HA) (present naturally in connective tissue) ... 63
Alginate (Obtained from Seaweed) ... 63
Collagen and Gelatin (obtained from animal tissue) ... 64
FUTURE OF NATURAL POLYMERS IN BIOMEDICAL APPLICATIONS ... 64
CONCLUSION ... 67
REFERENCES ... 68

CHAPTER 4 PLANT-DERIVED POLYMERS AND THEIR CONTRIBUTION TO THE MANAGEMENT OF INFLAMMATORY BOWEL DISEASE. ... 74
Sakshi Gupta, Nidhi Agrawal, Mohammad Akbar Siddiqui, Meenakshi Jaiswal and *S.K. Lanjhiyana*
INTRODUCTION ... 75
Basic Introduction to Plant-derived Polymers ... 76
Pectin ... 76
Inulin ... 76
Cyclodextrin ... 78
Guar Gum ... 79
Cellulose ... 80
Carrageenan ... 81
Alginate ... 82
ROLE OF PLANT-DERIVED POLYMERS IN THE MANAGEMENT OF IBD ... 83
Pectin in IBD ... 83
Inulin in IBD ... 84
Cyclodextrin (CDs) in IBD ... 84
Guar gum in IBD ... 85
Cellulose in IBD ... 86
Carrageenan in IBD ... 86
Alginate in IBD ... 87

CONCLUSION 90
REFERENCES 90

CHAPTER 5 EXPLORING THE ROLE OF POLYMERS DERIVED FROM ANIMALS IN THE TREATMENT OF INFLAMMATORY BOWEL DISEASE 95
Rashmi Dewangan, Nidhi Agrawal, S.K. Lanjhiyana, Sanjay Kumar Bharti and *Meenakshi Jaiswal*
INTRODUCTION 96
THE IMPORTANCE OF ANIMAL-DERIVED POLYMERS IN IBD 97
Chitosan 98
Gelatin 100
Collagen 101
Hyaluronic Acid 103
Albumin 105
Chondroitin 106
ETHICAL CONSIDERATIONS IN OBTAINING ANIMAL-DERIVED POLYMERS 107
Safety Considerations in Sourcing Animal-derived Polymers 108
CONCLUSION 108
DISCLOSURE (ARTIFICIAL INTELLIGENCE) 108
REFERENCES 108

CHAPTER 6 MICROBIAL-DERIVED POLYMERS: REVOLUTIONIZING INFLAMMATORY BOWEL DISEASE TREATMENT 117
Rashmi Dewangan and *Nikita Verma*
INTRODUCTION 118
MICROBIAL-DERIVED POLYMERS 119
Ideal Characteristics of Microbial-derived Polymers for IBD Treatment 120
Biocompatibility and Biodegradability 120
pH-responsive 120
Enzyme-responsive Behaviour 120
Mucus-Penetrating Ability 120
Stability During GI Transit 120
Controlled and Sustained Release 120
Anti-inflammatory and Prebiotic Properties 120
Adhesion and Retention inside the Colon 121
Ease of Functionalization 121
Scalable and Economical Production 121
Classification of Microbial-derived Polymers 121
Cationic Polymers 122
Anionic Biopolymers 122
Non-Ionic Biopolymers 122
Bacteria-derived Polymers 122
Fungal-derived Polymers 123
Algae-derived Polymers 123
ROLE OF MICROBIAL-DERIVED POLYMERS IN IBD 124
Alginate 124
Hyaluronic Acid 127
Xanthan Gum 129
Poly-γ-Glutamic Acid (PGA) 130
β-glucan 131
Algae Polysaccharides 132
Red Algae Polysaccharides 132

Ulva Polysaccharide ... 132
ANIMAL-DERIVED POLYMERS IN IBD: INDUSTRIAL AND BIOPHARMACEUTICAL APPLICATIONS ... 133
CONCLUSION ... 133
DIRECTIONS FOR FUTURE RESEARCH ... 134
REFERENCES ... 134

CHAPTER 7 ADVANCEMENTS IN NANO DRUG DELIVERY SYSTEMS USING NATURAL POLYMERS ... 143
Nidhi Agrawal, Rashmi Dewangan, Mohammad Akbar Siddiqui, Sakshi Gupta, S.K. Lanjhiyana and *Meenakshi Jaiswal*
INTRODUCTION ... 143
NATURAL POLYMERS USED IN NANO DD SYSTEMS ... 145
Cyclodextrins ... 145
Cellulose ... 145
Starch ... 146
Inulin ... 146
Pectin ... 147
Guar Gum ... 147
Chitosan ... 148
Gelatine ... 149
Alginate ... 149
MECHANISM OF DRUG RELEASE FROM NANO FORMULATIONS ... 150
RECENT PATENTS AND MARKETED NANOFORMULATIONS USING NATURAL POLYMERS ... 151
CONCLUSION ... 153
REFERENCES ... 153

CHAPTER 8 NATURAL POLYMERS IN COMBINATION THERAPIES FOR INFLAMMATORY BOWEL DISEASE MANAGEMENT ... 160
Mohammad Akbar Siddiqui, Nidhi Agrawal, Sakshi Gupta, Meenakshi Jaiswal and *S.K. Lanjhiyana*
INTRODUCTION ... 160
Overview of Inflammatory Bowel Disease (IBD) ... 160
Pathophysiology of UC and CD ... 161
Diagnosis ... 161
Challenges in Current IBD Treatments ... 162
ROLE OF COMBINATION THERAPY IN IBD ... 163
COMBINATION THERAPIES USING NATURAL POLYMERS ... 163
Combination Therapy with Small Molecules ... 164
Combination Therapy with Probiotic ... 164
Combination Therapy with Biologics ... 165
Combination Therapy with Antibiotics ... 166
CONCLUSION AND FUTURE PERSPECTIVES ... 167
REFERENCES ... 168

CHAPTER 9 ADVANCEMENT IN BIOENGINEERED NATURAL POLYMERS FOR COMBATING IBD: CURRENT PROGRESS AND FUTURE PROSPECTS ... 173
Shibangi Mukhopadhyay, Yogesh Vaishnav, Achal Mishra, Sanjay Kumar Bharti, Rajkumar and *Meenakshi Jaiswal*
INTRODUCTION ... 173

TYPES OF SYNTHETIC POLYMERS USED TO UPHOLD CONVENTIONAL METHODS TO TREAT IBD 176
Poly Lactic-co-glycolic Acid (PLGA) 177
Polyethylene Glycol (PEG) 178
Polyphenols 178
Polyacrylates 179
Polylactic Acid (PLA) 179
FROM FACING CHALLENGES TO INNOVATION: THE RISE OF REVOLUTIONIZING NATURAL POLYMERS WITH ENGINEERED SOLUTIONS TO COMBAT IBD 180
Challenges in Scale-up and Manufacturing 181
Polymeric Drug Delivery Systems 183
Polymer-drug Conjugate 183
Physical Encapsulation of the Drug in Polymeric Nanoparticles 184
Polymer Microparticles and Hydrogels 185
Smart Polymer-based Systems 185
Smart Hydrogels 185
Smart Nanoparticles 186
Smart Nanofibers 186
Smart Hybrid Bionanomaterials 186
Smart Probiotics 187
PATENT-BASED NEWER TECHNOLOGY TO TREAT IBD 187
MARKETED FORMULATIONS USING ENGINEERED NATURAL POLYMERS 187
Iron-sequestering Polymers for the Treatment of Iron Overload Disorders 193
Azopolymers used as Colon-specific Drug Delivery 193
Eudragit-coated Formulations 193
Certolizumab Pegol (Cimzia) 193
Programmable Polymers for Tissue Healing 194
CONCLUSION 194
REFERENCES 194

CHAPTER 10 CLINICAL APPLICATIONS OF NATURAL POLYMERS IN INFLAMMATORY BOWEL DISEASE: CHALLENGES IN TRANSLATING RESEARCH INTO PRACTICE 200
Prashant Tiwari and *Sunil Kumar Kadiri*
INTRODUCTION 201
Overview of Inflammatory Bowel Disease 201
Need for Novel Therapeutic Approaches 201
NATURAL POLYMERS: PROPERTIES AND POTENTIAL 202
Types of Natural Polymers Relevant to IBD 202
Polysaccharides 202
Proteins 203
Biocompatibility and Functional Characteristics 204
Biodegradation 204
Mucoadhesion 205
Controlled Drug Release 205
Anti-Inflammatory and Immunomodulatory Effects 205
Gut Microbiota Modulation 205
Biological Activity and Healing Properties 205
THERAPEUTIC APPLICATIONS IN IBD 206
Targeted Drug Delivery Systems 207

Polysaccharide-based Systems 207
Micro- and Nanoparticles 208
Biodegradable Polymers for Controlled Release 208
Mucosal Healing and Tissue Repair 208
Collagen-based Scaffolds 208
Hyaluronic acid in Tissue Regeneration 209
Hydrogel-based Systems for Local Application 209
Modulation of Gut Microbiota 209
Prebiotic Polysaccharides 210
Modulation of Gut Microbiota by Chitosan 210
Encapsulation of Probiotics 210
CHALLENGES IN CLINICAL TRANSLATION 210
Stability and Formulation Challenges 210
Degradation of Natural Polymers 211
Challenges in Formulating 211
Variations in Patient Response 211
Personalized Treatment Plans 211
Effectiveness and Side Effects 212
Regulatory and Manufacturing Hurdles 212
Regulatory Issues 213
Challenges in Manufacturing 213
Standardization Challenges 213
FUTURE DIRECTIONS 214
Advances in Polymer Science and Technology 214
Modification of Polymers for Enhanced Targeting 214
Multifunctional Polymers 214
Biodegradable and Bioactive Polymers 214
Nanotechnology and Personalized Medicine 215
Nanotechnology in Drug Delivery 215
Nanostructured Hydrogels 215
Personalized Medicine 215
Microbiome-based Therapies 216
Collaborative Pathways for Clinical Translation 216
Interdisciplinary R&D 216
Regulatory Support and Guidelines 216
Design of Clinical Trial and Recruitment of Patients 217
Cost-Effectiveness and Patient Compliance 218
CONCLUSION 218
AUTHORS CONTRIBUTION 219
DISCLOSURE 219
REFERENCES 219

SUBJECT INDEX 225

FOREWORD

In the edited book "Natural Polymers for Inflammatory Bowel Disease Therapy", the authors explored a new frontier with enormous promise to improve the management of Inflammatory Bowel Diseases (IBD). The increased interest in natural, biocompatible polymers as drug delivery vehicles reflects not just a shift toward more sustainable materials, but also a vital requirement to enhance patient outcomes via precision medicine. This collection is especially useful because of its interdisciplinary approach that connects fundamental research with preclinical and clinical applications. The contributors provided an in-depth investigation of the ways in which innovative drug delivery systems can address the unmet requirements in IBD therapy. This research will surely be an invaluable resource for scientists, doctors, and pharmaceutical experts working to develop the area of targeted drug delivery in IBD. The combination of theoretical knowledge, cutting-edge research, and practical application ensured that readers have a thorough grasp of the potential of natural polymers in IBD treatment.

Rajiv Gupta
Principal and Dean
School of Pharmacy
Babu Banarasi Das University
Lucknow 226028
Uttar Pradesh, India

PREFACE

Inflammatory Bowel Disease (IBD), which includes Crohn's disease and ulcerative colitis, is a chronic and severe disease that affects millions of people worldwide. The ongoing challenge of managing IBD comes from the disease's complex pathophysiology, the recurrent nature of the condition, and the necessity of long-term therapeutic strategies that are both safe and effective. Despite substantial progress in comprehending the molecular mechanisms of IBD, a critical challenge remains in developing innovative drug delivery systems that can improve the efficacy and specificity of treatments.

This book, "Natural Polymers for Inflammatory Bowel Disease Therapy," seeks to illuminate the promising potential of natural polymers in transforming the treatment of IBD. The provided contents investigate the application of naturally derived polymers in the development of sophisticated drug delivery systems, highlighting their potential for biocompatibility, biodegradability, and personalized therapeutic release in inflamed tissues.

In recent decades, synthetic polymers have predominated in medication delivery. However, natural polymers are rapidly being recognized for their distinct features, which can overcome some of the limitations of synthetic equivalents. Natural polymers offer a safer profile for prolonged use, enhanced imitation of the body's components, and the possibility of more accurate targeting of inflammatory areas in the gastrointestinal system. These attributes are especially vital for the management of IBD, as reducing systemic side effects and enhancing localized medication efficacy are imperative for improved patient outcomes.

This book is an invaluable resource for academics, medical practitioners, students, and pharmaceutical professionals working in the domains of drug delivery and gastrointestinal disorders. Each chapter discusses the most recent advances in polymer-based drug delivery methods, emphasizing their applicability to IBD and offering insights into the future prospects of this exciting field. This effort bridges the gap between scientific innovation and practical application, ranging from theoretical polymer chemistry investigations to clinical assessments of medicinal effectiveness.

This collection aims to encourage ongoing creativity and interdisciplinary collaboration in the exploration of the many functions of natural polymers in IBD therapy, thereby enhancing the development of more effective and customized treatment methods for individuals with IBD.

Meenakshi Jaiswal
Department of Pharmacy
Guru Ghasidas Vishwavidyalaya
Bilaspur 495009, Chhattisgarh
India
&
S.K. Lanjhiyana
Department of Pharmacy
Guru Ghasidas Vishwavidyalaya
Bilaspur 495009, Chhattisgarh
India

List of Contributors

Arvinder Kaur	Akash Institute of Pharmacy, Bangalore-562110, India
Achal Mishra	Department of Pharmacy, Guru Ghasidas Vishwavidyalaya, Bilaspur 495009, India
Bina Gidwani	Department of Pharmaceutical Quality Assurance, Columbia Institute of Pharmacy, Raipur 493111, India
Mohit Rajak	Department of Pharmacy, Guru Ghasidas Vishwavidyalaya, Bilaspur 495009, India
Meenakshi Jaiswal	Department of Pharmacy, Guru Ghasidas Vishwavidyalaya, Bilaspur 495009, India
Mayank Garhewal	Department of Pharmacy, Guru Ghasidas Vishwavidyalaya, Bilaspur 495009, India
Mohammad Akbar Siddiqui	Department of Pharmacy, Guru Ghasidas Vishwavidyalaya, Bilaspur 495009, India
Naresh Sahu	Department of Pharmacy, Guru Ghasidas Vishwavidyalaya, Bilaspur 495009, India
Neha Dubey	Department of Pharmaceutics, Columbia Institute of Pharmacy, Raipur 493111, India
Nikita Verma	MATS School of Pharmacy, MATS University, Raipur-493441, India
Nidhi Agrawal	Department of Pharmacy, Guru Ghasidas Vishwavidyalaya, Bilaspur 495009, India
Prashant Tiwari	Department of Pharmacology, College of Pharmaceutical Sciences, Dayananda Sagar University, Karnataka-562112, India
Rahul Goswami	Department of Pharmaceutical Chemistry, Columbia Institute of Pharmacy, Raipur 493111, India
Ravindra Kumar Pandey	Department of Pharmacognosy, Columbia Institute of Pharmacy, Raipur 493111, India
Rajkumar	Department of Pharmacy, Guru Ghasidas Vishwavidyalaya, Bilaspur 495009, India
Rashmi Dewangan	Department of Pharmacy, Guru Ghasidas Vishwavidyalaya, Bilaspur 495009, India
Shekhar Verma	Department of Pharmacy, Guru Ghasidas Vishwavidyalaya, Bilaspur 495009, India
Shilpa Sahu	Department of Pharmaceutical Quality Assurance, Columbia Institute of Pharmacy, Raipur 493111, India
Sagar Sahu	Department of Pharmaceutical Chemistry, Columbia Institute of Pharmacy, Raipur 493111, India
Shiv Shankar Shukla	Department of Pharmaceutical Quality Assurance, Columbia Institute of Pharmacy, Raipur 493111, India

Sakshi Gupta	Department of Pharmacy, Guru Ghasidas Vishwavidyalaya, Bilaspur 495009, India
S.K. Lanjhiyana	Department of Pharmacy, Guru Ghasidas Vishwavidyalaya, Bilaspur 495009, India
Shibangi Mukhopadhyay	Department of Pharmacy, Guru Ghasidas Vishwavidyalaya, Bilaspur 495009, India
Sunil Kumar Kadiri	Department of Pharmacology, College of Pharmaceutical Sciences, Dayananda Sagar University, Karnataka-562112, India
Vaishali Bharat	Department of Pharmacy, Guru Ghasidas Vishwavidyalaya, Bilaspur 495009, India
Yogesh Vaishnav	Department of Pharmacy, Guru Ghasidas Vishwavidyalaya, Bilaspur 495009, India

CHAPTER 1

Inflammatory Bowel Disease: Overview, Variants, and Underlying Mechanisms

Vaishali Bharat[1], **Mohit Rajak**[1], **Nidhi Agrawal**[1], **S.K. Lanjhiyana**[1], **Meenakshi Jaiswal**[1] and **Sanjay Kumar Bharti**[1,*]

[1] *Department of Pharmacy, Guru Ghasidas Vishwavidyalaya, Bilaspur 495009, Chhattisgarh, India*

Abstract: Chronic inflammatory diseases of the Gastrointestinal tract (GI tract) are collectively called Inflammatory Bowel Disease (IBD). These diseases include Crohn's Disease (CD) and Ulcerative Colitis (UC). IBD is an autoimmune disease characterized by persistent and recurrent inflammation of the intestinal tract. It has emerged as a major problem in the field of medicine on a global scale, with its frequency steadily growing. One theory proposes that IBD is caused by an inappropriate and persistent immune response to intestinal microorganisms, which is controlled by the genetic predisposition of a person, originating from the interaction between the host and the microorganisms. An imbalance in the homeostasis of microorganisms leads to colonization and invasion of the gut by opportunistic pathogens, which, in turn, increases the likelihood of a host immunological response and promotes the development of IBD. It is essential to identify the particular pathogens that contribute to the development of IBD to facilitate early detection of the illness. Although the etiology of IBD is largely unclear, it is known that it is caused by a complex interplay of genetic, environmental, and microbial factors, in addition to immunological interventions. This chapter discusses the epidemiology, variants, and underlying mechanisms of IBD, with a particular emphasis on the complex interplay of a large number of factors that are responsible for the pathogenesis of the disease. In addition to this, we talk about the many different therapy choices that are available to combat the condition.

Keywords: Crohn's disease, Gastrointestinal tract, Inflammation, Inflammatory bowel disease, Intestinal barrier, Microorganisms, Pathogens, Ulcerative colitis.

[*] **Corresponding author Sanjay Kumar Bharti:** Department of Pharmacy, Guru Ghasidas Vishwavidyalaya, Bilaspur 495009, Chhattisgarh, India; E-mail: skbharti.ggu@gmail.com

Meenakshi Jaiswal & S.K. Lanjhiyana (Eds.)

INTRODUCTION

IBD is a blanket term for a bunch of conditions that cause inflammation and swelling of the GI tract. IBD is characterized by stomach discomfort, diarrhea bloody stools, weight loss, and the influx of neutrophils and macrophages that create cytokines, proteolytic enzymes, and free radicals, leading to intestinal mucosa inflammation and ulceration [1]. Two major types of IBD are Crohn's disease and Ulcerative colitis [2]. The initial instance of IBD resembling what is now termed ulcerative colitis was documented in the late 1700s, and the name was coined in 1859 [3]. Subsequently, in 1932, CD was acknowledged as a separate condition from ulcerative colitis owing to its transmural and frequently patchy inflamed pattern that can impact any segment of the GI system [4]. Conversely, ulcerative colitis is confined to the colon, usually commencing at the rectum and extending proximally to the cecum in several cases [5]. Patients suffering from UC are at a higher risk of developing colorectal cancer throughout their lives [6]. A comparison of symptoms and cytokine profiles between CD and UC is presented in Table **1**.

UC is a nonspecific, diffuse inflammation of unknown origin that consistently damages the colonic mucosa from the rectal side, frequently resulting in erosions and ulcers [7]. CD is a chronic inflammatory disease of unknown etiology that is characterized by non-contiguous all-stratified granulomatous inflammation and fistulae [8].

Although IBD mostly affects young individuals, it can manifest at any age, with roughly 25% of patients presenting before the age of 20. The highest occurrence of IBD in childhood occurs during adolescence; nevertheless, over 20% of children with IBD will manifest symptoms before the age of 10, and roughly 5% will do so before the age of 5. The prevalence of IBD, particularly childhood-onset IBD, is rising globally. Recent studies indicate a swift increase in very early onset IBD in certain regions with historically high rates of both pediatric and adult-onset IBD [9].

Recent epidemiological research reveals that IBD has shown significant rises in frequency across all continents. The yearly incidence of IBD varies from 10.5 to 46.1 per 100,000 in Europe, 7.3 to 30.2 per 100,000 in North America, 23.7 to 39.8 per 100,000 in Oceania, and 1.37 to 1.5 per 100,000 in Asia and the Middle East [10].

Microbiomes are present in every human ecological niche studied, including the mouth cavity, skin surface, digestive system, oesophagus, lungs, and others [11]. The microbiome consists of bacteria, Archaea, viruses, phages, and fungi. Bacteria are the predominant microbiome in terms of species diversity [12].

Among the areas, the gut microbiota is the most examined because it has the most diverse microbial population. The human digestive system has roughly 1000 types of bacteria, amounting to 100 trillion microorganisms, which are likely important in controlling host homeostasis [13]. Any underlying factor that induces dysbiosis of the gut microbiota may result in immunological compromise and trigger or exacerbate IBD. For instance, the overuse of antibiotics, changes in diet, and non heritable factors, such as environmental factors, smoking, and so forth, may modify the makeup of the gut microbiota, potentially leading to the development of IBD, and thus must be considered in the etiopathogenesis of these diseases [14]. The gut microbial makeup differs between individuals with IBD and healthy individuals [15].

Although IBD is primarily linked to an imbalance of gut microbiota and its impact on the immune system, the underlying cause of dysbiosis and pathogenesis remains unclear. In recent years, advancements have been made in elucidating the pathophysiology of this illness [16]. Research indicates that the development of IBD is linked to a combination of the host's genetic vulnerability, intestinal microbiota, various environmental factors, and immunological anomalies [17]. Fig. (**1**) shows the role of gut dysbiosis in the pathogenesis of IBD. The combination of a compromised intestinal barrier and gut dysbiosis is likely to perpetuate mucosal inflammation and potentially result in IBD [18].

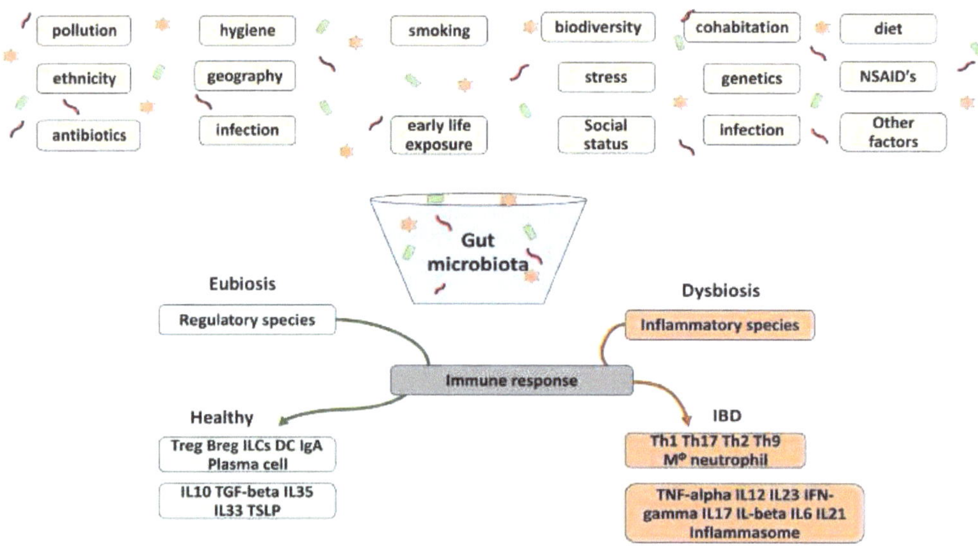

Fig. (1). Role of gut dysbiosis in the pathogenesis of IBD.

Table 1. Comparison between symptoms and cytokine profiles of UC and CD.

Symptom	Ulcerative colitis	Crohn's disease	References
Area affected	Any area in the innermost lining of the colon, continuous with no patches of normal tissue	Most commonly, the lower ileum, but can flare up anywhere, including the colon; patches of normal tissue between affected areas; can affect the entire intestinal wall	[19, 20]
Abdominal pain/cramping	Lower abdominal cramping, mild tenderness	Moderate to severe abdominal tenderness in the right lower quadrant	[21]
Diarrhea	Typically, four episodes per day	Typically, four episodes per day	[21, 22]
Blood in stool	Present	Present	[23]
Fever	Low grade in severe cases	Low grade in severe cases	[23]
Physical examination	A rectal exam may show peri-anal irritation, fissures, hemorrhoids, fistulas, and abscesses	Peritoneal irritation, abdominal or pelvic mass	[24]
Appetite	Often decreased during periods of disease exacerbation	Often decreased during periods of disease exacerbation	[25]

MECHANISMS IN INFLAMMATORY BOWEL DISEASE

IBD, such as CD and UC, are long-term conditions that cause inflammation in the gastrointestinal tract. These conditions are associated with major morbidity and mortality, resulting in substantial patient burden and costs to healthcare systems [26]. This chronic condition results from a complex interplay among several factors outlined in Fig. (**2**). These factors include genetic, environmental, and pollution-related impacts, which are further discussed in this section.

There are different factors affecting IBD: -

Genetic Factor

Our comprehension of the genetic factors in IBD has experienced a transformation, mostly due to innovative genotyping and sequencing technology [27]. Recent advancements in DNA analysis and sequencing have facilitated Genome-Wide Association Studies (GWAS) for inflammatory bowel disease IBD, discovering Single Nucleotide Polymorphisms (SNPs). These studies have found 163 IBD-associated loci: 110 are linked to both UC and CD, 30 are specific to CD, and 23 are specific to UC [28].

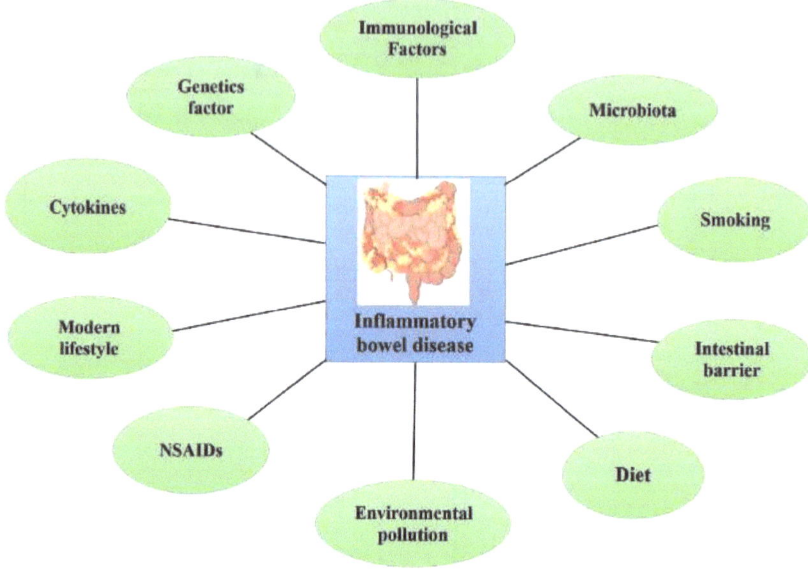

Fig. (2). Pathophysiology of Inflammatory Bowel Disease.

The Nucleotide-binding Oligomerization Domain 2 (NOD2) gene is frequently mutated in CD patients, occurring in about one-third of cases. NOD2, part of the Nod-Like Receptor (NLR) family, detects microbial invaders, recognizing a peptidoglycan fragment called Muramyl Dipeptide (MDP) found in bacterial cell walls. When NOD2 binds MDP, it activates pathways that stimulate the immune response, including Nuclear Factor kappa B (NF-κB), leading to the secretion of proinflammatory cytokines [29].

Additionally, NOD2 mutations are linked to issues with autophagy, which helps trap and eliminate bacteria. Another associated gene, ATG16L1, is crucial for autophagy, and its polymorphisms can disrupt T-cell responses, leading to inflammation and mucosal barrier disruption. Current investigations using advanced genetic analysis techniques, such as GWAS and SNPs, have identified a significant connection between the IL23R gene and IBD. Both UC and CD have been linked to specific genetic locations, including IL23R, IL12B, JAK2, and STAT3. The disease mechanisms of IBD involve the Th17 and IL-23 pathways [30].

Modern Lifestyle

Lifestyle factors such as physical activity, obesity, stress, sleep, and smoking have varying effects on CD and UC and can influence the risk and outcomes of IBD [31]. The impact of alcohol consumption and the influence of sleep on IBD require further research. A study using data from the UK Biobank to explore the interaction between genetic risk and lifestyle factors suggests that a healthy lifestyle can mitigate the genetic risk of developing IBD [32].

Environmental Pollution

Exposure to air pollution has been linked to IBD. Short-term exposure to high levels of airborne particles can increase gut permeability and immune response [33], while chronic exposure can lead to inflammation and changes in the gut microbiota [34]. Some studies indicate a connection between air pollution components (NO_2, SO_2, CO, and fine particulate matter) and IBD. For instance, higher NO_2 levels are linked to Crohn's disease in young individuals, and higher SO_2 levels are linked to ulcerative colitis. In areas with high air pollution emissions, there is a significant increase in IBD hospitalizations [35].

Diet

Dietary changes in modern society have been linked to IBD, as they can alter gut microbiota, leading to an abnormal immune response. People with IBD often have reduced microbial diversity, with more harmful bacteria and fewer beneficial ones. Studies suggest diet can influence IBD risk; for example, high fiber intake, especially from fruits and vegetables, reduces the risk of Crohn's disease, while certain fats (n3 PUFAs) can lessen the severity of colitis. Conversely, a diet high in animal protein increases the risk of IBD. These effects are observed both before and after the onset of IBD [36].

Microbiota

The intestinal microbiota is essential for both maintaining health and regulating illness [34]. IBD is associated with an imbalance in gut bacteria; there is a decrease in diversity and an increase in harmful bacteria like Proteobacteria, while helpful bacteria such as *Faecalibacterium prausnitzii* and *Roseburia* decrease. This imbalance causes inflammation and damages the gut's protective layer, allowing bacteria to spread into deeper tissue and create a cycle of damage. Beneficial bacteria that produce butyrate, like *Faecalibacterium*, help reduce inflammation, and their decline is linked to IBD. Harmful bacteria like *Escherichia coli* alter inflammation and cause IBD [37].

Smoking

Smoking is a risk factor in IBD, with differing effects on CD and UC. Smoking is linked to an increased risk of CD, leading to more severe disease [38, 39]. On the other hand, smoking appears to have a protective effect against UC, with smokers experiencing less severe disease. However, quitting smoking in UC patients can worsen disease outcomes. Studies also show that smoking has a high impact on CD, and smoke can have similar negative effects as active smoking. Smoking cessation benefits CD patients, lowering relapse risk, while nicotine may help induce remission in UC, despite mild side effects [40].

Smoking affects the immune system, both in terms of immune responses and the production of mucus in the colon. Nicotine, a key substance in cigarettes, inhibits the function of T-helper type 2 cells (Th2 cells) but does not affect Th1 cell function. There is also evidence suggesting that smoking impacts autophagy, a process that is thought to play a significant role in Crohn's disease [17].

Intestinal Barrier

The intestinal barrier, made up of physical, chemical, immune, and microbial defenses, plays an essential role in maintaining the gastrointestinal tract [41]. Defects in the intestinal epithelial barrier cause IBD, affecting protective mechanisms such as Pattern Recognition Receptors (PRRs), antimicrobial peptides, the mucus layer, autophagy, and barrier permeability [42]. These defects increase microbial contact with the epithelium, triggering excessive immune responses that contribute to chronic inflammation. IBD primarily affects heavily colonized gut areas like the distal ileum and colon, indicating the involvement of the microbiota in the disease. Studies show that CD is linked to luminal contents and the microbial role in inflammation. Despite extensive research, no specific pathogen has been identified; however, microbial defects play a crucial role in IBD pathogenesis [43].

Immunological Factors

The pathogenesis of IBD involves dysfunctions in both innate and adaptive immune systems. Recent investigations have identified immune factors, particularly T-cell responses, in IBD. Ulcerative Colitis (UC) has been associated with Th1 and Th2 responses, whereas Th17 cells are implicated in the pathogenesis of IBD. Innate responses like epithelial function, the microbiota, and phagocytosis are the main factors in different types of IBD [29]. The epidemiology of IBD is characterized by a decrease in goblet cells, which secrete substances important for innate immunity and mucus that protects the gut lining. This leads to an impaired intestinal barrier and increased exposure to antigens, triggering the innate immune response. Various immune cells and cytokines are involved, with Antigen-Presenting Cells (APCs) connecting innate and adaptive immune responses. An imbalance of pro-inflammatory factors at the expense of anti-inflammatory processes leads to chronic inflammation and damage to the intestinal barrier [44].

The IBD involves a complex interplay of immune cells (like dendritic cells, T cells, and macrophages) and cytokines that drive tissue damage and inflammation. Pro-inflammatory cytokines (*e.g.*, TNF-α, IL-1, IL-6) contribute to disease progression, while anti-inflammatory cytokines (*e.g.*, TGF-β, IL-10) help control IBD. Understanding these immune pathways is crucial for developing effective treatments for IBD [45].

NSAIDs

NSAIDs are commonly used as anti-inflammatory agents but are associated with gastric ulcers and the development of IBD [46]. Their mechanism involves the inhibition of protective prostaglandins through nonselective COX inhibition, leading to damage of the intestinal mucosal layer. Long-term or frequent NSAID use increases the risk of CD and UC. Humans using NSAIDs for at least 15 days per month show a higher risk of both conditions. COX-1 inhibitor drugs lead to a reduction in protective prostaglandins, which results in an increased risk of IBD, but selective COX-2 inhibitors like celecoxib do not increase IBD [34]. Although IBD is not directly caused by anxiety or depression, these conditions can affect the development of the disease . A study found that both CD and UC disease can lead to mental health issues in patients. Anxiety and depression can cause psychological stress that can worsen IBD symptoms and trigger recurrence. The relationship between IBD and mental health is complicated, as the gut-brain axis, inflammation, and alterations in gut microbiota are some of the ways that both disorders can affect other physiological systems. Anxiety and depression can have significant effects on a patient's quality of life and the progression of their illness [47].

TREATMENT OF INFLAMMATORY BOWEL DISEASE

IBD has seen some advancements in treatment in recent years. Traditional treatments given in Table **2**, like aminosalicylates, corticosteroids, immunomodulators, and biologics, are still used [48]. Various medications used in the treatment of IBD are mentioned in Table **2**. New strategies are emerging, such as small-molecule therapies and apheresis (a process that removes certain components from the blood). Biologic therapies, especially TNF inhibitors, have been successful in helping many patients achieve long-term remission of IBD. New approaches like improving gut health (intestinal microecology) and cell therapy have become popular in recent times. The treatment goal for IBD has evolved from controlling symptoms and healing the mucosal layer [49].

For moderate to severe IBD, biological agents, such as small-molecule medicines, are currently the preferred treatment, either individually or combined with immunomodulatory medications [50]. Fig. (**3**) illustrates the various treatment options for IBD.

Table 2. Medication for inflammatory bowel disease.

Sr. No.	Class	Example	MOA & Adverse effect	References
01.	**5-Amino salicylic acid (5-ASA)**	Sulfasalazine (SALAZOPYRI)	Inhibit COX and LOX pathways, Inhibition of cytokine, PAF, TNFα, and NFκB. **AE:** Oligozoospermia, male infertility	[51]
		Mesalazine (MESACOL)	Inhibit COX and LOX pathways. **AE:** Leucopenia, nephrotoxicity, and hypersensitivity reactions	[52]
		Balsalazide (COLOREX)	Prostaglandins and leukotrienes; Inhibiting their production in the intestines. **AE**: Abdominal pain or cramping and leukopenia	[53]
		Olsalazine (DIPENTUM)	Inhibiting the production of pro-inflammatory chemicals. **AE:** Allergic reactions, nausea	[51]
02.	**Corticosteroids**	Prednisolone (MILLIPRED)	Prednisolone binds to glucocorticoid receptors, modulating the expression of genes that control inflammation and immune response. **AE:** Foetal abnormalities, Cushing's habitus	[54]
		Hydrocortisone (CORTEF)	It inhibits **phospholipase A2**, an enzyme that releases arachidonic acid, which is involved in the production of inflammatory mediators. **AE:** Muscular weakness, cleft palate, and osteoporosis	[55]
03.	**Immunosuppressants**	Azathioprine (AZASAN)	They inhibit the conversion of inosine monophosphate to adenine and guanine nucleotides, which are the building blocks for RNA and DNA. **AE:** Bone marrow depression, nausea, and vomiting	[56]
		Methotrexate (TREXALL)	Inhibiting dihydrofolate reductase (DHFRase)-blocking the conversion of dihydrofolic acid to tetrahydrofolic acid. **AE:** Megaloblastic anaemia and pancytopenia	[57]

(Table 2) cont.....

Sr. No.	Class	Example	MOA & Adverse effect	References
		Cyclosporine (GENGRAF)	It inhibits T lymphocyte proliferation, IL-2 cytokine production, and calcineurin. **AE:** Nephrotoxicity and excessive hair growth	[58]

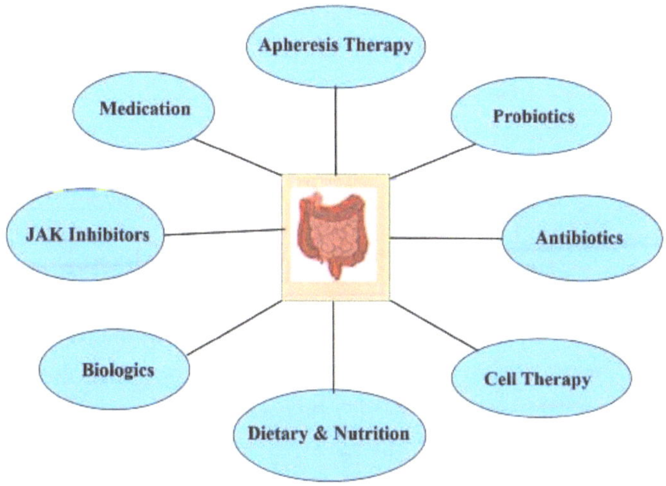

Fig. (3). The treatment options for inflammatory bowel disease.

Biologics

Anti-TNF Therapy

Tumour Necrosis Factor alpha (TNF-α) is a family of cytokines that have an important role in inflammation, apoptosis, and tissue damage. Its overexpression can lead to autoimmune diseases [59]. Anti-TNF-α monoclonal antibodies like Infliximab and Adalimumab have reduced inflammation and tissue damage in conditions such as UC and CD in recent years. Numerous studies have shown that Infliximab reduces the need for surgery and hospitalizations in UC and promotes healing of CD. Monitoring serum levels and anti-drug antibodies is recommended for optimal treatment of IBD [60].

Anti-IL-12/23 Therapy

Interleukin-12/23 (IL-12/23) is a pro-inflammatory cytokine in intestinal inflammation that causes IBD pathogenesis. IL-23/23 inhibitors are recommended as a treatment therapy for IBD patients. Mirikizumab has been used for the treatment of UC, with higher potency at low doses [61].

JAK Inhibitors

A novel oral treatment for IBD, JAK inhibitors have a rapid clinical response [62]. JAK inhibitors block multiple signalling pathways and target JAK1, JAK2, JAK3, and TYK2, which are involved in the pathophysiology of IBD. Tofacitinib, an oral JAK inhibitor that primarily targets JAK1 and JAK3, is approved for treating IBD, particularly moderate to severe UC [63]. JAK inhibitors may enhance the effectiveness of treatment by targeting cytokines that cause various inflammatory diseases [64].

Apheresis Therapy

Apheresis therapy is a new IBD treatment approach developed in Japan. It targets and removes specific leukocytes (like granulocytes, monocytes, and activated lymphocytes) from peripheral blood to reduce local inflammation [48]. The characteristic features of IBD are leukocyte infiltration and the subsequent production of interleukins and cytokines. Non-pharmacologic treatments like Granulocyte-Monocyte Apheresis (GMA) and Leukocyte Apheresis (LCAP) are emerging as effective alternatives. GMA has a strong safety profile, especially in pediatric and pregnant patients, and shows promise for UC. LCAP entraps leukocytes and suppresses cytokine release, thus leading to better disease remission and reducing reliance on steroids and immunosuppressants. Both treatments have mild side effects and are popular as non-pharmacological options for IBD [65, 66].

Probiotics

Probiotics are of particular interest as a potential treatment option for IBD. Probiotics show potential benefits for patients with mild to moderate UC. Studies have demonstrated that strains like *E. coli Nissle*, *Lactobacillus rhamnosus GG*, and *S. boulardii* can help induce UC. Probiotics are especially beneficial for patients with 5-ASA intolerance, but they should be used in severe UC due to their potential effects [67].

Cell Therapy

There are many studies on the role of Mesenchymal Stem Cells (MSCs) in intestinal fibrosis. Studies suggest that MSCs can treat IBD, such as collagen deposition and epithelial-to-mesenchymal transition, in models of colitis. MSCs help control fibrogenesis by regulating extracellular matrix turnover and decreasing profibrotic gene expression through the release of hepatocyte growth factor and tumor necrosis factor-stimulated gene 6. These anti-fibrotic effects of

MSCs are also observed in other fibrosis models. This is a novel stem cell therapy for the treatment of IBD [68, 69].

Dietary and Nutrition

Diet and nutrition have traditionally played a minor role in IBD management due to limited knowledge and clinical practice constraints. For patients with IBD, the significance of individualized diets lies in catering to their unique nutrient requirements and medical circumstances. However, recent interest has grown in the impact of diet on IBD, especially with a better understanding of the microbiome. Dietary recommendations for CD treatment include insights from emerging fields like nutrigenomics, with main objective being the improvement of patient health [70]. To fully understand the role of diet in the development and progression of IBD, more studies have been conducted. The effect of nutrition on the risk of IBD has been the subject of numerous investigations [71].

Antibiotics

Many studies suggest that antibiotics could play a role in IBD treatment by altering gut microbiota. While antibiotics may help reduce infections in CD patients, their importance in inducing remission is limited. Overuse of antibiotics may increase the risk of developing IBD, particularly in children, and is associated with higher risks of infections like *Clostridium difficile* in IBD patients. Numerous studies have examined the benefits of antibiotics in IBD treatment [72, 73].

CONCLUSION

This chapter demonstrated that IBD is fundamentally a chronic inflammatory illness of the gastrointestinal tract, marked by symptoms like diarrhea, weight loss, and hematochezia. We discussed two principal variants of inflammatory bowel disease, ulcerative colitis and Crohn's disease, and how these illnesses differ in terms of their symptoms and cytokine profiles. Crohn's disease can affect any segment of the gastrointestinal system; however, its manifestations predominantly occur in the ileum. Conversely, ulcerative colitis is confined to the colon and rectum. This chronic illness arises from a complex interaction among numerous factors, including genetic, environmental, and pollution-related influences. All these factors, in turn, disturb the gut microbiome, leading to dysbiosis and, eventually, a damaged intestinal barrier, persistent inflammation, and tissue damage. Effective management of IBD involves many therapeutic choices, including drugs such as aminosalicylates, biologics, and cell therapy. By comprehending the interconnections among these elements, researchers can develop enhanced and targeted pharmacological therapy, thereby establishing more effective management strategies for IBD in patients.

REFERENCES

[1] Szałwińska P, Włodarczyk J, Spinelli A, Fichna J, Włodarczyk M. Ibs-symptoms in ibd patients—manifestation of concomitant or different entities. J Clin Med 2020; 10(1): 31. [http://dx.doi.org/10.3390/jcm10010031] [PMID: 33374388]

[2] Qiu P, Ishimoto T, Fu L, Zhang J, Zhang Z, Liu Y. The gut microbiota in inflammatory bowel disease. Front Cell Infect Microbiol 2022; 12(February): 733992. [http://dx.doi.org/10.3389/fcimb.2022.733992] [PMID: 35273921]

[3] Mulder DJ, Noble AJ, Justinich CJ, Duffin JM. A tale of two diseases: The history of inflammatory bowel disease. Journal of Crohn's and Colitis Elsevier 2014; 8: 341-1.

[4] Cushing K, Higgins PDR. Management of crohn disease: A review. JAMA - Journal of the American Medical Association American Medical Association 2021; 325: 69-80.

[5] Shan Y, Lee M, Chang EB. The gut microbiome and inflammatory bowel diseases. Annu Rev Med 2022; 73(1): 455-68. [http://dx.doi.org/10.1146/annurev-med-042320-021020] [PMID: 34555295]

[6] Fanizzi F, Allocca M, Fiorino G, *et al.* Raising the bar in ulcerative colitis management. Therap Adv Gastroenterol 2024; 17: 17562848241273066. [http://dx.doi.org/10.1177/17562848241273066] [PMID: 39600566]

[7] Jaiswal M, Agrawal N, Kumar Y, Lanjhiyana SK. *In vivo* models of chemically induced colitis for inflammatory bowel diseases: An overview. Challenges and Advances in Pharmaceutical Research 2022; 10(21): 141-9.

[8] Nakase H, Uchino M, Shinzaki S, *et al.* Evidence-based clinical practice guidelines for inflammatory bowel disease 2020. J Gastroenterol 2021; 56(6): 489-526. [http://dx.doi.org/10.1007/s00535-021-01784-1] [PMID: 33885977]

[9] Borowitz SM. The epidemiology of inflammatory bowel disease: Clues to pathogenesis? Front Pediatr 2023; 10(January): 1103713. [http://dx.doi.org/10.3389/fped.2022.1103713] [PMID: 36733765]

[10] Caron B, Honap S, Peyrin-Biroulet L. Epidemiology of inflammatory bowel disease across the ages in the era of advanced therapies. J Crohn's Colitis 2024; 18 (Suppl. 2): ii3-ii15. [http://dx.doi.org/10.1093/ecco-jcc/jjae082] [PMID: 39475082]

[11] Jaiswal M, Lanjhiyana SK. A critical review on colon targeted drug delivery systems for management of inflammatory bowel disease. Int J Pharm Sci Res 2019; 10(3): 985. [http://dx.doi.org/10.13040/IJPSR.0975-8232.10]

[12] Manos J. The human microbiome in disease and pathology. Acta Pathol Microbiol Scand Suppl 2022; 130(12): 690-705. [http://dx.doi.org/10.1111/apm.13225] [PMID: 35393656]

[13] Quaglio AEV, Grillo TG, Oliveira ECSD, Stasi LCD, Sassaki LY. Gut microbiota, inflammatory bowel disease and colorectal cancer. World J Gastroenterol 2022; 28(30): 4053-60. [http://dx.doi.org/10.3748/wjg.v28.i30.4053] [PMID: 36157114]

[14] Haneishi Y, Furuya Y, Hasegawa M, Picarelli A, Rossi M, Miyamoto J. Inflammatory bowel diseases and gut microbiota. Int J Mol Sci 2023; 24(4): 3817. [http://dx.doi.org/10.3390/ijms24043817] [PMID: 36835245]

[15] Glassner KL, Abraham BP, Quigley EMM. The microbiome and inflammatory bowel disease. J Allergy Clin Immunol 2020; 145(1): 16-27. [http://dx.doi.org/10.1016/j.jaci.2019.11.003] [PMID: 31910984]

[16] Nishida, A., Inoue, R., Inatomi, O. et al. Gut microbiota in the pathogenesis of inflammatory bowel disease. Clin J Gastroenterol 2018. 11: 1-10. [http://dx.doi.org/10.1007/s12328-017-0813-5]

[17] Guan Q. A Comprehensive review and update on the pathogenesis of inflammatory bowel disease. J Immunol Res. 2019; 7247238. [http://dx.doi.org/10.1155/2019/7247238] [PMID: 31886308]

[18] Santana PT, Rosas SLB, Ribeiro BE, Marinho Y, de Souza HSP. Dysbiosis in inflammatory bowel disease: pathogenic role and potential therapeutic targets. Int J Mol Sci 2022; 23(7): 3464. [http://dx.doi.org/10.3390/ijms23073464] [PMID: 35408838]

[19] Segal JP, Jean-Frédéric LeBlanc A, Hart AL. Ulcerative colitis: An update. Clinical Medicine. J R Coll Physicians Lond 2021; 21(2): 135-9.

[20] Gajendran M, Loganathan P, Jimenez G, *et al.* A comprehensive review and update on ulcerative colitis. Dis Mon 2019; 65(12): 100851. [http://dx.doi.org/10.1016/j.disamonth.2019.02.004] [PMID: 30837080]

[21] Tontini GE, Vecchi M, Pastorelli L, Neurath MF, Neumann H. Differential diagnosis in inflammatory bowel disease colitis: State of the art and future perspectives. World J Gastroenterol 2015; 21(1): 21-46. [http://dx.doi.org/10.3748/wjg.v21.i1.21] [PMID: 25574078]

[22] Tiwari A, Jain A, Verma A, Jain SK. Exploitable signaling pathways for the treatment of inflammatory bowel disease. Curr Signal Transduct Ther 2018; 12(2): 76-84. [http://dx.doi.org/10.2174/1574362412666170330145342]

[23] Feuerstein JD, Cheifetz AS. Crohn disease: Epidemiology, diagnosis, and management. Mayo Clin Proc 2017; 92(7): 1088-103. [http://dx.doi.org/10.1016/j.mayocp.2017.04.010] [PMID: 28601423]

[24] Ouyang Q, Tandon R, Goh KL, *et al.* Management consensus of inflammatory bowel disease for the Asia–Pacific region. J Gastroenterol Hepatol 2006; 21(12): 1772-82. [http://dx.doi.org/10.1111/j.1440-1746.2006.04674.x] [PMID: 17074013]

[25] Head KA, Jurenka JS. Inflammatory bowel disease Part 1: Ulcerative colitis-pathophysiology and conventional and alternative treatment options. Altern Med Rev. 2003; 8(3): 247-83. [PMID: 12946238]

[26] Ramos GP, Papadakis KA. Mechanisms of disease: Inflammatory bowel diseases. Mayo Clin Proc 2019; 94(1): 155-65. [http://dx.doi.org/10.1016/j.mayocp.2018.09.013] [PMID: 30611442]

[27] Graham DB, Xavier RJ. Pathway paradigms revealed from the genetics of inflammatory bowel disease. Nature Nature Research. 2020; Vol. 578: pp. 527-39. [http://dx.doi.org/10.1038/s41586-020-2025-2] [PMID: 32103191]

[28] Schirmer M, Garner A, Vlamakis H, Xavier RJ. Microbial genes and pathways in inflammatory bowel disease. Nat Rev Microbiol 2019; 17(8): 497-511. [http://dx.doi.org/10.1038/s41579-019-0213-6] [PMID: 31249397]

[29] Ananthakrishnan AN. Epidemiology and risk factors for IBD. Nat Rev Gastroenterol Hepatol 2015; 12(4): 205-17. [http://dx.doi.org/10.1038/nrgastro.2015.34] [PMID: 25732745]

[30] Jang J, Jeong S. Inflammatory bowel disease: Pathophysiology, treatment, and disease modeling. Biochip J 2023; 17(4): 403-30. [http://dx.doi.org/10.1007/s13206-023-00118-y]

[31] Rozich JJ, Holmer A, Singh S. Effect of lifestyle factors on outcomes in patients with inflammatory bowel diseases. Am J Gastroenterol 2020; 115(6): 832-40.

[http://dx.doi.org/10.14309/ajg.0000000000000608] [PMID: 32224703]

[32] Sun Y, Yuan S, Chen X, *et al.* The contribution of genetic risk and lifestyle factors in the development of adult-onset inflammatory bowel disease: A prospective cohort study. Am J Gastroenterol 2023; 118(3): 511-22.
[http://dx.doi.org/10.14309/ajg.0000000000002180] [PMID: 36695739]

[33] Li FR, Wu KY, Fan WD, Chen GC, Tian H, Wu XB. Long-term exposure to air pollution and risk of incident inflammatory bowel disease among middle and old aged adults. Ecotoxicol Environ Saf 2022; 242: 113835.
[http://dx.doi.org/10.1016/j.ecoenv.2022.113835] [PMID: 35816845]

[34] Mentella MC, Scaldaferri F, Pizzoferrato M, Gasbarrini A, Miggiano GAD. Nutrition, IBD and Gut Microbiota: A Review. Nutrients NLM (Medline). 2020; 12.
[http://dx.doi.org/10.3390/nu12040944] [PMID: 32235316]

[35] Ananthakrishnan AN, Bernstein CN, Iliopoulos D, *et al.* Environmental triggers in IBD: a review of progress and evidence. Nat Rev Gastroenterol Hepatol 2018; 15(1): 39-49.
[http://dx.doi.org/10.1038/nrgastro.2017.136] [PMID: 29018271]

[36] Chiba M, Nakane K, Komatsu M. Westernized diet is the most ubiquitous environmental factor in inflammatory bowel disease. Perm J 2019; 23(1): 18-107.
[http://dx.doi.org/10.7812/TPP/18-107] [PMID: 30624192]

[37] Veauthier B, Hornecker JR. Crohn's disease: Diagnosis and management. Am Fam Physician. 2018; 98(11): 661-669.
[PMID: 30485038]

[38] Thomas T, Chandan JS, Li VSW, *et al.* Global smoking trends in inflammatory bowel disease: A systematic review of inception cohorts. PLoS One 2019; 14(9): e0221961.
[http://dx.doi.org/10.1371/journal.pone.0221961] [PMID: 31545811]

[39] Papoutsopoulou S, Satsangi J, Campbell BJ, Probert CS. Review article: impact of cigarette smoking on intestinal inflammation—direct and indirect mechanisms. Alimentary Pharmacology and Therapeutics Blackwell Publishing Ltd;. 2020; 51: pp. 1268-85.

[40] Vedamurthy A, Ananthakrishnan AN. Influence of environmental factors in the development and outcomes of inflammatory bowel disease. Gastroenterol Hepatol (N Y) 2019; 15(2): 72-82.
[PMID: 31011301]

[41] Chen Y, Cui W, Li X, Yang H. Interaction between commensal bacteria, immune response and the intestinal barrier in inflammatory bowel disease. Frontiers in Immunology Frontiers Media SA. 2021; Vol. 12.
[http://dx.doi.org/10.3389/fimmu.2021.761981] [PMID: 34858414]

[42] Schoultz I, Keita ÅV. Cellular and molecular therapeutic targets in inflammatory bowel disease—focusing on intestinal barrier function. Cells MDPI. 2019; Vol. 8.
[http://dx.doi.org/10.3390/cells8020193] [PMID: 30813280]

[43] Antoni L, Nuding S, Wehkamp J, Stange EF. Intestinal barrier in inflammatory bowel disease. World J Gastroenterol 2014; 20(5): 1165-79.
[http://dx.doi.org/10.3748/wjg.v20.i5.1165] [PMID: 24574793]

[44] Kałużna A, Olczyk P, Komosińska-Vassev K. The role of innate and adaptive immune cells in the pathogenesis and development of the inflammatory response in ulcerative colitis. J Clin Med 2022; 11(2): 400.
[http://dx.doi.org/10.3390/jcm11020400] [PMID: 35054093]

[45] Tatiya-aphiradee N, Chatuphonprasert W, Jarukamjorn K. Immune response and inflammatory pathway of ulcerative colitis. J Basic Clin Physiol Pharmacol 2018; 30(1): 1-10.
[http://dx.doi.org/10.1515/jbcpp-2018-0036] [PMID: 30063466]

[46] Narula N, Wong ECL, Pray C, *et al.* Associations of antibiotics, hormonal therapies, oral

contraceptives, and long-term nsaids with inflammatory bowel disease: Results from the Prospective Urban Rural Epidemiology (PURE) study. Clin Gastroenterol Hepatol 2023; 21(10): 2649-2659.e16. [http://dx.doi.org/10.1016/j.cgh.2022.11.037] [PMID: 36528284]

[47] Hu S, Chen Y, Chen Y, Wang C. Depression and anxiety disorders in patients with inflammatory bowel disease. Front Psychiatry 2021; 12(October): 714057. [http://dx.doi.org/10.3389/fpsyt.2021.714057] [PMID: 34690829]

[48] Gordon H, Minozzi S, Kopylov U, *et al.* ECCO guidelines on therapeutics in Crohn's Disease: Medical treatment. J Crohn's Colitis 2024; 18(10): 1531-55. [http://dx.doi.org/10.1093/ecco-jcc/jjae091] [PMID: 38877997]

[49] Cai Z, Wang S, Li J. Treatment of inflammatory bowel disease: A comprehensive review. Front Med (Lausanne) 2021; 8(December): 765474. [http://dx.doi.org/10.3389/fmed.2021.765474] [PMID: 34988090]

[50] Triantafillidis JK, Zografos CG, Konstadoulakis MM, Papalois AE. Combination treatment of inflammatory bowel disease: Present status and future perspectives. World J Gastroenterol 2024; 30(15): 2068-80. [http://dx.doi.org/10.3748/wjg.v30.i15.2068] [PMID: 38681984]

[51] Tripathi KD. Essentials of medical pharmacology. Jaypee Brothers medical publishers; 2018.

[52] Park H, Kim W, Kim D, Jeong S, Jung Y. Mesalazine activates adenosine monophosphate-activated protein kinase: implication in the anti-inflammatory activity of this anti-colitic drug. Curr Mol Pharmacol 2019; 12(4): 272-80. [http://dx.doi.org/10.2174/1874467212666190308103448] [PMID: 30848228]

[53] Swami D, Siddiqui S, Kumar U, Devarajan S, Aich J. One of the 5-aminosalicylates drug, mesalamine as a drug repurposing lead against breast cancer. Bull Natl Res Cent 2022; 46(1): 249. [http://dx.doi.org/10.1186/s42269-022-00939-1]

[54] Calméjane L, Laharie D, Kirchgesner J, Uzzan M. Review article: Updated management of acute severe ulcerative colitis: From steroids to novel medical strategies. United European Gastroenterol J 2023; 11(8): 722-32. [http://dx.doi.org/10.1002/ueg2.12442] [PMID: 37475143]

[55] Bruscoli S, Febo M, Riccardi C, Migliorati G. Glucocorticoid therapy in inflammatory bowel disease: mechanisms and clinical practice. Front Immunol 2021; 12: 691480. [http://dx.doi.org/10.3389/fimmu.2021.691480] [PMID: 34149734]

[56] Mallick B, Malik S. Use of azathioprine in ulcerative colitis: a comprehensive review. Cureus 2022; 14(5): e24874. [http://dx.doi.org/10.7759/cureus.24874] [PMID: 35698683]

[57] Demase K, Monitto CK, Little RD, Sparrow MP. The role of low-dose oral methotrexate in increasing anti-TNF drug levels and reducing immunogenicity in IBD. J Clin Med 2023; 12(13): 4382. [http://dx.doi.org/10.3390/jcm12134382] [PMID: 37445417]

[58] Cohen NA, Dalal SR, Choi D, Rubin DT. Ozanimod maintenance therapy after cyclosporine induction in acute severe ulcerative colitis. ACG Case Rep J 2022; 9(7): e00832. [http://dx.doi.org/10.14309/crj.0000000000000832] [PMID: 35919406]

[59] Berg DR, Colombel JF, Ungaro R. The role of early biologic therapy in inflammatory bowel disease. Inflamm Bowel Dis. 2019. [http://dx.doi.org/10.1093/ibd/izz059]

[60] Anjie SI, Hanzel J, Gecse KB, D'Haens GR, Brandse JF. Anti-drug antibodies against anti-TNF in patients with inflammatory bowel disease: an evaluation of possible strategies. Scand J Gastroenterol 2024; 59(2): 169-75. [http://dx.doi.org/10.1080/00365521.2023.2278424] [PMID: 37961895]

[61] Danese S, Peyrin-Biroulet L. Evolution of IL-23 blockade in inflammatory bowel disease. J Crohn's

Colitis 2022; 16 (Suppl. 2): ii1-2.
[http://dx.doi.org/10.1093/ecco-jcc/jjab188] [PMID: 35553668]

[62] Honap S, Agorogianni A, Colwill MJ, *et al.* JAK inhibitors for inflammatory bowel disease: recent advances. Frontline Gastroenterol 2024; 15(1): 59-69.
[http://dx.doi.org/10.1136/flgastro-2023-102400] [PMID: 38487554]

[63] Herrera-deGuise C, Serra-Ruiz X, Lastiri E, Borruel N. JAK inhibitors: A new dawn for oral therapies in inflammatory bowel diseases. Front Med (Lausanne) 2023; 10(March): 1089099.
[http://dx.doi.org/10.3389/fmed.2023.1089099] [PMID: 36936239]

[64] Tian Z, Zhao Q, Teng X. Anti-IL23/12 agents and JAK inhibitors for inflammatory bowel disease. Front Immunol 2024; 15(July): 1393463.
[http://dx.doi.org/10.3389/fimmu.2024.1393463] [PMID: 39086483]

[65] De Vita E. Clinical cases. Psicoter Sci Um 2021; 8960(3): 516-8.
[http://dx.doi.org/10.3280/PU2021-003009]

[66] Iizuka M, Etou T, Sagara S. Efficacy of cytapheresis in patients with ulcerative colitis showing insufficient or lost response to biologic therapy. World J Gastroenterol 2022; 28(34): 4959-72.
[http://dx.doi.org/10.3748/wjg.v28.i34.4959] [PMID: 36160647]

[67] Akutko K, Stawarski A. Probiotics, prebiotics and synbiotics in inflammatory bowel diseases. J Clin Med 2021; 10(11): 2466.
[http://dx.doi.org/10.3390/jcm10112466] [PMID: 34199428]

[68] Wang Y, Huang B, Jin T, Ocansey DKW, Jiang J, Mao F. Intestinal fibrosis in inflammatory bowel disease and the prospects of mesenchymal stem cell therapy. Front Immunol 2022; 13(March): 835005.
[http://dx.doi.org/10.3389/fimmu.2022.835005] [PMID: 35370998]

[69] Ko JZH, Johnson S, Dave M. Efficacy and safety of mesenchymal stem/stromal cell therapy for inflammatory bowel diseases: an up-to-date systematic review. Biomolecules 2021; 11(1): 82.
[http://dx.doi.org/10.3390/biom11010082] [PMID: 33440772]

[70] Caio G, Lungaro L, Caputo F, Zoli E, Giancola F, Chiarioni G, *et al.* Nutritional treatment in crohn's disease. Nutrients 2021; 1-23.
[PMID: 34066229]

[71] de Castro MM, Pascoal LB, Steigleder KM, *et al.* Role of diet and nutrition in inflammatory bowel disease. World J Exp Med 2021; 11(1): 1-16.
[http://dx.doi.org/10.5493/wjem.v11.i1.1] [PMID: 33585174]

[72] Fenneman AC, Weidner M, Chen LA, Nieuwdorp M, Blaser MJ. Antibiotics in the pathogenesis of diabetes and inflammatory diseases of the gastrointestinal tract. Nat Rev Gastroenterol Hepatol 2023; 20(2): 81-100.
[http://dx.doi.org/10.1038/s41575-022-00685-9] [PMID: 36258032]

[73] Fenneman AC, Weidner M, Chen LA, Nieuwdorp M, Blaser MJ. Antibiotics in the pathogenesis of diabetes and inflammatory diseases of the gastrointestinal tract. Nat Rev Gastroenterol Hepatol 2023; 20(2): 81-100.
[http://dx.doi.org/10.1038/s41575-022-00685-9] [PMID: 36258032]

CHAPTER 2

Microenvironment in IBD: Implications for Drug Release and Nano-Based Targeting Strategies

Mayank Garhewal[1], **Achal Mishra**[1], **Shekhar Verma**[1], **Naresh Sahu**[1], **Arvinder Kaur**[2] and **Yogesh Vaishnav**[1,*]

[1] *Department of Pharmacy, Guru Ghasidas Vishwavidyalaya, Bilaspur 495009, Chhattisgarh, India*

[2] *Akash Institute of Pharmacy, Prasannahalli, Bangalore 562110, Karnataka, India*

Abstract: The microenvironment of Inflammatory Bowel Disease (IBD) presents unique opportunities and obstacles for targeted treatment and drug administration. These include altered gut microbiota, dysregulated immune responses, and chronic inflammation. This chapter explores the detailed connections between the development of advanced drug delivery systems and the IBD microenvironment, with a focus on nano-based targeting strategies. The effects of the pathogenic features of IBD, such as elevated levels of pro-inflammatory cytokines, reactive oxygen species, and intestinal epithelial permeability, on drug release kinetics and biodistribution are investigated. The chapter shows how these pathological changes can be targeted using nanotechnology to improve therapeutic outcomes, reduce systemic toxicity, and deliver medications to specific locations. Developing stimuli-responsive nanocarriers that release drugs in response to pH, redox potential, or enzymatic activity, as well as using ligand-functionalized nanoparticles for active targeting of immune cells or inflammatory tissues, are significant topics. The potential for nanoformulations driven by the microbiome and the role of the gut microbiota in controlling the effectiveness of medications are also examined. In order to bridge the gap between preclinical research and clinical application, interdisciplinary approaches are essential. The chapter concludes with a summary of the translational challenges and possible avenues for nano-based therapy in IBD.

Keywords: Dysbiosis, Fibrosis, Immune cell, Markers, Microbiota, Multifunctional targeting.

INTRODUCTION

Inflammatory Bowel Disease (IBD), which includes persistent diseases such as Crohn's disease and ulcerative colitis, is caused by long-lasting inflammation of

* **Corresponding author Yogesh Vaishnav:** Department of Pharmacy, Guru Ghasidas Vishwavidyalaya, Bilaspur 495009, Chhattisgarh, India; E-mail: yogesh446688@gmail.com

the gastrointestinal tract resulting from multiple mechanisms, including immune dysregulation, epithelial barrier dysfunction, dysbiosis, and ongoing remodeling of tissues. The pathological environment in which IBD lesions occur is particularly unique because of the acidic microenvironment, overproduction of relatively pro-inflammatory Reactive Oxygen Species (ROS), increased enzymatic activity, and heightened influx of immune cells, all of which affect drug release, absorption, and dosing efficacy [1, 2].

The utilization of nanotechnology is a promising breakthrough that allows for smart drug delivery strategies to be designed for the specific challenges generated by the IBD microenvironment. Nano-based systems such as pH-sensitive polymers, ROS-responsive nanoparticles, enzyme-degradable coatings, and ligand-targeted nanoparticles can be designed to only release drug payload in response to specific local stimuli (*e.g.*, pH drop, ROS surge, or total enzyme overexpression) within hyperinflammatory microenvironments. For example, pH-sensitive formulations like Eudragit-coated mesalamine tablets preferentially release active drug under acidic conditions in the colon, while others like ROS-responsive nanoparticles containing siRNA or anti-inflammatory agents can take advantage of local oxidative stress to deliver drug payloads in a more site-selective manner. Nano-carriers also improve drug mucoadhesion and increase cellular uptake to improve drug retention and efficacy and limit side effects [3, 4].

Distinct pathological features of the IBD environment, such as localized pH changes, concentrations of Reactive Oxygen Species (ROS), and increased levels of digestive or inflammatory enzymes, will determine the manner and timing of drug release from advanced delivery devices. For example, inflammation-induced acidification of gut segments can trigger pH-sensitive polymers to release their payload in the inflamed regions, while healthy regions remain largely unaffected. Elevated levels of ROS at inflamed sites can trigger specific nanoparticles designed to respond to oxidative stress, which also deliver drugs exactly where they are needed, all while minimizing often undesirable off-target effects. Similarly, enzymes overexpressed in IBD lesions that are distinct from those in healthy tissues, such as lysozyme and colonic bacterial azoreductase, can trigger localized activation of therapeutics (*e.g.*, prodrugs or nanocarrier coatings) without unwanted degradation in healthy tissues. By utilizing these features of the local microenvironment, nano-based drug delivery systems can achieve device-mediated, targeted, responsive, and precise therapeutic effects in the management of IBD [1, 3, 5].

There is an increasing number of *in vivo* studies showing the clinical utility of nano-formulations in models of Inflammatory Bowel Disease (IBD), suggesting translational progress. For example, ROS-sensitive thioketal nanoparticles encapsulating siRNA for delivery to colitic mice can significantly reduce inflammatory burden and disease severity. Some enzyme-, pH-, and ligand-responsive nanosystems demonstrate promising biodistribution and therapeutic efficacy, including budesonide-loaded PEGylated nanoparticles, folate-decorated liposomes targeting activated macrophages, and dual-responsive hydrogels promoting the regrowth of colonic tissues. Multifunctional nanocarriers that incorporate passive targeting of disease tissues, ligand-mediated delivery to specific cells, and microenvironment-responsive release systems are moving past laboratory research into clinical testing, and several of these therapeutic approaches are demonstrating a greater degree of symptom control and mucosal healing in IBD animal models and early patient cohorts [6, 7].

Continuing challenges include variability among patients, stability of carriers during gastrointestinal transit, and regulatory issues with synthetic polymers; however, interdisciplinary partnerships are forging ahead with continued creativity in the field of individual, efficient, and biomarker-guided nanotherapeutics. This paradigm shift represents a new chapter for precision medicine in IBD and hopefully renewed hope for optimally treating this condition and enhancing the quality of life of patients.

THE IBD MICROENVIRONMENT: PATHOLOGICAL FEATURES

Inflammatory Bowel Disease (IBD), which includes Crohn's disease and ulcerative colitis, is typified by persistent, recurrent inflammation of the gastrointestinal tract. A complicated interplay between immune system failure, environmental variables, gut microbiota abnormalities, and genetic predisposition characterizes the multifactorial pathophysiology of IBD. Within the gastrointestinal tract's impacted areas, these interactions provide a very dynamic and unique milieu. Developing targeted and efficient therapies, especially those that make use of drug delivery systems and nanotechnology, requires an understanding of the pathogenic characteristics of this microenvironment [8, 9].

Inflammatory and Immune Dysregulation

Chronic, dysregulated inflammation is the central component of the IBD microenvironment. To guard against pathogens and prevent unwarranted immune reactions against commensal bacteria, the immune system in healthy people strikes a careful balance between tolerance and immune activation. But this equilibrium is upset in IBD. T cells, macrophages, dendritic cells, neutrophils, and other immune cells are drawn to the site of inflammation as a result of the gut's mucosal immune system being overly reactive [10].

The inflammatory pathway is maintained in large part by the secretion of pro-inflammatory cytokines such as TNF-α, IL-1β, IL-6, and IL-17. As part of the disease's systemic impacts, this cytokine storm not only sustains local inflammation but also damages distant organs and tissues. These inflammatory mediators are overproduced, which damages tissue, compromises the epithelial barrier, and results in ulcers and other clinical characteristics that are typical of IBD [11 - 13].

Altered Gut Microbiota (Dysbiosis)

Dysbiosis, or an imbalance in the gut microbiota's makeup, is a defining characteristic of IBD. A stable and varied microbiome is essential for immune system modulation, gut homeostasis, and the growth inhibition of harmful microorganisms in healthy people. The microbial ecology is disturbed in IBD, with an overabundance of potentially harmful species like *Proteobacteria* and *Enterobacteriaceae* and a decline in beneficial bacteria like *Firmicutes* and *Bacteroidetes* [14, 15].

By generating metabolites and signalling molecules that can change immune cell activity and increase intestinal permeability, this microbial imbalance makes inflammation worse. Additionally, the dysbiotic microbiota may exacerbate the pathophysiology of the disease by directly inciting immunological responses and promoting the persistence of inflammation [16].

Epithelial Barrier Dysfunction

A single layer of Intestinal Epithelial Cells (IECs) makes up the epithelial barrier, which is crucial for preserving gut integrity and blocking the entry of harmful substances like infections, toxins, and allergens. IBD significantly impairs this barrier. Intestinal permeability is increased when tight junctions, which link neighboring epithelial cells, are disrupted; this condition is known as “leaky gut” [17, 18].

Because of this compromised barrier function, toxins, microbal components, and luminal antigens can enter the underlying tissue, further activating the immune system and prolonging the inflammatory cycle. Further compromising defensive mechanisms against infections, the loss of epithelial integrity is linked to changes in mucus production and a decrease in antimicrobial peptide output [19, 20].

Tissue Remodeling and Fibrosis

Chronic inflammation in IBD causes fibrosis and tissue remodeling over time [21]. The gut wall thickens and scars due to the formation of extracellular matrix proteins and fibroblast proliferation triggered by chronic stimulation of inflammatory pathways [22]. Fibrosis is especially noticeable in Crohn's disease and can result in strictures, which are small sections of the intestine that impede regular bowel movements and may need surgery.

The dysregulated immunological response in IBD is the primary cause of fibrosis, with collagen-producing fibroblasts and inflammatory mediators like TGF-β playing important roles. Fibrosis can eventually lead to decreased motility, which exacerbates the illness and makes therapy more difficult [23].

Changes in pH and Enzyme Activity

Changes in the gut's inflammatory areas, including altered biochemical conditions, are another distinctive aspect of the IBD microenvironment [24]. Because infiltrating immune cells and bacteria boost the generation of lactic acid and other metabolites, inflammation can cause localized pH alterations. Areas of active disease often exhibit an acidic environment. The effectiveness of treatments that depend on particular pH-dependent mechanisms may be impacted by this acidic pH's effects on medication solubility and release. Enzymes like Matrix Metalloproteinases (MMPs), which aid in tissue remodeling and destruction, are also frequently activated in the inflammatory milieu of IBD [25]. Certain proteases, such as calpains and cathepsins, can also change the intestinal epithelium's structure, which could jeopardize the gut barrier's integrity and open up new therapeutic targets [26].

Vascular Changes and Angiogenesis

Chronic inflammation also causes angiogenesis, or the growth of new blood vessels, in the affected areas. Vascular Endothelial Growth Factor (VEGF) and other angiogenic factors are upregulated, which enhances the inflammatory response by encouraging immune cell infiltration while simultaneously providing oxygen and nutrition to the inflammatory tissues [27, 28].

Increased blood vessel permeability brought on by the aberrant vasculature linked to IBD exacerbates tissue damage and causes edema. When creating drug delivery systems, this changed vascular architecture is a crucial factor to take into account because it may have an impact on how therapeutic chemicals are distributed and accumulated in inflammatory tissues [28, 29].

IMPLICATIONS FOR DRUG RELEASE

A dynamic and diverse gut milieu makes the treatment of Inflammatory Bowel Disease (IBD), which includes Crohn's disease and ulcerative colitis, difficult.

Pathophysiological variables like oxidative stress, disruption of mucus barriers, immune cell infiltration, enzyme overexpression, and altered pH all have a substantial impact on drug release in IBD. There are unique opportunities to develop responsive and intelligent medication delivery systems due to these microenvironmental cues [30, 31].

Because of early degradation, off-target effects, or inadequate penetration at the site of inflammation, the effectiveness of treatment medicines in IBD may be challenged. The complex nature of the sick colon, in which inflammation alters the biochemical, physical, and immunological milieu, is not addressed by conventional drug delivery techniques. Researchers are now able to leverage particular characteristics of the IBD microenvironment for site-specific and regulated medication release thanks to recent developments in nanotechnology and biomaterials. The key microenvironmental alterations in IBD are discussed in this chapter, along with how these characteristics affect and facilitate tailored medication delivery techniques [31, 32].

THE IBD MICROENVIRONMENT AFFECTING DRUG RELEASE

Altered pH Implication for Drug Delivery with Example

The pH normally falls between 6.5 and 7.0 in a healthy colon. However, due to the accumulation of acidic metabolites, bacterial dysbiosis, and reduced bicarbonate secretion, the pH falls to about 5.0–6.0 in IBD, particularly during active inflammation [33]. Implications for drug delivery are the use of pH-sensitive polymers, such as Eudragit® S100, which dissolves above pH 7, and Eudragit® L100, which dissolves above pH 6 [34, 35]. This ensures targeted release in the irritated colon [34]. For example, the active ingredient in eudragit-coated mesalamine tablets (like Asacol®) is released in the colon and terminal ileum, reducing absorption in the upper gastrointestinal tract [36, 37].

Elevated Reactive Oxygen Species (ROS) — Implications for Drug Delivery with Example

Excessive generation of ROS, including superoxide, hydroxyl radicals, and hydrogen peroxide, by immune cells (neutrophils and macrophages) invading the body is a sign of IBD pathogenesis. ROS worsen inflammation and result in oxidative damage [38].

Implications for Drug Deliver: Under oxidative conditions, materials that are sensitive to ROS (such as thioketal linkers) undergo degradation, thereby releasing the medication at the site of inflammation [38, 39]. For example, in mice affected by colitis caused by Dextran Sulfate Sodium (DSS), thioketal-based nanoparticles loaded with TNF-α siRNA showed selective release in inflammatory colonic regions, significantly reducing local inflammation [39 - 41].

ROS-Responsive drug delivery in IBD: Thioketal nanoparticles have been shown to release TNF-α siRNA in the ROS-rich region of DDS-induced colitis in mice, reducing local inflammation.

Enzyme Overexpression — Implication for Drug Delivery with Example

Enzymes linked to digestion and immunity, including Matrix Metalloproteinases (MMPs), esterases, and azoreductases, are increased in the colon as a result of inflammation [42]. Implications for drug delivery include prodrugs and nanoparticle coatings that contain enzyme-sensitive links that can cleave selectively in inflammatory regions, causing the release of the drugs [43]. For example, Azoreductase from colonic bacteria cleaves azo-linked prodrugs of 5-Aminosalicylic Acid (5-ASA), such as sulfasalazine, to release the drug's active ingredient locally [42, 44, 45].

Immune Cell Infiltration — Implication for Drug Delivery with Example

Mucosal infiltration by T lymphocytes, neutrophils, and macrophages is a characteristic of IBD [46]. Receptors like CD44, scavenger receptors, and folate receptor-β are increased in these immune cells [47].

Implication for Drug Delivery: Delivery to inflammatory immune cells can be selectively achieved *via* active targeting through ligand-receptor interactions [48, 49]. For example, Dexamethasone-delivering folate-decorated liposomes demonstrated greater anti-inflammatory activity in colitis models due to increased absorption by activated macrophages [50].

Disrupted Mucosal Barrier — Implications for Drug Delivery with Example

Because of decreased mucin synthesis and damage to the epithelial cells, the mucus layer is thinner and more porous in IBD, which increases the penetration of pathogens and foreign particles [51].

Implications for Drug Delivery: Mucus-penetrating nanoparticles, such as PEGylated nanoparticles, can pass through mucus and gather in the submucosa or epithelial layer [52]. Fig. (**12**) shows the disrupted mucosal barrier and PEGylated nanoparticle delivery in IBD. For example, in mice treated with Dextran Sodium Sulfate (DSS) to induce colitis, PEGylated PLGA nanoparticles containing budesonide showed improved penetration and retention in inflammatory colonic regions [52, 53].

Dysbiosis and Microbial Enzymes

IBD modifies the nature of the gut microbiota, thereby affecting enzyme activity and microbial metabolism. One can use specific bacterial enzymes to break down carriers or activate prodrugs [54, 55].

Implications for Drug Delivery: Enzyme-cleavable coatings can be used to target bacterial enzyme-rich areas, causing colon-specific delivery [56]. For example, in the distal colon, the drug is released when polysaccharide-based coatings (such as guar gum and pectin) break down in reaction to microbial enzymes [57].

MULTIFUNCTIONAL NANOCARRIER SYSTEMS: HARNESSING THE IBD MICROENVIRONMENT

Precision therapy is becoming possible as more nanoformulations are developed to respond to multiple IBD-related stimuli [58]. Among the examples are:

Dual pH- and ROS-Responsive Nanoparticles

Poly(β-amino ester) nanoparticles containing curcumin provide a novel formulation approach for targeted drug delivery [59]. Site-specific drug release is made possible by the mechanism of action, which involves pH-dependent swelling of the nanoparticle matrix and breakdown caused by Reactive Oxygen Species (ROS) [58, 59]. By releasing curcumin, particularly in oxidative and acidic environments, considerable therapeutic benefits were observed in mouse models of colitis, consequently lowering the degree of inflammation associated with colitis [58].

Enzyme and pH Dual-Sensitive Hydrogels

To deliver probiotics or anti-inflammatory medications, a hydrogel-based formulation combining gelatin and Matrix Metalloproteinase (MMP)-cleavable linkers has been designed [60 - 62]. Thus, to ensure targeted and responsive medication release, this innovative hydrogel is designed to expand in acidic pH environments and break down in the presence of inflammatory mucosa that is high in MMPs [63]. As a result, it makes it possible for therapeutic drugs to be delivered continuously and aids in the gut microbiome regeneration, which may help treat inflammatory bowel disorders [62, 63].

CLINICAL IMPLICATIONS AND TRANSLATIONAL CONSIDERATIONS

Despite the fact that numerous stimuli-responsive systems have shown promise in preclinical models, a number of obstacles need to be overcome before they can be used in clinical settings [64, 65]:

- Stimulus strength is affected by heterogeneity in disease severity and place (*e.g.*, ROS levels differ amongst individuals).
- Without early activation, stability during GI transit must be guaranteed.
- Reproducibility and scalability in the development of smart nanocarriers.
- Synthetic polymers and nanoparticles enhance safety and regulatory concerns.

Nonetheless, a new era of precision IBD treatment may be ushered in by the success of certain formulations that are making progress in clinical studies [65].

IBD's inflammatory milieu provides a variety of physiological and biochemical indicators that can be used to improve smart drug delivery. These characteristics, which range from immune cell activity and enzymatic overexpression to pH changes and ROS abundance, make it possible to create responsive, site-specific drug release systems, as shown in Table **1**. Advanced drug delivery solutions hold great promise for improving therapeutic outcomes in IBD as nanotechnology and biomaterials continue to evolve [45].

Table 1. Microenvironmental features and corresponding delivery strategies.

Microenvironmental Feature	Example Formulation	Delivery Strategy
Acidic pH	Eudragit-coated mesalamine [36]	pH-sensitive polymers
High ROS levels	Thioketal nanoparticles with siRNA [66]	ROS-responsive linkers
MMPs/Proteases	Gelatin-based hydrogels [67]	Enzyme-cleavable polymers
Immune cell markers	Folate-liposomes with dexamethasone [69]	Ligand-targeted nanocarriers
Mucus disruption	PEGylated PLGA NPs [70]	Mucus-penetrating particles
Dysbiosis and enzymes	Azo-linked sulfasalazine [42]	Microbial-degradable coatings

- Systems that respond to several inputs for higher specificity.
- Platforms for personalized therapy based on each patient's unique microbiota and illness indicators.
- Biodegradable and bioinspired carriers to improve functionality and safety.
- Integration with theranostic methods' diagnostic tools [71].

TARGETING STRATEGIES IN NANO-BASED DELIVERY

Passive Targeting

Passive targeting exploits the Enhanced Permeability and Retention (EPR) effect induced by abnormal blood vessel formation and increased permeability at inflammatory locations [72].

Enhanced Permeability and Retention (EPR) Effect

Nanoparticles, which are usually 100–200 nm in size, can aggregate specifically in inflammatory intestinal tissues due to leaky vasculature and reduced lymphatic drainage [72, 73].

Mucosal Adhesion

Certain nanoparticles are made with mucoadhesive polymers (such as pectin and chitosan) that prolong their residence time in the colon and improve local drug availability [74].

Example: PLGA nanoparticles coated with chitosan [70] and loaded with dexamethasone show enhanced mucosal adhesion and long-lasting anti-inflammatory effects in mouse models of colitis [69].

Active Targeting Strategies

Active targeting is the process by which ligands bind to overexpressed cell markers or receptors in inflamed intestinal regions [72].

Targeting Immune Cells

a. Targeting Macrophages

Activated macrophages that express mannose receptors (CD206) are abundant in inflammatory areas [75].

Strategy: Attaching mannose or mannose derivatives to the surface of nanoparticles [76]. For example, in DSS-induced colitis, mannosylated solid lipid nanoparticles loaded with budesonide demonstrated enhanced macrophage uptake and decreased colonic inflammation [77].

b. Dendritic Cell Targeting

Anti-DEC-205 antibodies can be used for targeted delivery [78], which can guide nanoparticles to dendritic cells and alter immune responses [79].

Targeting Epithelial Cells

a. Folate Receptor Targeting

The inflammatory colonic epithelium overexpresses folate receptors [80, 81]. Strategy: Nanoparticles coupled with folate for receptor-mediated endocytosis [82]. For example, 5-Aminosalicylic Acid (5-ASA) incorporated into folate-functionalized PLGA nanoparticles enhanced localized drug release and cellular absorption in epithelial cells [83]. Inhibiting cell trafficking to the gut mucosa can be achieved by targeting α4β7 integrin, which is expressed on active leukocytes [84].

Adhesion Molecule Targeting

In IBD, adhesion molecules ICAM-1 and VCAM-1 are increased. Strategy: Selective binding using antibody-functionalized nanoparticles. For example, as shown in Fig. (**1**), in inflammatory colon tissues, liposomes containing siRNA and tagged with an anti-ICAM-1 antibody showed excellent specificity and efficient gene silencing.

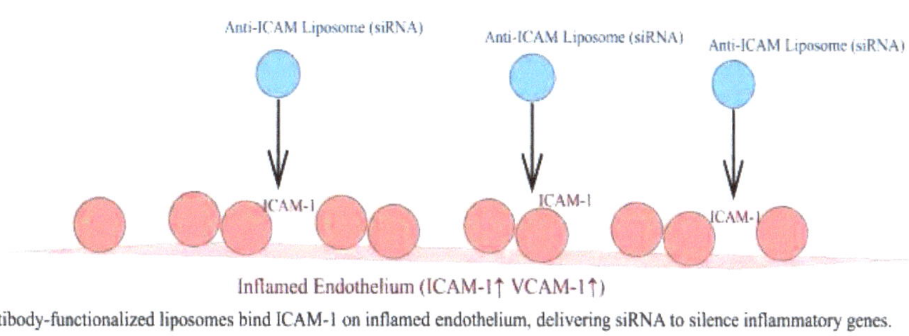

Fig. (1). Targeting ICAM-1 in IBD using Antibody-Functionalized Liposomes [84].

Targeting That Responds to Stimuli

For regulated drug release, nanoparticles can be designed to react to IBD-specific stimuli such as pH, enzymes, and Reactive Oxygen Species (ROS), as illustrated in Fig. (**2**) [85].

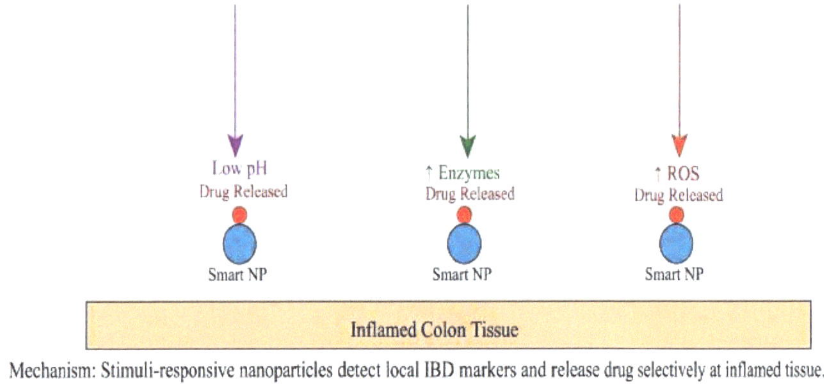

Fig. (2). Stimule-Responsive Nanoparticle Mechanism in IBD.

Delivery that is sensitive to pH

The pH of inflammatory colonic areas is frequently lower (5.0–6.0) [86].

Strategy: Employ pH-sensitive polymers such as poly(methacrylic acid) or Eudragit S100 [36]. For example, curcumin-encapsulated pH-sensitive liposomes improved local anti-inflammatory effects by releasing their payload in the acidic environment of inflammatory tissues [36, 86].

Delivery that is Enzyme-responsive

In IBD, there is an increase in proteases, glycosidases, and Matrix Metalloproteinases (MMPs) [63].

Strategy: Prodrugs may be activated or degraded by disease-specific enzymes [87]. For example, 5-ASA was released in the sick tissues *via* dextran-based nanoparticles that were broken down by colonic glycosidases [42].

ROS-responsive Delivery

Excess ROS are produced by inflammatory tissues [58].

Strategy: Include ROS-cleavable linkers (diselenide, thioketal) in nanocarriers [66]. For example, in colitis models, thiolated silica nanoparticles reduced inflammation by releasing dexamethasone in response to oxidative stress [66].

Strategies for Dual or Multifunctional Targeting

As shown in Fig. (**3**), combining different targeting methods improves accuracy and effectiveness [51, 52]. For example, Budesonide administration using mannose and pH-responsive nanoparticles improved therapeutic efficacy and decreased systemic toxicity by targeting both macrophages and acidic environments [52, 53]. In TNBS-induced colitis [58], folate-functionalized, ROS-sensitive liposomes loaded with siRNA [88] and anti-inflammatory medications produced synergistic benefits [89].

Translational Aspects and *in vivo* Examples

As summarized in Table **2**, nano-based strategies have shown significant promise in preclinical models of IBD, with multiple *in vivo* studies demonstrating improved therapeutic outcomes.

Table 2. Multi-responsive Nanocarriers for Drug Delivery.

Nanocarrier Type	Drug Loaded	Model	Outcomes	Reference
PLGA NPs	Budesonide	TNBS-induced colitis (rat)	Reduced inflammation, increased drug accumulation	[70]
Liposomes	Patchouli alcohol	DSS-induced colitis (mouse)	Decreased disease activity, body weight loss	[65]
Chitosan NPs	Curcumin	DSS-induced colitis (mouse)	Attenuated clinical symptoms, colon damage	[38]
ROS-responsive NPs	Genistein	DSS-induced colitis (mouse)	Reduced DAI, increased colon length	[58]
Hyaluronic Acid NPs	Lysine-Proline-Valine tripeptide	DSS-induced colitis (mouse)	Decreased colitis signs, mucosa healing	[88]
Folate-functionalized NPs	6-Shogaol	DSS-induced colitis (mouse)	Soothed colitis symptoms, bowel regeneration	[89]

These examples (Table **2**) show the potential of nano-based strategies to enhance drug delivery, reduce systemic side effects, and improve therapeutic outcomes in IBD. Future research should focus on developing multi-responsive nanocarriers that can simultaneously target multiple pathological features of IBD, paving the way for more effective and personalized treatments.

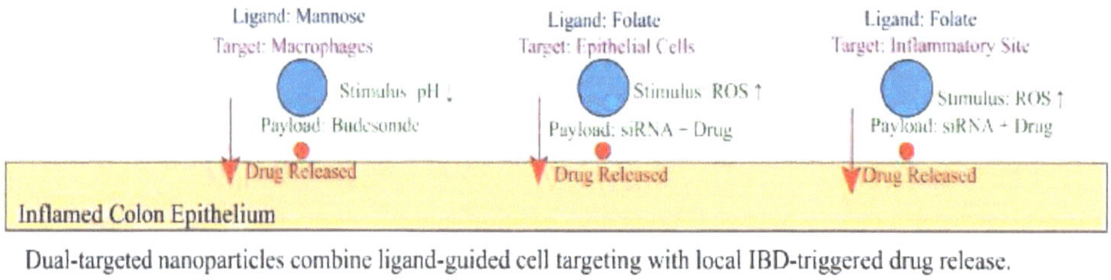

Fig. (3). Dual/Multifunctional Targeting Nanoparticles in IBD.

CONCLUSION

This chapter examines how drug delivery is impacted by the distinct and pathological milieu of Inflammatory Bowel Disease (IBD) and how nanotechnology can be used to enhance therapeutic results. IBD, which includes Crohn's disease and ulcerative colitis, is characterized by immunological dysregulation, fibrosis, epithelial barrier failure, disturbed microbiota (dysbiosis), chronic inflammation, and changes in biochemical parameters such as pH and enzyme activity. The pathological features of IBD include alterations in the intestinal microenvironment and immune dysregulation, with overproduction of cytokines (*e.g.*, TNF-α and IL-6) leading to persistent inflammation.

Dysbiosis: Changes in the gut microbiota result in an increase in harmful bacteria and a decrease in protective species.

Barrier Dysfunction: Immune activation is promoted by a leaky gut, caused by the loss of tight junction integrity.

Fibrosis: Prolonged inflammation impairs intestinal motility and leads to tissue scarring.

Acidic pH and Enzyme Activity: Inflammation alters drug solubility and metabolism by inducing local acidosis and upregulating enzymes such as Matrix Metalloproteinases (MMPs).

Vascular Changes: Increased vascular permeability and angiogenesis influence drug accumulation in inflamed intestinal regions.

Implications for Drug Release: Conventional therapeutics struggle in the complex IBD microenvironment, while nanotechnology offers prospects for intelligent, site-specific drug delivery. Environmental cues like these can be used to customize responsive delivery systems.

pH variations: pH-sensitive coatings enable regulated drug release in response to local acidity.

ROS levels: In oxidative environments, Reactive Oxygen Species (ROS) trigger the degradation of ROS-sensitive linkers or carriers, resulting in targeted drug release.

Enzyme sensitivity: Drug carriers that respond to overexpressed enzymes can achieve site-specific release in tissues with elevated enzymatic activity.

Ligand-receptor interactions: Nanoparticles decorated with specific ligands can selectively target immune cells, such as macrophages, *via* receptor-mediated uptake.

Mucus penetration: Nanoparticles designed to penetrate mucus can reach deeper tissue layers, particularly where mucus structure is disrupted during inflammation.

Multifunctional Nanocarriers: Advanced systems, such as enzyme/pH-sensitive hydrogels and dual pH- and ROS-sensitive nanoparticles, react to a variety of stimuli. These offer enhanced therapeutic efficacy, prolonged release, and localization.

Targeting Techniques for Delivery using Nanotechnology:

- The Enhanced Permeability and Retention (EPR) effect in inflammatory tissues is used in passive targeting.
- Active Targeting uses ligand-conjugated nanoparticles to target adhesion molecules such as ICAM-1, immune cells, or epithelial cells.
- Stimuli-Responsive Targeting allows for regulated release according to enzymes, ROS, or local pH.
- Multifunctional targeting combines several strategies to increase treatment synergy and specificity.

Preclinical research is encouraging, but issues, including patient variability, medication stability, manufacturing scalability, and regulatory safety, need to be resolved. Future developments can include customized nanoformulations based on illness profiles and microbiota, bioinspired and biodegradable carriers, and integration with diagnostic tools (theranostic).

DISCLAIMER (ARTIFICIAL INTELLIGENCE)

Partial use of artificial intelligence tools (Perplexity AI) was employed solely to enhance the language and improve clarity of the manuscript. The scientific content, interpretations, and conclusions presented in this chapter are entirely the responsibility of the authors.

REFRENCES

[1] Gan R, Ni E, Li G, Chen W. A new paradigm for precision drug delivery in inflammatory bowel disease: Effective transfer, enhanced retention, and pathology-targeting treatment *via* biomaterials and engineered platforms. MedComm – Biomaterials and Applications 2025; 4(3): e70022. [http://dx.doi.org/10.1002/mba2.70022]

[2] Yasmin F, Najeeb H, Shaikh S, *et al.* Novel drug delivery systems for inflammatory bowel disease. World J Gastroenterol 2022; 28(18): 1922-33. [http://dx.doi.org/10.3748/wjg.v28.i18.1922] [PMID: 35664964]

[3] Mohajeri S, Moayedi S, Mohajeri S, Yadegar A, Haririan I. Targeting pathophysiological changes using biomaterials-based drug delivery systems: A key to managing inflammatory bowel disease. Front Pharmacol 2022; 13: 1045575. [http://dx.doi.org/10.3389/fphar.2022.1045575] [PMID: 36438794]

[4] Huang W, Hsu JC, Zhou J, *et al.* Stimuli-responsive nanomaterials for targeted drug delivery in inflammatory bowel disease: Advances and emerging directions. Matter 2025; 8(9): 102249. [http://dx.doi.org/10.1016/j.matt.2025.102249] [PMID: 41200039]

[5] Gao J, Li J, Luo Z, Wang H, Ma Z. Nanoparticle-based drug delivery systems for inflammatory bowel disease treatment. Drug Des Devel Ther 2024; 18: 2921-49. [http://dx.doi.org/10.2147/DDDT.S461977] [PMID: 39055164]

[6] Wang H, Zhou F, Shen M, Ma R, Yu Q. Classification of nanomaterial drug delivery systems for inflammatory bowel disease. Int J Nanomedicine 2025; 20: 1383-99. [http://dx.doi.org/10.2147/IJN.S502546] [PMID: 39925683]

[7] Kiilerich KF, Andresen T, Darbani B, *et al.* Advancing inflammatory bowel disease treatment by targeting the innate immune system and precision drug delivery. Int J Mol Sci 2025; 26(2): 575. [http://dx.doi.org/10.3390/ijms26020575] [PMID: 39859291]

[8] Yan PG, Li JN. Advances in the understanding of the intestinal micro-environment and inflammatory bowel disease. Chin Med J (Engl) 2020; 133(7): 834-41. [http://dx.doi.org/10.1097/CM9.0000000000000718] [PMID: 32106123]

[9] Colgan SP, Curtis VF, Campbell EL. The inflammatory tissue microenvironment in IBD. Inflamm Bowel Dis 2013; 19(10): 2238-44. [http://dx.doi.org/10.1097/MIB.0b013e31828dcaaf] [PMID: 23702808]

[10] Long A, Kleiner A, Looney RJ. Immune dysregulation. J Allergy Clin Immunol 2023; 151(1): 70-80. [http://dx.doi.org/10.1016/j.jaci.2022.11.001] [PMID: 36608984]

[11] Pedersen J, Coskun M, Soendergaard C, Salem M, Nielsen OH. Inflammatory pathways of importance for management of inflammatory bowel disease. World J Gastroenterol 2014; 20(1): 64-77. [http://dx.doi.org/10.3748/wjg.v20.i1.64] [PMID: 24415859]

[12] Wei J, Feng J. Signaling pathways associated with inflammatory bowel disease. Recent Pat Inflamm Allergy Drug Discov 2010; 4(2): 105-17. [http://dx.doi.org/10.2174/187221310791163071] [PMID: 20001899]

[13] Bamias G, Pizarro TT, Cominelli F. Pathway-based approaches to the treatment of inflammatory bowel disease. Transl Res 2016; 167(1): 104-15. [http://dx.doi.org/10.1016/j.trsl.2015.09.002] [PMID: 26408803]

[14] Walker WA. Dysbiosis. InThe microbiota in gastrointestinal pathophysiology. Academic Press 2017; 1: 227-32.

[15] Weiss GA, Hennet T. Mechanisms and consequences of intestinal dysbiosis. Cell Mol Life Sci 2017; 74(16): 2959-77. [http://dx.doi.org/10.1007/s00018-017-2509-x] [PMID: 28352996]

[16] Carding S, Verbeke K, Vipond DT, Corfe BM, Owen LJ. Dysbiosis of the gut microbiota in disease.

Microb Ecol Health Dis 2015; 26(1): 26191.
[http://dx.doi.org/10.3402/mehd.v26.26191] [PMID: 25651997]

[17] Celebi Sözener Z, Cevhertas L, Nadeau K, Akdis M, Akdis CA. Environmental factors in epithelial barrier dysfunction. J Allergy Clin Immunol 2020; 145(6): 1517-28.
[http://dx.doi.org/10.1016/j.jaci.2020.04.024] [PMID: 32507229]

[18] Lee J, Wasinger V, Yau Y, Chuang E, Yajnik V, Leong R. Molecular pathophysiology of epithelial barrier dysfunction in inflammatory bowel diseases. Proteomes 2018; 6(2): 17.
[http://dx.doi.org/10.3390/proteomes6020017] [PMID: 29614738]

[19] McGuckin MA, Eri R, Simms LA, Florin THJ, Radford-Smith G. Intestinal barrier dysfunction in inflammatory bowel diseases. Inflamm Bowel Dis 2009; 15(1): 100-13.
[http://dx.doi.org/10.1002/ibd.20539] [PMID: 18623167]

[20] Dai T, Fang W, Zhu W, *et al.* Atractylenolide III ameliorates DSS-induced colitis by improving intestinal epithelial barrier *via* suppressing the NF-κB-Mediated MLCK-pMLC signaling pathway. Food Chem Toxicol 2025; 196: 115158.
[http://dx.doi.org/10.1016/j.fct.2024.115158] [PMID: 39613239]

[21] Ahn JH, da Silva Pedrosa M, Lopez LR, *et al.* Intestinal E. coli-produced yersiniabactin promotes profibrotic macrophages in Crohn's disease. Cell Host Microbe 2025; 33(1): 71-88.e9.
[http://dx.doi.org/10.1016/j.chom.2024.11.012] [PMID: 39701098]

[22] Acharjee A, Shivaji U, Santacroce G, *et al.* Novel transcriptomic signatures in fibrostenotic crohn's disease: Dysregulated pathways, promising biomarkers, and putative therapeutic targets. Inflamm Bowel Dis 2025; 31(6): 1502-13.
[http://dx.doi.org/10.1093/ibd/izaf021] [PMID: 39977234]

[23] Chen Y, Li J, Zhang X, *et al.* Mesenteric adipose-derived exosomal TINAGL1 enhances intestinal fibrosis in Crohn's Disease *via* SMAD4. J Adv Res 2025; 70: 139-58.
[http://dx.doi.org/10.1016/j.jare.2024.05.016] [PMID: 38750695]

[24] Nugent SG, Kumar D, Rampton DS, Evans DF. Intestinal luminal pH in inflammatory bowel disease: possible determinants and implications for therapy with aminosalicylates and other drugs. Gut 2001; 48(4): 571-7.
[http://dx.doi.org/10.1136/gut.48.4.571] [PMID: 11247905]

[25] Kjærgaard S, Damm MMB, Chang J, *et al.* Altered structural expression and enzymatic activity parameters in quiescent ulcerative colitis: are these potential normalization criteria? Int J Mol Sci 2020; 21(5): 1887.
[http://dx.doi.org/10.3390/ijms21051887] [PMID: 32164249]

[26] Siddique I, Khan I. Mechanism of regulation of Na-H exchanger in inflammatory bowel disease: role of TLR-4 signaling mechanism. Dig Dis Sci 2011; 56(6): 1656-62.
[http://dx.doi.org/10.1007/s10620-010-1524-7] [PMID: 21221801]

[27] Pousa ID, Maté J, Gisbert JP. Angiogenesis in inflammatory bowel disease. Eur J Clin Invest 2008; 38(2): 73-81.
[http://dx.doi.org/10.1111/j.1365-2362.2007.01914.x] [PMID: 18226040]

[28] Zoroddu S, Di Lorenzo B, Paliogiannis P, Mangoni AA, Carru C, Zinellu A. Vascular endothelial growth factor in inflammatory bowel disease: A systematic review and meta-analysis. Eur J Clin Invest 2025; 55(3): e14361.
[http://dx.doi.org/10.1111/eci.14361] [PMID: 39545600]

[29] Wang S, Jiang Q, Liu Y, Zhang X, Huang Y, Zhang H. The role of immune cells in moyamoya disease. Brain Sci 2025; 15(2): 137.
[http://dx.doi.org/10.3390/brainsci15020137] [PMID: 40002470]

[30] Kiilerich KF, Andresen T, Darbani B, *et al.* Advancing inflammatory bowel disease treatment by targeting the innate immune system and precision drug delivery. Int J Mol Sci 2025; 26(2): 575.

[http://dx.doi.org/10.3390/ijms26020575] [PMID: 39859291]

[31] Singh D, Srivastava S, Pradhan M, Kanwar JR, Singh MR. Inflammatory bowel disease: pathogenesis, causative factors, issues, drug treatment strategies, and delivery approaches. Critical Reviews™ in Therapeutic Drug Carrier Systems 2015; 32(3) [http://dx.doi.org/10.1615/CritRevTherDrugCarrierSyst.2015011095]

[32] Kotla NG, Singh R, Baby BV, *et al.* Inflammation-specific targeted carriers for local drug delivery to inflammatory bowel disease. Biomaterials 2022; 281: 121364. [http://dx.doi.org/10.1016/j.biomaterials.2022.121364] [PMID: 35066288]

[33] Gvozdeva Y, Staynova R. pH-dependent drug delivery systems for ulcerative colitis treatment. Pharmaceutics 2025; 17(2): 226. [http://dx.doi.org/10.3390/pharmaceutics17020226] [PMID: 40006593]

[34] Zeeshan M, Ali H, Khan S, Khan SA, Weigmann B. Advances in orally-delivered pH-sensitive nanocarrier systems; an optimistic approach for the treatment of inflammatory bowel disease. Int J Pharm 2019; 558: 201-14. [http://dx.doi.org/10.1016/j.ijpharm.2018.12.074] [PMID: 30615925]

[35] Kshirsagar SJ, Bhalekar MR, Umap RR. *In vitro in vivo* comparison of two pH sensitive Eudragit polymers for colon specific drug delivery. Journal of pharmaceutical sciences and research 2009; 1(4): 61.

[36] Heikal EJ, Kaoud RM, Gad S, *et al.* Development of Novel pH-sensitive eudragit coated beads containing curcumin-mesalamine combination for colon-specific drug delivery. Gels 2023; 9(4): 264. [http://dx.doi.org/10.3390/gels9040264] [PMID: 37102876]

[37] Patil PB, Hajare AA, Awale RP. Development and evaluation of mesalamine tablet formulation for colon delivery. Research Journal of Pharmacy and Technology 2011; 4(11): 1751-6.

[38] Xiong T, Xu H, Nie Q, *et al.* Reactive oxygen species triggered cleavage of thioketal-containing supramolecular nanoparticles for inflammation-targeted oral therapy in ulcerative colitis. Adv Funct Mater 2025; 35(1): 2411979. [http://dx.doi.org/10.1002/adfm.202411979]

[39] Shrestha P, Duwa R, Lee S, Kwon TK, Jeong JH, Yook S. ROS-responsive thioketal nanoparticles delivering system for targeted ulcerative colitis therapy with potent HDAC6 inhibitor, tubastatin A. Eur J Pharm Sci 2024; 201: 106856. [http://dx.doi.org/10.1016/j.ejps.2024.106856] [PMID: 39032536]

[40] Regmi S, Pathak S, Nepal MR, *et al.* Inflammation-triggered local drug release ameliorates colitis by inhibiting dendritic cell migration and Th1/Th17 differentiation. J Control Release 2019; 316: 138-49. [http://dx.doi.org/10.1016/j.jconrel.2019.11.001] [PMID: 31689461]

[41] Fukata T, Mizushima T, Nishimura J, *et al.* The supercarbonate apatite-MicroRNA complex inhibits dextran sodium sulfate-induced colitis. Mol Ther Nucleic Acids 2018; 12: 658-71. [http://dx.doi.org/10.1016/j.omtn.2018.07.007] [PMID: 30092402]

[42] Wang W, Chen Y, Wang Y, *et al.* Azo-linked 5-ASA-coumarin prodrug: Fluorescent tracking for colonic drug release in UC treatment. Talanta 2025; 284: 127277. [http://dx.doi.org/10.1016/j.talanta.2024.127277] [PMID: 39608145]

[43] Nedelcu A, Mosteanu O, Pop T, Mocan T, Mocan L. Recent advances in nanoparticle-mediated treatment of inflammatory bowel diseases. Appl Sci (Basel) 2021; 11(1): 438. [http://dx.doi.org/10.3390/app11010438]

[44] Suneela D, Gaurav V, Samuel S. Azo reductase- activated colon- targeting prodrugs of aminosalicylates for inflammatory bowel disease: preparation, pharmacokinetic and pharmacodynamic profile. Inflamm Allergy Drug Targets 2013; 12(6): 419-32. [http://dx.doi.org/10.2174/1871528112666131122103940] [PMID: 24266686]

[45] Rajput IB, Khan D, Mirza R, *et al.* Inflammatory bowel disease: Exploring pathogenesis,

epidemiology, conventional therapies, and advanced nanoparticle based drug delivery systems. Bionanoscience 2025; 15(1): 206.
[http://dx.doi.org/10.1007/s12668-025-01809-6]

[46] Zhou GX, Liu ZJ. Potential roles of neutrophils in regulating intestinal mucosal inflammation of inflammatory bowel disease. J Dig Dis 2017; 18(9): 495-503.
[http://dx.doi.org/10.1111/1751-2980.12540] [PMID: 28857501]

[47] Gerami M. Folate receptor beta as an imaging target for inflammatory bowel disease. Immune Netw 2016; 16(6): 337-43.

[48] Kiilerich KF, Andresen T, Darbani B, *et al.* Advancing inflammatory bowel disease treatment by targeting the innate immune system and precision drug delivery. Int J Mol Sci 2025; 26(2): 575.
[http://dx.doi.org/10.3390/ijms26020575] [PMID: 39859291]

[49] Yasmin F, Najeeb H, Shaikh S, *et al.* Novel drug delivery systems for inflammatory bowel disease. World J Gastroenterol 2022; 28(18): 1922-33.
[http://dx.doi.org/10.3748/wjg.v28.i18.1922] [PMID: 35664964]

[50] Kumar A, Husain N, Anbazhagan AN, *et al.* Dexamethasone upregulates the expression of the human SLC26A3 (DRA, *D* own- *R* egulated in *A* denoma) transporter (an IBD Susceptibility Gene) in intestinal epithelial cells and attenuates gut inflammation. Inflamm Bowel Dis 2025; 31(3): 625-35.
[http://dx.doi.org/10.1093/ibd/izae271] [PMID: 39657154]

[51] Mansouri P, Mansouri P, Behmard E, Najafipour S, Kouhpayeh A, Farjadfar A. Novel targets for mucosal healing in inflammatory bowel disease therapy. Int Immunopharmacol 2025; 144: 113544.
[http://dx.doi.org/10.1016/j.intimp.2024.113544] [PMID: 39571265]

[52] Shakeri R, Mirjalili SZ, Karakus CO, Safavi M. Therapeutic and pharmaceutical applications of pegylated nano-carriers. InPEGylated nanocarriers in medicine and pharmacy. Singapore: Springer Nature Singapore 2025; 1: 555-602.
[http://dx.doi.org/10.1007/978-981-97-7316-9_18]

[53] Jackson K, Galipeau H, Hann A, *et al.* Lytic phage attenuates colitis severity in gnotobiotic mice colonized with ibd-associated *E. coli* NRG857C. Inflamm Bowel Dis 2025; 31 (Suppl. 1): S4-5.
[http://dx.doi.org/10.1093/ibd/izae282.012]

[54] Martell M, Quarnstrom CF, Khoruts A, Vezys V, Staley C, Shmidt E. Chronic intestinal inflammation and microbial dysbiosis are associated with female reproductive outcomes in a mouse model of inflammatory bowel disease. Gastro Hep Advances 2025; 3: 100670.
[http://dx.doi.org/10.1016/j.gastha.2025.100670]

[55] Fernández-Veledo S, Grau-Bové C, Notararigo S, Huber-Ruano I. The role of microbial succinate in the pathophysiology of inflammatory bowel disease: mechanisms and therapeutic potential. Curr Opin Microbiol 2025; 85: 102599.
[http://dx.doi.org/10.1016/j.mib.2025.102599] [PMID: 40132355]

[56] Zhao S, Yu N, Han H, Guo S, Murthy N. Advances in acid-degradable and enzyme-cleavable linkers for drug delivery. Curr Opin Chem Biol 2025; 84: 102552.
[http://dx.doi.org/10.1016/j.cbpa.2024.102552] [PMID: 39642424]

[57] Udaipuria N, Bhattacharya S. Novel carbohydrate polymer-based systems for precise drug delivery in colon cancer: Improving treatment effectiveness with intelligent biodegradable materials. Biopolymers 2025; 116(1): e23632.
[http://dx.doi.org/10.1002/bip.23632] [PMID: 39340194]

[58] Wan X, Zhang C, Lei P, *et al.* Precision therapeutics for inflammatory bowel disease: advancing ROS-responsive nanoparticles for targeted and multifunctional drug delivery. J Mater Chem B Mater Biol Med 2025; 13(10): 3245-69.
[http://dx.doi.org/10.1039/D4TB02868F] [PMID: 39905851]

[59] Markovic MD, Panic VV, Pjanovic RV. Polymeric nanosystems: A breakthrough approach to treating

inflammation and inflammation related diseases. Biopolymers 2025; 116(3): e70012.
[http://dx.doi.org/10.1002/bip.70012] [PMID: 40104970]

[60] Zhang Q, Lv B, Li M, *et al.* Recent advances in the application of hydrogels as drug carriers in inflammatory bowel disease: A review. Int J Mol Sci 2025; 26(7): 2894.
[http://dx.doi.org/10.3390/ijms26072894] [PMID: 40243468]

[61] Zhang S, Kang L, Hu S, *et al.* Carboxymethyl chitosan microspheres loaded hyaluronic acid/gelatin hydrogels for controlled drug delivery and the treatment of inflammatory bowel disease. Int J Biol Macromol 2021; 167: 1598-612.
[http://dx.doi.org/10.1016/j.ijbiomac.2020.11.117] [PMID: 33220374]

[62] Abed OA, Attlassy Y, Xu J, Han K, Moon JJ. Emerging nanotechnologies and microbiome engineering for the treatment of inflammatory bowel disease. Mol Pharm 2022; 19(12): 4393-410.
[http://dx.doi.org/10.1021/acs.molpharmaceut.2c00222] [PMID: 35878420]

[63] Long J, Liang X, Ao Z, *et al.* Stimulus-responsive drug delivery nanoplatforms for inflammatory bowel disease therapy. Acta Biomater 2024; 188: 27-47.
[http://dx.doi.org/10.1016/j.actbio.2024.09.007] [PMID: 39265673]

[64] Nicolò S, Faggiani I, Errico C, *et al.* Translational characterization of immune pathways in inflammatory bowel disease: insights for targeted treatments. Expert Rev Clin Immunol 2025; 21(1): 55-72.
[http://dx.doi.org/10.1080/1744666X.2024.2400300] [PMID: 39313992]

[65] Prasad S, Cross RK, Monroe MB, *et al.* Challenges in IBD research 2024: Novel technologies. Inflamm Bowel Dis 2024; 30 (Suppl. 2): S30-8.
[http://dx.doi.org/10.1093/ibd/izae082] [PMID: 38778625]

[66] Wilson DS, Dalmasso G, Wang L, Sitaraman SV, Merlin D, Murthy N. Orally delivered thioketal nanoparticles loaded with TNF-α–siRNA target inflammation and inhibit gene expression in the intestines. Nat Mater 2010; 9(11): 923-8.
[http://dx.doi.org/10.1038/nmat2859] [PMID: 20935658]

[67] Zhu Y, Wang Q, Chen Y, *et al.* Living probiotics-loaded hydrogel microspheres with gastric acid resistance and ROS triggered release for potential therapy of inflammatory bowel disease. ACS Appl Polym Mater 2023; 5(1): 957-67.
[http://dx.doi.org/10.1021/acsapm.2c01893]

[68] Raj S. Biomaterials for manipulating mast cell activity. Doctoral dissertation, University of Alberta 2021.

[69] Poh S, Chelvam V, Ayala-López W, Putt KS, Low PS. Selective liposome targeting of folate receptor positive immune cells in inflammatory diseases. Nanomedicine 2018; 14(3): 1033-43.
[http://dx.doi.org/10.1016/j.nano.2018.01.009] [PMID: 29410110]

[70] Shrestha N, Xu Y, Prévost JRC, *et al.* Impact of PEGylation on an antibody-loaded nanoparticle-based drug delivery system for the treatment of inflammatory bowel disease. Acta Biomater 2022; 140: 561-72.
[http://dx.doi.org/10.1016/j.actbio.2021.12.015] [PMID: 34923097]

[71] Shrivastava S, Jain S, Kumar D, Soni SL, Sharma M. A review on theranostics: an approach to targeted diagnosis and therapy. Asian Journal of Pharmaceutical Research and Development 2019; 7(2): 63-9.
[http://dx.doi.org/10.22270/ajprd.v7i2.463]

[72] Neurath MF. Current and emerging therapeutic targets for IBD. Nat Rev Gastroenterol Hepatol 2017; 14(5): 269-78.
[http://dx.doi.org/10.1038/nrgastro.2016.208] [PMID: 28144028]

[73] Li S, Zhang F, Zhang Q. Pathological features-based targeted delivery strategies in IBD therapy: A mini review. Biomed Pharmacother 2022; 151: 113079.

[http://dx.doi.org/10.1016/j.biopha.2022.113079] [PMID: 35605297]

[74] Thomas S, Baumgart DC. Targeting leukocyte migration and adhesion in Crohn's disease and ulcerative colitis. Inflammopharmacology 2012; 20(1): 1-18. [http://dx.doi.org/10.1007/s10787-011-0104-6] [PMID: 22205271]

[75] Na YR, Stakenborg M, Seok SH, Matteoli G. Macrophages in intestinal inflammation and resolution: a potential therapeutic target in IBD. Nat Rev Gastroenterol Hepatol 2019; 16(9): 531-43. [http://dx.doi.org/10.1038/s41575-019-0172-4] [PMID: 31312042]

[76] Mydock-McGrane LK, Cusumano ZT, Janetka JW. Mannose-derived FimH antagonists: a promising anti-virulence therapeutic strategy for urinary tract infections and Crohn's disease. Expert Opin Ther Pat 2016; 26(2): 175-97. [http://dx.doi.org/10.1517/13543776.2016.1131266] [PMID: 26651364]

[77] Pinheiro do Nascimento L, Tsapis N, Reynaud F, *et al.* Mannosylation of budesonide palmitate nanoprodrugs for improved macrophage targeting. Eur J Pharm Biopharm 2022; 170: 112-20. [http://dx.doi.org/10.1016/j.ejpb.2021.12.001] [PMID: 34890789]

[78] Bourque J, Hawiger D. Applications of antibody-based antigen delivery targeted to dendritic cells *in vivo*. Antibodies (Basel) 2022; 11(1): 8. [http://dx.doi.org/10.3390/antib11010008] [PMID: 35225867]

[79] Klaska IP, Yu T, Fordyce R, *et al.* Targeted delivery of autoantigen to dendritic cells prevents development of spontaneous uveitis. Front Immunol 2023; 14: 1227633. [http://dx.doi.org/10.3389/fimmu.2023.1227633] [PMID: 37727784]

[80] Ye X, Chen T, Du Y, *et al.* Folic acid-based hydrogels co-assembled with protocatechuic acid for enhanced treatment of inflammatory bowel disease. Colloids Surf B Biointerfaces 2025; 246: 114367. [http://dx.doi.org/10.1016/j.colsurfb.2024.114367] [PMID: 39541908]

[81] Poh S, Chelvam V, Ayala-López W, Putt KS, Low PS. Selective liposome targeting of folate receptor positive immune cells in inflammatory diseases. Nanomedicine 2018; 14(3): 1033-43. [http://dx.doi.org/10.1016/j.nano.2018.01.009] [PMID: 29410110]

[82] Gardey E, Brendel JC, Stallmach A. Pathophysiology of IBD as a key strategy for polymeric nanoparticle development. Adv Ther (Weinh) 2025; 8(3): 2400439. [http://dx.doi.org/10.1002/adtp.202400439]

[83] Liu Y, Huang J, Li S, *et al.* Advancements in hydrogel-based drug delivery systems for the treatment of inflammatory bowel disease: a review. Biomater Sci 2024; 12(4): 837-62. [http://dx.doi.org/10.1039/D3BM01645E] [PMID: 38196386]

[84] Cancino C, Horn V, Obermayer B, *et al.* P0010 Characterization of proliferating memory $CD4^+$ T cells reveals a distinct immune signature in anti-$\alpha 4\beta 7$ integrin therapy non-responders Inflammatory Bowel Disease patients. J Crohn's Colitis 2025; 19 (Suppl. 1): i346. [http://dx.doi.org/10.1093/ecco-jcc/jjae190.0184]

[85] Parvin N, Joo SW, Mandal TK. Biodegradable and stimuli-responsive nanomaterials for targeted drug delivery in autoimmune diseases. J Funct Biomater 2025; 16(1): 24. [http://dx.doi.org/10.3390/jfb16010024] [PMID: 39852580]

[86] Gvozdeva Y, Staynova R. pH-dependent drug delivery systems for ulcerative colitis treatment. Pharmaceutics 2025; 17(2): 226. [http://dx.doi.org/10.3390/pharmaceutics17020226] [PMID: 40006593]

[87] Dahan A, Markovic M, Keinan S, *et al.* Computational modeling and *in-vitro/in-silico* correlation of phospholipid-based prodrugs for targeted drug delivery in inflammatory bowel disease. J Comput Aided Mol Des 2017; 31(11): 1021-8. [http://dx.doi.org/10.1007/s10822-017-0079-5] [PMID: 29101519]

[88] De Leo V, Catucci L, Maurelli AM, Daniello V, Conese M, Di Gioia S. Liposomes and exosome-like nanoparticles for curcumin delivery to the gut and to treat inflammatory bowel disease. In advances in

novel phytopharmaceuticals. CRC Press. 2025; pp. 134-59.

[89] Dryden GW, Dryden SM. Synergistic benefits of dietary strategies in the management of IBD. Curr Gastroenterol Rep 2025; 27(1): 8.
[http://dx.doi.org/10.1007/s11894-024-00949-1] [PMID: 39702516]

CHAPTER 3

Sources and Biomedical Utilization of Natural Polymers

Neha Dubey[1], **Shilpa Sahu**[2], **Sagar Sahu**[3], **Rahul Goswami**[3], **Shiv Shankar Shukla**[2], **Ravindra Kumar Pandey**[4] and **Bina Gidwani**[2,*]

[1] *Department of Pharmaceutics, Columbia Institute of Pharmacy, Raipur 493111, Chhattisgarh, India*

[2] *Department of Pharmaceutical Quality Assurance, Columbia Institute of Pharmacy, Raipur 493111, Chhattisgarh, India*

[3] *Department of Pharmaceutical Chemistry, Columbia Institute of Pharmacy, Raipur 493111, Chhattisgarh, India*

[4] *Department of Pharmacognosy, Columbia Institute of Pharmacy, Raipur 493111, Chhattisgarh, India*

Abstract: Natural polymers are derived from diverse biological sources such as plants, animals, microbes, and marine organisms. They have gained immense attention in biomedical research due to their biocompatibility, biodegradability, and inherent bioactivity. This chapter explores the various sources of natural polymers like cellulose, starch, chitosan, collagen, and alginate. This chapter also highlights their unique physicochemical properties and ecological sustainability. Furthermore, it delves into their multifaceted applications in the biomedical field, such as drug delivery systems, tissue engineering scaffolds, wound healing materials, and orthopedic and cardiovascular devices. The versatility of natural polymers lies in their structural tunability, which allows for the development of tailored solutions for complex medical challenges. By exploring current trends and challenges in the utilization of natural polymers, this chapter underscores their pivotal role in advancing sustainable and effective biomedical technologies. The limitations of traditional dosage systems, alongside enhanced and targeted drug delivery techniques, are mitigated by the use of polymers that exhibit superior bioavailability, biocompatibility, and reduced toxicity. Consequently, nanomedicines are regarded as a novel category of pharmaceuticals. This book chapter rigorously evaluates the application of natural polymers and their drug delivery methods for localised or targeted, regulated, and prolonged medication release in the treatment of life-threatening disorders.

Keywords: Biodegradability, Biomedical, Natural polymer, Physiochemical property.

* **Corresponding author Bina Gidwani**, Department of Pharmaceutical Quality Assurance, Columbia Institute of Pharmacy, Raipur 493111, Chhattisgarh, India; E-mail: beenagidwani@gmail.com

Meenakshi Jaiswal & S.K. Lanjhiyana (Eds.)

INTRODUCTION

The initial phase of the era, spanning much of historical and ancient times, commenced thousands of years ago with the utilization of wood and natural fibers. Between the sixteenth and seventeenth centuries, rubber was discovered, serving as a quintessential example of a natural polymer. Proteins, nucleic acids, and polysaccharides exemplify natural polymers integral to biological systems, performing many essential functions. Certain natural polymers, such as chitin and cellulose, are crucial for preserving the structural integrity of cells in both plants and animals, whilst others, like lysozyme, offer biological protection against environmental factors. These natural polymers possess distinct physicochemical and biological properties that can be advantageous across several fields due to their compositional and origin diversity [1]. Organic polymers and their derivatives are utilized throughout various industries, including textile and paper manufacturing, food additives, functional foods and nutraceuticals, and the biomedical sector (*e.g.*, medication delivery and cosmetic applications). The utilization of polymers derived from renewable resources is beneficial due to their natural abundance, renewability, and low carbon footprint, making them essential for the development of innovative materials such as hydrogels, films, membranes, coatings, and micro and nanoparticle systems [2].

Polymers are large molecules characterized by high molecular weights, commonly referred to as macromolecules. They are composed of several smaller molecules, known as monomers. Natural polymers are those that occur naturally or are produced through biological polymerization processes, rather than synthetic methods such as insertion or distillation polymerization. Herbal polymers are derived from plants and animals. Our body is composed of proteins, nucleic acids, and other natural polymers. Furthermore, natural polymers may be employed to revitalize and replenish the skin [3]. Natural polymers are derived from sources such as flora, microorganisms, and fauna. They consist of proteins and carbohydrates that provide structural support to both plants and animals. The six principal categories of natural polymers are proteins, polysaccharides, polynucleotides, polyisoprenes, polyesters, and lignin [4]. Due to their origin, natural polymers are more cost-effective, readily available, potentially biodegradable, and biocompatible compared to the other two groups. Besides being a prevalent element of our everyday nutrition, numerous polymers possess significant uses in the food, pharmaceutical, cosmetic, prosthetic, and medical industries. Numerous frequently utilized natural polymers are derived from proteins and carbohydrates [5].

Origin of Natural Polymer

The term "polymer" is derived from the Greek words "*poly*," meaning "many," and "*meros*," meaning "parts" or "units." This illustrates the composition of polymers, which consist of several repeating units. One reason for the growing interest in natural polymers is their availability from abundant and renewable natural sources, which are also easily accessible. Polysaccharides are prevalent in nature and can be readily sourced from several organisms, including bacteria (*e.g.*, dextran, xanthan gum), plants (*e.g.*, pectin, guar gum, mannan), animals (*e.g.*, chitosan, chondroitin), and algae (*e.g.*, alginates). They may also be generated by recombinant DNA methods. The various beneficial properties of monosaccharide polymers include their high stability, non-toxicity, hydrophilicity, biodegradability, gel-forming abilities, and ease of chemical modification [6]. The structural composition of plant polysaccharides exhibits significant variability, depending on the plant and the specific plant parts from which they originate, such as leaves, seeds, roots, and tubers. Two unique structural features contribute to the richness and diversity of polysaccharides: firstly, monosaccharides can be linked in multiple configurations, either α or β; secondly, the presence of branched side chains is notable. Fig. (**1**) illustrates the categories of natural polymers.

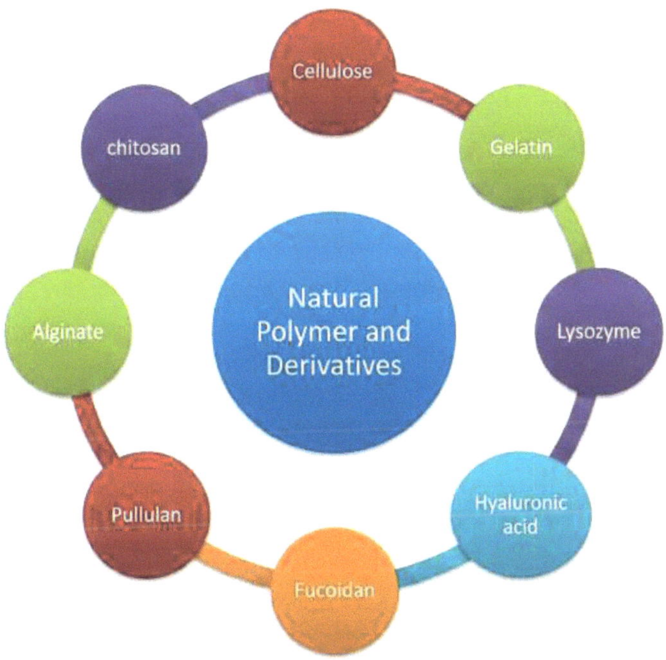

Fig. (1). Natural polymers and derivatives.

Characteristics/ Importance of Natural Polymers

Renewable Source, Biocompatible, and Non-toxic

All of these naturally occurring polymers are composed of repeating monosaccharide units and are carbohydrates. They are therefore non-toxic, unlike manufactured polymers.

Economic

Compared to synthetic polymers, natural polymers are less expensive and have lower production costs.

Biodegradable

Since natural polymers are made by living things, neither the environment nor people are negatively impacted by them. Synthetic polymers, on the other hand, are created using chemicals that have a negative environmental impact.

Easily Accessible

These polymers are herbal, produced in several nations, are less expensive than synthetic polymers, and have no negative side effects. Large amounts of natural polymers are produced since they are utilized in several sectors [7].

Tailored Properties with Modification in Functional Group

Depending on the need, it is possible to chemically alter its mechanical strength, solubility, and other attributes. The polymer chain contains particular chemical groups that facilitate interactions with other molecules.

Low Toxicity

When used, there are few negative effects on the environment or body.

Good Mechanical Strength and Process Ability

Adequate tensile strength, flexibility, and resilience depending on the desired use. These can be easily processed into different shapes and forms using various manufacturing techniques [8].

Advancements in Natural polymer

Natural Polymers

Advancements in natural polymers represent a promising frontier in materials science, offering sustainable, biodegradable alternatives to synthetic polymers. From cellulose to chitosan and collagen, natural polymers exhibit desirable properties for a wide range of applications, especially in the medical domain, packaging, and textiles. However, challenges such as slow production rates, microbial contamination, and batch variability must be overcome to fully harness the potential of these materials. With continued research and innovation, natural polymers are poised to play a significant role in the development of more sustainable and eco-friendly materials for the future [9 - 15]. Some of these polymers are discussed below -

Cellulose

Found in large quantities in plants, cellulose's high fibre strength makes it useful for paper, textiles, and bioplastics.

Chitosan

Made from the exoskeleton of crustaceans, chitin, this substance has antibacterial qualities and is utilized in medication delivery and wound dressings.

Collagen

A protein found in connective tissues, used in medical implants due to its biocompatibility and capacity to enhance tissue regeneration.

Alginate

Extracted from seaweed, forms gels when mixed with calcium ions, used in drug delivery and tissue engineering.

Starch

is a carbohydrate that is present in many foods, including potatoes and cereal grains. It constitutes a polymer composed of thousands of glucose monomers, and during its production, it produces water molecules.

Proteins or Polypeptides

DNA is a common example of this, as proteins are made up of amino acid units that are connected by peptide bonds [10].

Role of Natural Polymers in Pharmaceuticals

Natural polymers serve various roles, such as binder, matrix former, film coater, thickener, stabilizer, *etc.*, depending on the concentration used [16, 17]. The roles are listed in Table **1**.

Table 1. Various roles of natural polymers as excipients.

Sr. No	Role	Application
1.	Binder	To hold ingredients together
2.	Matrix formers	To control drug release
3.	Film coating formers	To protect drugs and improve appearance
4.	Thickeners/Viscosity enhancers	To improve stability and control the release
5.	Stabilizers	To prevent degradation of active ingredients
6.	Disintegrants	To aid in the breakdown of tablets
7.	Solubilizers	To enhance drug solubility
8.	Emulsifiers	To stabilize mixtures of oil and water
9.	Suspending agents	To keep solid particles suspended in liquids
10.	Gelling agents	To form gels for various applications
11.	Bioadhesive	To adhere to biological surfaces for localized drug delivery

CLASSIFICATION OF POLYMERS BASED ON THEIR SOURCE OF ORIGIN

Classification is based on the biochemical origin:

Proteins

These are vital components of living organisms, forming structures like muscles, hair, and enzymes. They are polymers of amino acids.

Cellulose

This is the most prevalent organic molecule on Earth, found in plant cell walls. It provides structural support and is a major component of wood and cotton.

Starch

This is a Carbohydrate used by Plants to Store Energy. It is a Polymer of Glucose.

Resins

These are sticky substances produced by plants, often used for defense or to seal wounds. They have complex structures and vary widely in composition [16].

Semi-synthetic Polymers

These are derived from natural polymers through chemical modifications to alter their properties.

Example: Cellulose derivatives

Cellulose

A natural polymer found in plant cell walls.

Cellulose Derivatives

Cellulose acetate: Used in making films, fibers (like rayon), and photographic film.

Cellulose nitrate: Previously used in explosives and lacquers (now largely replaced by safer alternatives).

Carboxymethyl Cellulose (CMC): Used as a thickener, stabilizer, and emulsifier in food and other industries [16].

Starch Derivatives

Modified Starches

Used in food processing to improve texture, stability, and shelf life.

Important Note: Silicones are **not** derived from natural polymers. They are synthetic polymers based on silicon and oxygen [17].

3.7 Synthetic Polymers:

These are polymers produced in laboratories through chemical polymerization of simple molecules.

Examples include:

Nylon: Used in fibers, plastics, and engineering materials.

Polyethylene: Widely used in packaging, plastic bags, and containers.

Polystyrene: Used in packaging, insulation, and disposable cutlery.

Synthetic Rubber: Used in tires, automotive parts, and other applications.

PVC (Polyvinyl Chloride): Used in pipes, construction materials, and flooring.

Teflon: Known for its non-stick properties, used in cookware and industrial applications [17].

Herbal/Natural Polymers

Natural polymers possess certain limitations/disadvantages as mentioned below. Table **2** lists the polysaccharides obtained from plant, animal, and vegetable origins, along with their sources, compositions, and applications.

Table 2. Polysaccharides obtained from plant, animal, and vegetable origins, along with their sources, compositions, and applications.

S. No	Name of polymer	Description	Biosynthesis	Biomedical applications	References
1.	**Hyaluronic Acid**	Hyaluronic acid or Hyaluronan, a naturally occurring chemical, is a high-molecular-weight polysaccharide that is widely distributed in the connective tissue extracellular matrix. It belongs to a group of substances called mucopolysaccharides, belonging to the glycosaminoglycans (GAGs) family.	Hyaluronic acid is the only mucopolysaccharidethat is not synthesized in the Golgi apparatus. There are three HA synthases, which are responsible for its formation (Has1, Has2, and Has3). All of these are located in the cell membrane with the active end facing the inside of the cell. Synthesis occurs on the inner side of the cell membrane and keeps the individual polymer segments from emerging into the cell.	**♦Dermal Filler** Dermal fillers are used for facial rejuvenation and to temporarily eliminate the appearance of rhytides and skin folds. Hyaluronan transports vital nutrients to these fibers and forms bonds with collagen and elastin. Due to the ability of HA to effectively augment soft tissue in a comprehensive nonsurgical facial rejuvenation approach, physicians utilize it to restore the durability of skin. **♦Tissue Engineering** The field of tissue engineering (TE) is broad and primarily concerned with the regeneration of lost or damaged tissues. By developing biological substitutes, TE allows for the replacement of damaged tissues, both structurally and functionally, while promoting tissue growth in vivo. Owing to its broad availability, non-immunogenic properties, and ease of adjusting chain length, HA is a flexible macromolecule with enormous potential for use in TE applications. Hyaluronan hydrogels have the ability to exchange nutrients, oxygen, and metabolic waste while simulating the water content of individual tissues. **♦Orthopaedic applications** HA plays a vital role in the development of cartilage and the maintenance of synovial fluid. Viscosupplementation with HA products helps improve the physiological environment in an osteoarthritic joint by supplementing the shock absorption and lubrication properties of osteoarthritic synovial fluid. **♦Ophthalmology** HA, a natural component of the vitreous humor of the eye, has found many successful applications in ophthalmologic surgery. HA is particularly useful as a space-filling matrix in the eye; thus, intraocular injection of HA during surgery is used to maintain the shape of the anterior chamber. **♦Cardiovascular application** HA has also proven effective in improving the blood compatibility of cardiovascular implants, such as vascular grafts and stents. For example, biomaterial surfaces treated with cross-linked HA have been associated with reduced platelet adhesion and thrombus formation. HA derivatives with higher degrees of sulfation are associated with increased ability to prevent blood coagulation. **♦Cancer Therapy** It has been reported that HA significantly alters a number of signaling pathways linked to cancer. The majority of its effects are mediated by interactions with cell surface receptors (TLR-2, TLR-4, RHAMM, LYVE, and CD44), which bind and react to HA when they are activated. The main ligand for CD44 is HA. CD44 is overexpressed in a variety of malignancies, such as pancreatic, breast, lung, ovarian, prostate, and so forth.	[53, 54]

(Table 2) cont.....

S. No	Name of polymer	Description	Biosynthesis	Biomedical applications	References
2.	**Chondroitin Sulfate**	Chondroitin sulfate (CS) is a natural substance found in cartilage, tendons, and connective tissues. It is a polysaccharide that is made up of sulfated and unsulfated sugars. Repeating disaccharide units of glucuronic acid and N-acetyl-D-galactosamine that have been sulphated, whether at the 4- or 6-hydroxyl of the galactosamine residues, make up chondroitin sulphate (CS). CS consists of a sequence of glucuronic acid (GlcA) and N-acetyl galactosamine (GalNAc) linked by alternating β-(1→4) and β-(1→3) glycosidic bonds. The sulfate groups are important because they contribute to the molecule's negative charge, which attracts water and contributes to the flexibility and cushioning properties of cartilage. Here is a simplified version of the repeating disaccharide unit of chondroitin sulfate: **→ β-D-glucuronic acid (GlcA) → β-D-N-acetylgalactosamine (GalNAc) 4-sulfate →**	Chondroitin sulfate (CS) is a Glycosaminoglycan (GAG) polymer that is synthesized through a process that involves sulfating sugar residues. The process is catalyzed by chondroitin sulfotransferases, which are enzymes found in the Golgi apparatus.	**♦Osteoarthritis Treatment** As a supplement, chondroitin sulfate is often used to help manage symptoms of osteoarthritis, such as joint pain and stiffness. It is believed to work by promoting the health of cartilage, improving joint function, and reducing inflammation. In some cases, chondroitin sulfate is administered in combination with glucosamine to enhance its effects, though studies on its efficacy have yielded mixed results. **♦Cartilage Repair and Regeneration** Chondroitin sulfate is a key component of the extracellular matrix in cartilage and is involved in maintaining its structure and function. In regenerative medicine, it is being investigated for its potential to aid in the repair of damaged cartilage, particularly in conditions like arthritis or after joint injuries. There is research on the use of chondroitin sulfate in tissue engineering, where it could be incorporated into scaffolds or used with stem cells to encourage the regeneration of cartilage. **♦Drug Delivery Systems** Due to its bioactivity and ability to bind to certain proteins, chondroitin sulfate has also been explored for use in drug delivery systems. For instance, it can be modified to create nanoparticles that help deliver drugs directly to the site of injury or disease, such as inflamed or damaged joints. These drug delivery systems can improve the precision and effectiveness of treatments, potentially reducing side effects. **♦Wound Healing** Chondroitin sulfate has been investigated for its role in wound healing, especially in cases of tissue damage. Some studies suggest that it could help promote tissue repair by stimulating cell growth and extracellular matrix formation. **♦Biomedical Coatings** In medical devices and implants, chondroitin sulfate is sometimes used in coatings or surface treatments to improve biocompatibility. It can enhance the integration of implants with the body and reduce the risk of rejection or inflammation. **♦Gene Therapy and Cartilage Engineering** Researchers are exploring the use of chondroitin sulfate in gene therapy approaches to promote cartilage regeneration. By combining it with genetic material or growth factors, they aim to stimulate the repair or regeneration of cartilage in patients with conditions like osteoarthritis.	[55, 56]
3.	**Chitin and Chitosan**	Chitin is the second-most abundant natural polysaccharide in the world, exceeded in mass only by cellulose. Chitin is a polymer composed of β-1,4-linked N-acetyl-D-glucosamine. Chitosan is the partially deacetylated form of chitin, where a fraction of the N-acetyl-D-glucosamine has been converted into D-glucosamine. Chitin is a polysaccharide made up of repeating units of N-acetylglucosamine (GlcNAc), an amino sugar. The monomers are linked by β-1,--glycosidic bonds. It is structurally similar to cellulose but with an amide group (-NHCOCH□) attached to each monomer, which gives it unique properties, whereas chitosan is derived from chitin through a process called deacetylation, which involves removing some of the acetyl groups (CH□CO) from the chitin molecule. The extent of deacetylation determines the properties of chitosan. The result is a polysaccharide made up of glucosamine (GlcN) units connected by β-1,4-glycosidic bonds.	The biosynthesis of chitin starts with glucose, which is converted into UDP-N-acetylglucosamine (UDP- GlcNAc). Glucokinase and phosphoglucoisomerase are enzymes involved in this initial conversion, where glucose is first converted into glucose-6-phosphate and then into glucose-1 -phosphate. Glucose-1-phosphate is then acetylated by the enzyme glucosamine---phosphate N-acetyltransferase to form N-acetylglucosamine-6- phosphate, and then converted into UDP-N- acetylglucosamine by the action of UDP-glucose dehydrogenase and uridyltransferase. UDP-GlcNAc is used as a substrate by chitin synthase enzymes to polymerize and form chitin. Chitosan is derived from chitin through a process called deacetylation, in which the acetyl groups (CH_3CO) are removed from the N- acetylglucosamine units.	**♦Chitosan as a Drug Delivery Agent:** • Beneficial Properties: o Bioadhesion: Sticks well to mucosal surfaces. o Polycationic Surface: Enables strong interactions with drugs. o Biocompatibility: Safe for use within the body. **♦Chitin from Marine Sponges:** • Source: Skeletons of sponges like *Ianthella flabelliformis*. Study by Kovalchuk et al.: o Fabric-like chitin scaffolds from *Ianthella flabelliformis* showed potential for drug delivery. o Scaffolds retained antiseptic decamethoxine and released it to inhibit bacterial growth. **♦Chitin-Based Microspheres:** Study by Zheng et al.: o Developed carboxymethyl chitin microspheres (CMCH-Ms) encapsulated in thermosensitive hydrogels. o Utilized physical cross-linking (temperature increase) to maintain the structure of the microspheres. o High acetylation levels of carboxymethyl chitins are crucial for this temperature-sensitive cross-linking. **♦Application of Chitin and Chitosan in Cancer Therapy** Carboxymethyl chitin (CMC) nanoparticles as a drug delivery system for the anticancer drug 5-fluorouracil (5-FU). **Key Points:** **• CMC Nanoparticles** These nanoparticles are water-soluble and created by cross-linking with $CaCl_2$ and $FeCl_3$. They are then loaded with the anticancer drug, 5-Fu. **• Chemical Modification of Chitin:** Modifying chitin (like carboxymethylation) significantly improves its properties, including water solubility, biocompatibility, and reactivity. **• Carboxymethylation:** • This process enhances chitin's water solubility while maintaining biocompatibility and avoiding immune responses. It involves a reaction between chitin powder and monochloroacetic acid, using isopropyl alcohol as a solvent. **♦Potential Benefits:** • **Improved Drug Delivery:** CMC nanoparticles could potentially improve the targeted delivery of 5-Fu to cancer cells, minimizing side effects in healthy tissues. • **Controlled Release:** The nanoparticles' structure may allow for controlled release of the drug, optimizing its effectiveness [57-58]. **♦Potential for Chitin and Chitosan in Wound Healing** • **Chitosan's Antimicrobial Properties:** Chitosan itself has antimicrobial properties, making it a suitable candidate for wound care applications. • **Liposomes for Skin Delivery:** Liposomes are effective carriers for poorly soluble drugs, as they interact more readily with the skin's lipid-rich environment. **• Chitosomes for Enhanced Delivery:** o Combining liposomes with chitosan creates "chitosomes," which enhance antimicrobial activity and improve drug delivery to the skin. o Chitosan coating can improve liposome retention at the wound site [57-58]. **• Study by Hemmingsen et al.:** o This study demonstrated that chitosomes loaded with Chlorhexidine (CHX) resulted in: ▪ Increased release of CHX. ▪ Sustained release of CHX compared to CHX formulations without chitosomes. **♦Implications:** • **Improved Treatment of Skin Infections:** Chitosan-coated liposomes offer a promising approach for the treatment of skin and soft tissue infections (SSTIs). • **Enhanced Drug Delivery:** The combination of chitosan's antimicrobial properties and liposomes' ability to deliver drugs effectively to the skin can lead to more efficient and targeted treatment. • **Sustained Release:** The sustained release of the antimicrobial drug from the chitosomes can provide prolonged antimicrobial activity at the wound site, potentially improving healing outcomes.	[57, 58]

(Table 2) cont.....

S. No	Name of polymer	Description	Biosynthesis	Biomedical applications	References
4.	**Alginic Acid**	Natural hydrophilic colloidal polysaccharide alginic acid is derived from different types of brown seaweed (Phaeophyceae). **Chemical Structure** Alginic acid is a co-polymer made up of repeating units of mannuronic acid (M) and guluronic acid (G), linked by β-1,4 and α-1,4 glycosidic bonds. The structure of alginic acid can vary depending on the ratio of mannuronic acid to guluronic acid in the polymer chain, which influences its properties (like viscosity and gelation). **Mannuronic Acid (M):** A C-5 epimer of glucose with a carboxyl group (-COOH) on the C-6 carbon. **Guluronic Acid (G):** A C-5 epimer of mannuronic acid, also with a carboxyl group (-COOH) on the C-6 carbon.	Biosynthesis begins with the production of activated sugar nucleqtides, which are the building blocks of the alginate chain. Mannose-1-phosphate is converted to GDP-mannose, and Mannose---phosphate is converted to GDP-gulose. These are the activated sugar nucleotide precursors. Alginate synthase enzymes use GDP-mannose and GDP-gulose to polymerize the sugar units into a growing alginate chain, linking mannuronic acid (M) and guluronic acid (G) in a repeating pattern.	Alginic acid, a natural polysaccharide extracted from brown seaweed, has a wide range of applications across various fields due to its unique properties, such as biocompatibility, biodegradability, and the ability to form gels. Here is a summary of its key applications. • Dental: Used in dental impressions to create accurate molds for dental prosthetics. • Biosensors: Explored for use in biosensors to detect biomolecules or pathogens. • Gastrointestinal: A key component of antacids to relieve heartburn by forming a protective gel layer. • Health Supplements: Used in some supplements to support digestive health. • Surgical Implants: Incorporated into surgical implants to provide support and enhance healing. • Tissue Engineering: Used to create biodegradable scaffolds for tissue regeneration. • Drug Delivery: Encapsulates drugs to protect them and enable controlled release.	[59, 60]
5.	**Cellulose**	Cellulose is a polysaccharide composed of several hundred to thousands of linearly connected β(1→4) D-glucose units. The molecular formula of cellulose is $(C\square H_{10}O_5)_n$. **Chemical Structure** Cellulose is a naturally occurring polysaccharide composed of β-D-glucopyranose units linked by β-1,4-glycosidic bonds. Monomer: The repeating unit of cellulose is glucose (C□H□□O□), specifically β--glucopyranose. Linkage: The glucose units are linked by β-1,--glycosidic bonds. → Glucose (β-D-glucopyranose) → Glucose → Glucose → (and so on)	Glucose is converted into UDP-glucose by the enzyme UDP-glucose pyrophosphorylase. The enzyme cellulose synthase uses UDP-glucose to polymerize glucose units into long chains through β-1,4-glycosidic bonds. The cellulose chains are extruded outside the cell and form microfibrils, which are stabilized by hydrogen bonding. The cellulose microfibrils are integrated into the plant cell wall, providing strength and rigidity.	♦**Wound Dressing:** Cellulose-based materials like cellulose acetate and CMC are used in wound dressings to: • Create a moist healing environment. • Absorb wound exudates. • Protect wounds from infection. • Promote faster healing. ♦**Artificial Tears:** Methyl cellulose and hydroxypropyl methylcellulose are used in artificial tears to: • Lubricate the eyes. • Relieve dryness and irritation. ♦**Diagnostic Devices:** Cellulose-based materials are used in diagnostic tests like pregnancy tests and rapid disease tests to: • Act as substrates for reagent flow. • Facilitate the detection of target molecules. ♦**Tissue Regeneration:** Nanocellulose, with its high surface area and biocompatibility, shows promise in: • Supporting cell growth. • Facilitating tissue regeneration. ♦**Colon Drug Delivery:** Cellulose derivatives like CMC are being investigated for: • Protecting drugs from stomach acid. • Enabling targeted drug release in the colon [17].	[61, 62]

Drawbacks of Herbal Polymers

Microbial Contamination:

- Natural polymers, being derived from natural sources, are susceptible to microbial contamination during production and storage.

Batch-to-Batch Variation

- The quality and properties of natural polymers can vary significantly between batches due to factors like environmental conditions, source variability, and processing methods. This inconsistency can pose challenges in consistent product manufacturing [18].

Uncontrolled Rate of Hydration

- The water content in natural polymers can vary depending on factors like source, harvesting time, and environmental conditions. This inconsistency can affect their physical and chemical properties [18].

Slow Process:

- The production of natural polymers often involves slower processes compared to the synthesis of many synthetic polymers [18].
- **Heavy Metal Contamination:**

- Biopolymers, particularly those originating from botanical sources, may be contaminated with heavy metals from the environment [19].

TYPES OF NATURAL POLYMERS AND THEIR APPLICATIONS IN THE BIOMEDICAL FIELD

Natural polymers have been developed for various uses such as drug delivery systems, tissue engineering, and wound dressings, and the fabrication of biological substitutes such as blood vessels, ear cartilage, and the esophagus. By modifying their chemical and physical properties, natural polymers can overcome their inferior properties and replace synthetic polymers in some cases [63]. They offer biocompatibility, non-toxicity, bioactivity, and specific activity for cells or tissues, and can be used in drug delivery systems [64]. Originating from ancient times, natural polymers have evolved through research and development. Currently, ten types of natural polymeric materials are important in medicine, agriculture, daily life, coatings, films, woven mats, wastewater treatment technology, and vehicle production [65]. Natural polymers have a variety of origins, such as polysaccharides, proteins, lipids, and nucleic acids. Most of the natural polymers originate from plants, fungi, bacteria, algae, and animals' exoskeletons, tissues, organs, waste materials, *etc*. In addition, these polymers can also be found in metabolic products, exosomes, and other animal and plant secretions.

Based on these sources and the technical methods for their isolation, natural polymers can be classified into the following groups-

Polysaccharides: Starch, cellulose, chitin, chitosan, agar, alginate, carrageenan, and pectin

Proteins: Gelatine, collagen, casein, and keratin; the small groups of polymeric lipids and polymeric nucleic acids are still being explored.

Animal origin: Keratin, silk, wool, casein, bees' wax, egg shells, gelatin, collagen, and fibrin.

Plants and fungi origin: Cellulose, chitin, lignin, pectin, agar, alginic acid, carrageenan, extract, seed, and others [71].

Polymers are crucial for health applications, including artificial organ repair, tissue regeneration, wound dressings, drug delivery, and biodegradable bio-plastics. Natural polymers, including polysaccharides like alginate, chitosan, cellulose, hyaluronic acid, and starch, are versatile biomaterials with excellent biocompatibility, non-toxicity, and biodegradability. They are ideal for biotechnological, pharmacy, agro-food, and environmental protection. However, these polymers have some identified problems and limitations:

i. Possible microbial contamination during isolation.
ii. Decreased tunability of their properties.
iii. Possible immunogenic reactions.
iv. Uncontrollable rate of the degradation process.
v. Insufficient mechanical strength and poor water stability.

The five principal natural polymers, namely hyaluronic acid, chondroitin sulfate, chitin and chitosan, alginic acid, and cellulose, are discussed along with their descriptions, chemical structures, physical/chemical properties, biosynthesis, and biomedical applications, as listed in Table **3**.

Table 3. Natural polymers along with their descriptions, chemical structures, physical/chemical properties, biosynthesis, and biomedical applications.

Name	Source	Composition	Biomedical Applications	References
Alginate	Alginates, with their exceptional gel-forming ability, are utilized in various medical fields, including cell culture, drug delivery, and NK vaccines, due to their versatility. **Source of origin-*Brown Seaweeds*:** The primary natural source, including species like: Laminaria japonica (Kelp) Macrocystis pyrifera (Giant Kelp) Ascophyllumnodosum (Knotted Wrack) Fucusvesiculosus (Bladderwrack) ***Bacteria:*** Some bacteria, such as Pseudomonas and Azotobacter, also produce alginate, though these microbial sources are less common for commercial extraction compared to seaweeds.	-	***Tissue Engineering:*** Alginates are used to create scaffolds for tissue regeneration. Their ability to form hydrogels allows for cell encapsulation, and their biodegradability ensures that they can gradually be replaced by natural tissue. However, challenges such as a lack of vascularization and integration with the host tissue remain. ***Regenerative Medicine:*** Alginates are used in regenerative medicine for applications like wound healing, organ repair, and tissue engineering. Research has explored combining alginate with other materials like polycaprolactone (PCL) and magnetic nanoparticles (MNPs) to improve growth factor release and scaffold performance. ***Controlled Drug Delivery:*** The ability to control the release of encapsulated drugs through the modulation of alginate's structure and cross-linking makes it an ideal candidate for controlled drug release systems	[72, 73]
Cellulose	Cellulose, a naturally occurring amphiphilic, biodegradable polymer, has significant potential in biomedical applications due to its structural and functional properties. Cellulose and its derivatives have unique structures based on their closely packed cellulose chains, with inter and intra-hydrogen bonding. They are available in various varieties and can be modified in different ways for better use. **Source of origin-*Plants (Primary Source)*-** Common sources of plant-based cellulose include: **Wood:** softwoods (pine, spruce) and hardwoods (oak, birch). **Cotton:** Cotton fibers are almost pure cellulose, making cotton one of the highest-quality sources. **Hemp:** Hemp fibers contain a significant amount of cellulose and have been used in textiles and paper products. **Flax:** The fibers from the flax plant (used to make linen) also contain high cellulose content. **Rice Straw, Wheat Straw, and Corn Stover:** Agricultural by-products that contain cellulose, often used for biofuels or other industrial applications. **Bamboo**: Another plant that is rich in cellulose, commonly used for textiles and paper [74]. *Algae:*-brown algae, Green Algae (Cladophora species) *Bacteria (Microbial Source)-* Acetobacterxylinum-One of the most well-known bacteria that produces high-quality cellulose and is used in medical applications (e.g., wound dressings) and for making biodegradable materials. *Fungal*species of Basidiomycetes	o Cellulose is an organic polysaccharide, meaning it is a complex carbohydrate made up of many sugar molecules linked together. o Specifically, it consists of a linear chain of glucose units connected by $\beta(1\rightarrow4)$ glycosidic bonds. o Its chemical formula is $(C_6H_{10}O_5)_n$, where 'n' represents the number of glucose units in the chain. In essence, cellulose is a major structural component of plant cell walls, providing strength and support.	**• Microcrystalline Cellulose (MCC):** o Primarily used as a diluent/binder in tablet formulations. o It is suitable for both granulation and direct compression processes, making it a versatile excipient. **• Carboxymethyl Cellulose (CMC):** o Widely used in drug formulations for various purposes: • **A binder** for holding drug particles together. • Film-coating agent to protect drugs from moisture and improve appearance. • **Ointment base** for topical drug delivery. **• Cellulose Acetate:** o Used in the manufacture of wound dressings. These examples demonstrate the diverse applications of cellulose and its derivatives in the pharmaceutical field, highlighting their importance in developing safe and effective drug delivery systems. Wound Healing and Dressings Cellulose-based wound dressings promote healing by creating a moist environment, absorbing exudates, and reducing the risk of infection. They can be infused with antimicrobial agents or bioactive cellulose, enhancing healing and infection prevention. Tissue Engineering Cellulose and its derivatives, like cellulose nanofibers and nanocrystals, can serve as scaffolds in tissue engineering, mimicking the extracellular matrix and supporting cell adhesion, proliferation, and differentiation. Drug Delivery Systems Cellulose and its derivatives are used in controlled drug delivery systems for extended drug release, improving therapeutic efficacy and reducing side effects. Nanocellulose-based delivery allows targeted delivery of bioactive agents like small molecules, proteins, and nucleic acids. Bone Regeneration Cellulose-based bone scaffolds, often combined with materials like hydroxyapatite or collagen, provide structural support and promote osteogenesis. Calcium carbonate and cellulose derivatives are being studied for bone healing properties. Hemostatic Agents Oxidized regenerated cellulose (ORC) and cellulose-based hemostats are used to control bleeding during surgery and trauma care, promoting blood coagulation and tissue adhesion.	[19, 75, 76, 77]

(Table 3) cont.....

Name	Source	Composition	Biomedical Applications	References
			Implants and Prosthetics Cellulose-based composites are being explored for biocompatible implants and prosthetics due to their lightweight, strong, and biodegradable nature, making them suitable for artificial limbs and joints, ensuring an environmentally friendly solution.	
			Biodegradable Sutures Cellulose-derived sutures are biodegradable surgical stitches and wound closures that degrade over time, minimizing inflammation. They are suitable for soft tissues and avoid long term irritation.	
			Hydrogels for Biomedical Applications Cellulose-based hydrogels are useful for biomedical applications like controlled drug delivery, wound healing, and tissue regeneration. Modifying these hydrogels to respond to environmental stimuli opens up possibilities for smart drug delivery systems.	
			Antimicrobial Applications Cellulose can be modified with antimicrobial agents to produce materials that inhibit microbial growth, which are useful in biomedical products such as wound dressings and catheters. Cellulose-based coatings provide additional protection against bacterial colonization.	
			Biosensors and Diagnostic Tools Cellulose-based electrodes and cellulose nanomaterials are being used in biosensors for medical diagnostics, with cellulose nanocrystals enhancing sensitivity and selectivity, making them ideal for point-of-care diagnostics and wearable health-monitoring devices.	
			Artificial Blood Vessels Modified cellulose materials are being explored for small-diameter vascular grafts, providing mechanical support and promotingendothelial cell growth, which is crucial for creating functional blood vessels during bypass surgery.	
			Drug Carriers for Cancer Therapy Cellulose nanoparticles, specifically cellulose nanocrystals and CNFs, are being explored for controlled cancer drug delivery due to their small size, biocompatibility, and functionalization with targeting moieties.	
Starches	• It's the primary carbohydrate storage form in plants. • Found abundantly in seeds (like corn, rice, wheat) and underground organs (like potatoes). • Occurs naturally as **granules**, which are microscopic structures.	Starch is a complex carbohydrate composed of two main polymers: amylose and amylopectin. Both are made up of long chains of glucose molecules, but they differ in their structure and properties. • **Amylose:** o Linear and unbranched chain of glucose molecules o Linked by α-1,4 glycosidic bonds o Forms a helical structure o Less soluble in water than amylopectin o Makes up about 20-30% of starch in plants • **Amylopectin:** o Branched chain of glucose molecules o Linked by α-1,4 glycosidic bonds with α-1,6 glycosidic bonds at branch points o Highly branched structure o More soluble in water than amylose o Makes up about 70-80% of starch in plants The ratio of amylose to amylopectin in starch varies depending on the plant source, which can affect the starch's properties. For example, starches with higher amylose content tend to form stronger gels when heated and cooled.	• Several types of starch derived from different plant sources are used in the pharmaceutical industry, including: o Maize starch o Rice starch o Wheat starch o Potato starch Thermoplastic starch (TPS) has gained significant attention as a promising alternative to traditional petroleum-based plastics. Here is a breakdown of its key applications: • **Packaging:** A major area where TPS shines. It can be used to create various packaging materials, including: o **Containers:** For food and other products. o **Wraps and Films:** For food preservation and protection. o **Bags:** For various applications. • **Mulch Films:** TPS-based mulch films can help retain soil moisture, suppress weeds, and improve crop yields in agriculture. • **Textile Sizing Agents:** Used to strengthen and protect textile fibers during weaving and other processing steps. • **Adhesives:** TPS can be formulated into biodegradable adhesives for various applications.	

(Table 3) cont.....

Name	Source	Composition	Biomedical Applications	References
Collagen	Collagen is a complex protein that plays a vital role in the structure and function of various tissues throughout the body. Collagen, a protein-amino acid polymer, is the most abundant protein in animals and a crucial component of connective tissues, providing structure, strength, and elasticity. Collagen exists in several types:- Type I is the most abundant and found in the skin, tendons, and bones. Other types include Type II (cartilage) Type III (skin and blood vessels) Type IV (basement membranes) Type V (hair, cornea). Source of Origin-Collagen originates from animals and is found in several forms across different tissues. Sources of collagen are: **Bovine (Cows):** It is a primary source. Bone and skin are common sources of collagen derived from cattle. Bovine collagen is commonly used in supplements and medical products like wound dressings. **Porcine (Pigs):** Collagen from pigs, especially from their skin and bones, is widely used in medical products and cosmetics. It is also used in food products like gelatin. **Marine (Fish):** Fish skin, scales, and bones are rich in collagen, particularly Type I collagen. Marine collagen is often considered superior due to its higher bioavailability when consumed as a supplement. **Chicken:** Chicken cartilage is another rich source of collagen, often used in supplements aimed at improving joint health. **Other Sources:** Collagen can also be extracted from the tissues of other mammals, such as sheep, goats, and horses. In addition, human collagen is occasionally sourced from cadavers for medical uses, but this is rare and regulated. • **Primary Protein of Connective Tissues:** Collagen is the most abundant protein in the human body, forming the basis of connective tissues like skin, bones, tendons, ligaments, cartilage, and blood vessels. • **Triple Helix Structure:** Collagen molecules have a unique triple-helix structure, providing them with exceptional strength and resilience. • **Animal Sources:** Common sources include: o **Pig Skin:** A widely used source for collagen extraction. o **Bovine Hide:** Another significant source for collagen products. o **Pork and Cattle Bones:** Also used as collagen sources. **Gelatin:** • **Derived from Collagen:** Gelatin is produced by denaturing or chemically modifying collagen. • **Properties:** It is a water-soluble protein composed of 19 amino acids. • **Uses:** Gelatin has various applications in food, pharmaceuticals, and other industries. **Other Animal Proteins:** • **Elastin:** A protein that provides elasticity to tissues like skin and blood vessels. • **Albumin:** A protein found in blood plasma, important for maintaining blood volume and pressure. • **Fibrin:** A protein involved in blood clotting.	• **Amino Acid Rich:** Collagen is primarily composed of three amino acids: o **Glycine:** Found at nearly every third position in the collagen sequence. o **Proline:** A significant component of collagen's structure. o **Hydroxyproline:** A modified form of proline, crucial for collagen stability. • **Multiple Types:** There are over 28 types of collagen, each with specific functions and distributions within the body.	***Wound Healing and Tissue Regeneration:*** -Collagen serves as structural support, making it essential for wound healing and tissue regeneration. Biomaterials made of collagen are utilized in wound dressings. Collagen-based dressings promote cell migration, proliferation, differentiation, and the regulation of inflammation. Burns, ulcers, and surgical wounds use collagen sheets and sponges. Tissue Engineering like collagen scaffolds aid skin, cartilage, bone, and nerve regeneration. These scaffolds allow cells to grow, organize, and create tissues in three dimensions. Collagen is ideal for tissue engineering due to its biocompatibility and biodegradability. ***Drug Delivery Systems*** Collagen is utilized in controlled drug release systems due to its biodegradability and biocompatibility. It forms hydrogels that encapsulate drugs and release them in a controlled manner. Collagen-based drug delivery systems are being explored for wound healing and cancer therapy. ***Bone and Cartilage Regeneration*** Collagen-based materials are utilized for bone and cartilage regeneration due to their structural similarities. They are often combined with inorganic materials like hydroxyapatite or calcium phosphate for bone substitutes and cartilage repair, supporting chondrocyte growth and maintaining cartilage's mechanical properties. ***Ophthalmic Applications*** Collagen, a key component of the cornea, is utilized in various ophthalmic procedures, including corneal implants, contact lenses, and drug delivery systems for eye conditions like glaucoma and macular degeneration, offering improved biocompatibility and oxygen permeability. ***Vascular and Cardiac Applications*** Collagen is a valuable material for cardiovascular applications due to its ability to promote cell attachment and provide mechanical support, making it useful in vascular graft fabrication and heart valve replacement. ***Cosmetic and Aesthetic Applications*** Collagen is utilized in cosmetic surgery and aesthetic medicine to improve skin elasticity, texture, and hydration. It is used in collagen injections for wrinkle treatment and in collagen-based creams and lotions for skin rejuvenation, boosting collagen production. ***Dental Applications*** Collagen is utilized in dental treatments for gum and bone regeneration, particularly in periodontal surgeries and bone grafting procedures, to treat alveolar bone loss and aid implant placement. ***Cancer Therapy and Diagnostics*** Collagen is being explored for cancer diagnosis and treatment, specifically in targeted drug delivery and tissue-specific therapy. Engineered nanoparticles or micro particles can encapsulate anticancer drugs, while collagen degradation products can serve as biomarkers.	[20, 21, 78]

Name	Source	Composition	Biomedical Applications	References
Wheat Gluten	Wheat gluten is a complex mixture of proteins found in wheat. It is what gives dough its elasticity and helps baked goods rise.	• **Gliadins:** These are low-molecular-weight proteins with a relatively simple structure. They contribute to the viscosity and extensibility of dough. • **Glutenins:** These are high-molecular-weight proteins with a more complex, three-dimensional structure. They provide dough with its elasticity and strength. **NOTE** – **Gluten Sensitivity:** While gluten is essential for the texture and structure of many baked goods, it can cause health problems for people with celiac disease or gluten sensitivity.	-	[22-24]
Soy Protein	Soy protein comes in different forms depending on the processing method. Here is a breakdown of the main categories: • **Soy Protein Isolate:** o This is the most refined form of soy protein. o It has the highest protein content (typically 90% or more), as most of the non-protein components (like carbohydrates and fats) have been removed. o Soy protein isolate is often used in protein powders, sports nutrition products, and as a food additive to increase protein content. • **Soy Protein Concentrate:** o This form has a slightly lower protein content than isolate (usually around 70%). o It retains some of the original soybean's nutrients, such as fiber and some carbohydrates. o Soy protein concentrate is commonly used in foods like meat substitutes, baked goods, and cereals. • **Degradation Pattern:** The polymer's degradation rate should be predictable and controlled to ensure consistent drug release.	-	-	[25]
Carrageenan	Carrageenans, high molecular weight polymers from red algae, have numerous pharmacological applications in the food industry, drug delivery systems, and tissue repair. Their sulfate content affects their anti-coagulant, anti-inflammatory, and immunomodulatory effects. Silver nanoparticles are effective antiseptics in inhibiting microorganism growth in PVA films. Source of origin-Carrageenan is a natural polymer primarily derived from red seaweed, specifically the species Chondrus crispus (commonly known as Irish moss), Eucheuma, and Kappaphycus. These seaweeds are harvested from both coastal areas and open ocean environments. Carrageenan is extracted from the cell walls of these red algae, where it functions as a thickening, gelling, and stabilizing agent.	-	Drug Delivery Systems Carrageenan, with its gel-forming ability, is used in controlled drug release systems, particularly in oral delivery, where it can encapsulate drugs over extended periods. Wound Healing Carrageenan, a biocompatible substance, is utilized in wound healing due to its hydrogel properties, potential for cell proliferation and tissue regeneration, and its biocompatibility. Tissue Engineering Carrageenan, a gel-like material, is utilized in tissue engineering for its ability to support cell adhesion, proliferation, and differentiation, making it suitable for regenerative medicine. Antibacterial, Antiviral, and Anti-inflammatory Applications Carrageenan's antibacterial properties and anti-inflammatory effects make it beneficial for biomedical applications, particularly in managing inflammation-related conditions and promoting injury healing.	[86-88]

(Table 3) cont.....

Name	Source	Composition	Biomedical Applications	References
			Oral and Nasal Formulations Carrageenan, with its gel-like properties, is used in some formulations to treat sore throats and nasal conditions by coating mucous membranes and potentially delivering active compounds directly.	
			Vaccines: Carrageenan has been studied for its use as an adjuvant in vaccines, helping to improve the immune response to antigens. Some types of carrageenan are being researched for their ability to enhance the effectiveness of vaccines by stimulating immune cells.	
			Cell Encapsulation in Biotechnology Due to its gelation properties, carrageenan is used to encapsulate living cells, protecting them from external stress and allowing them to be used in various biotechnological applications, such as biosensors or the production of therapeutic proteins.	
			Cancer Treatment Some studies suggest carrageenan's potential in cancer treatment, where it may inhibit the growth of cancer cells or support the delivery of anticancer drugs. However, this application is still under investigation, and more research is needed to establish its effectiveness.	
Pectin	The pectin polymer is primarily composed of galacturonic acid units and plays a key role in maintaining plant structural integrity and regulating water retention. Pectin, a carbohydrate found in plant cell walls, has potential applications in drug delivery systems and medical treatments. Its structure, consisting of galacturonic acid units linked by α-1,4 glycosidic bonds, allows for the release of various medicinal agents. **Source of Origin-** Pectin is a naturally occurring polysaccharide found in the cell walls of many plants, particularly in fruits. It is most commonly sourced from citrus fruits (like oranges and lemons) and apples. Pectin can also be found in smaller quantities in other fruits like strawberries, apricots, and grapes.	-	***Drug Delivery Systems*** Pectin, with its ability to form gels and exhibit controlled release properties, is commonly used in drug delivery systems like nanoparticles, microspheres, and hydrogels. Its degradability in acidic stomach or intestine environments makes it an ideal candidate for oral delivery. ***Wound Healing and Tissue Engineering*** Pectin's moisture-retaining and gel-forming properties aid in wound healing, skin regeneration, and tissue engineering, while also serving as a scaffold for cell growth and proliferation. ***Cancer Therapy*** Pectin has potential in cancer therapy as a drug carrier and direct therapeutic application, potentially inhibiting cancer cell growth or enhancing chemotherapy effects, especially through its interaction with galectin-3. ***Bioactive Molecule Delivery*** Pectin, with its gel-forming ability, is a useful carrier for bioactive molecules like antioxidants, peptides, and vitamins, ensuring their stable and sustained release in nutraceuticals for long-lasting effects. ***Biosensors and Diagnostic Applications*** Pectin-based biosensors detect biomolecules like glucose and DNA, offering potential applications in point-of-care diagnostics and continuous monitoring of conditions, thanks to their biocompatibility and ease of modification. ***Controlled Release of Growth Factors*** Pectin is utilized in tissue engineering for controlled growth factor release, promoting tissue regeneration and repair in regenerative medicine and damaged organs. ***Gastrointestinal Drug Delivery*** Pectin's gel-forming ability, particularly in the stomach's acidic conditions, aids in controlled drug delivery by protecting sensitive drugs from stomach acids and gradually releasing them in the intestines. ***Hydrogels for Medical Applications*** Pectin is utilized in the production of hydrogels for medical applications, such as tissue engineering, wound dressings, and controlled drug delivery, due to its excellent moisture retention properties. ***Antimicrobial Properties*** Pectin's antimicrobial properties and low toxicity make it ideal for developing dressings, gels, and films to prevent infection in wounds and surgical sites	[83-85]
Latex	Latex, a natural fiber, is primarily derived from the rubber tree, Hevea brasiliensis, native to the Amazon Basin in South America. Its cultivation has expanded to Southeast Asia, including Thailand, Indonesia, and Malaysia. Latex is extracted by tapping, a process in which a thin layer of bark is sliced to release the sap. Its composition includes polyisoprene, water, proteins, lipids, and sugars. **Source of origin-**Latex, derived from the sap of the rubber tree Hevea brasiliensis, is a valuable natural polymer with unique properties such as elasticity, biocompatibility, and ease of modification. Other plants that produce latex include Ficus species, guayule, dandelions, Euphorbia species, and Castillae lastica. These plants produce latex with varying degrees of non-rubber components and require more processing to isolate the rubber.	-	Medical Gloves Latex gloves, known for their flexibility, tactile sensitivity, and good fit, are widely used in healthcare settings due to their superior comfort and sensitivity, despite the development of alternatives like nitrile gloves. Catheters and Tubing Latex-based materials are used in flexible medical tubing and catheters, providing ease of insertion and a snug fit, though synthetic alternatives have replaced them due to allergic concerns. Wound Dressings Latex-based materials are used in wound care for elastic bandages and adhesive dressings due to their conformability and stretchability, and may be incorporated into hydrocolloid or hydrogel dressings. Prosthetics and Orthotics Latex elastomers are used in custom-made prosthetic components, enhancing patient comfort and mobility. Their elasticity, comfort, and resilience make them suitable for parts requiring flexibility and strength. Surgical Drapes and Mats Latex is utilized in surgical drapes and mats due to its flexibility, water resistance, and biocompatibility, ensuring cleanliness and integrity in sterile environments during operations. Drug Delivery Systems Latex polymers can be utilized in drug delivery systems for slow-release mechanisms, encapsulating drugs at controlled rates, and delivering them over extended periods, reducing the need for frequent dosing.	[81, 82]

(Table 3) cont.....

Name	Source	Composition	Biomedical Applications	References
			Tissue Engineering Latex, with its elasticity and chemical modification capabilities, is a promising material for tissue engineering, serving as a scaffold for cell growth and adhesion.	
			Dental Applications Latex is used in dental materials like dental dams and orthodontic appliances due to its biocompatibility, ease of handling, and moldability, making it suitable for direct contact with human tissues.	
			Latex-Based Hydrogels Latex-based hydrogels, water-absorbent polymers, are utilized in biomedical applications like wound care, drug delivery, and tissue engineering for moisture retention and controlled release.	
			Latex-Based Implants Latex, due to its biocompatibility, is often utilized in the creation of soft-tissue implants like breast implants, ensuring flexibility and a natural feel.	

The structures of these five natural polymers are shown in Fig. (**2**). The rapidly developing biomedical applications of natural polymers focus on their sources and utilization in various fields such as drug delivery systems, implantable scaffolds, tissue engineering, wound adhesives, dressings, and oral care. Natural polymers exhibit various physicochemical properties and molecular structures, and are increasingly used in food and drug coatings [66]. They are used in China, India, and the EU for their enhanced tablet strength, taste masking, and controlled release. Most of the time, bioink is made up of natural polymers, cells, drugs, growth factors, and other materials that can be deposited in a controlled manner. It is recommended that bioinks are safe, easy to print, nontoxic, and biodegradable. New developments in bioinks centre on making derivatives that improve their mechanical properties and cell affinity, as well as on sending signals to help cells grow, stick together, and differentiate [67].

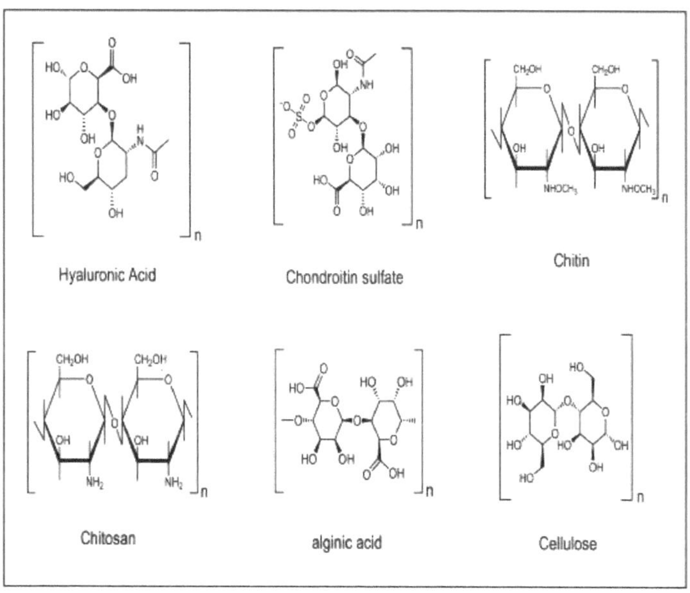

Fig. (2). Structures of natural polymers.

BIOMEDICAL APPLICATION OF NATURAL POLYMERS

The biomedical applications of these polymers are discussed as follows

Antibacterial Properties

The pharmaceutical industry is focusing on biomedicine based on antimicrobial materials to combat the rise in diseases caused by microorganisms. Multidrug-Resistant Bacteria (MDR) pose a significant threat to global health and food security, leading to severe infections like blood infections and pneumonia. Device-Related Infections (DRI) are common, particularly urinary catheter infections and central venous infections. To prevent these infections, antifouling or antimicrobial coatings have been employed, including polyethylene glycol, enzyme- or zwitterionic-based coatings, and superhydrophobic coatings. Modern tissue engineering aims to find the right fit for laboratory-created tissue to integrate into the body's matrix, aiding the healing of affected organs or tissue systems [28]. Tissue engineering is crucial for developing functional materials for scaffolding, as it helps prevent infections like chronic otitis, sinusitis, and endocarditis. Polymers with antibacterial or antimicrobial properties can be used in tissue engineering, with polyhydroxyalkanoates like polylactic acid, polyglycolic acid, and polyhydroxybutyrate being promising candidates. Thermoelectric applications require multifunctional composite materials, such as β-GP modified chitosan-based thermosensitive hydrogels for bone deformities and silk fibroin scaffolds for skin tissue engineering. Polyurethanes and 3D printing are also used in tissue engineering [29 - 31].

Hydrogel Preparation and Application

Hydrogels can be produced *via* various polymerization methods. A comprehensive review of each method exceeds the scope of this article; therefore, a succinct overview is provided instead. The fundamental premise in hydrogel preparation is the cross-linking of polymer chains. This can be achieved through chemical alteration with an external cross-linking agent or by irradiation with high-energy radiation. Researchers indicate that hydrogels can be synthesized utilizing two primary categories of cross-linking techniques: chemical cross-linking methods and physical cross-linking methods [32, 33]. Chemically crosslinked hydrogels utilize chemical means to create new covalent bonds between polymer chains, whereas physically crosslinked hydrogels rely on physical means to make connections between polymer chains. Both physical and chemical approaches possess distinct advantages and disadvantages. Various methods have been employed for hydrogel formation, including chemical, physical, and radiation cross-linking, as well as polymer grafting. Classical radical polymerization methods are highly controllable, yielding hydrogels with regulated compositions and morphologies, including the ability to modify size and create hollow core-shell particles. The functional macroinitiators and initiators facilitate the decorating of functional groups on the surface or within the hydrogels, hence promoting multivalent bioconjugation. Diverse crosslinking methodologies were employed for hydrogel synthesis, including amide crosslinking, click chemistry, and enzymatic crosslinking, photo-crosslinking, Schiff-base reactions, thiol-disulfide exchange, and more [34]. Common types of natural biodegradable polymers can be classified into four main groups for synthesising hybrid hydrogels, namely homopolysaccharides, heteropolysaccharides, polypeptides/proteins, and genetically engineered proteins. *in vivo*, these polymers are present as the constituents of the Extracellular Matrix (ECM), and their composition can vary with the source and processing of the polymer. In the field of protein/polysaccharide hybrid polymers, future work may involve natural polymers like fibrin/cellulose, collagen/HA (Hyaluronic Acid), gelatin/alginate, *etc*. In some cases, lignin is also utilized. Controlling their microstructures, characteristics, and reproducibility across experiments is tough [35].

Applications of Hydrogels Derived from Natural Sources

Due to the structure of hydrogels, their suitability as biomedical materials and their functional capabilities in numerous applications depend entirely on their structure. Several important factors define the network architecture of hydrogels: (1) polymer volume fraction in the swelled condition, (2) molecular weight between cross-links, and (3) density, along with mesh size, elastic modulus, and Flory–Huggins interaction parameter. The well-defined limits are reproducible and established through the application of rubber-elasticity theory and equilibrium-swelling. Hydrogels have special features that make them suitable for various purposes across multiple domains, such as tissue engineering, wound care, pharmaceutical delivery, sanitation, agriculture, and water purification [36].

Drug Delivery System

Polymer science is crucial for developing new DDSs, with future advancements focusing on modifying properties, creating innovative copolymers with targeting and bioresponsive components, and using new fabrication processes like molecular imprinting and nanoscale engineering. These polymers offer improved bioavailability, biocompatibility, lower toxicity, and mild side effects, making them valuable for maintaining human health. Over the past two decades, attention has increased on innovative drug delivery systems, particularly for controlled drug release, targeting techniques, effective methods, and disease prevention. These platforms, based on hydrophilic polymers, can modulate drug release characteristics, maintain high drug concentrations, and offer benefits in chemical stability, toxicity, and bio-distribution [68]. The applications of natural polymers in drug delivery systems include emulsification, suspension, sustained or controlled release, film coating, disintegration, solubilization, bioadhesion, gelling, thickening, and viscosity modulation. Additionally, they serve as bulking agents, in drug devices and modifications, for microencapsulation, and to provide mechanical reinforcement. These are increasingly being investigated to develop targeted therapies for specific chronic disorders [37, 38]. Natural polymers are increasingly used for drug delivery; however, the research and development of novel polymers for commercialization remain ongoing. However, the synthesis of pharmaceutical-grade natural polymers requires regulatory permission. Over several decades of formative treatments, numerous substances have demonstrated beneficial therapeutic benefits; yet, their bioavailability and pharmacokinetics are inadequate, resulting in undesirable systemic toxicity post-administration [39]. As a result, the delivery system of drug molecules through the use of hydrogels has become one of the most important strategies to enhance therapeutic potency. It is observed that the implementation of temperature-sensitive characteristics into hydrogel design represents an appropriate trigger for programming drug release. This strategy exploits local temperature differences and has great potential to improve drug release across most tissues. The drawbacks of hydrogels as drug delivery vehicles are their inability to use non-biocompatible and non-biodegradable monomers and crosslinkers as the monomers and crosslinkers, which can cause carcinogenic, teratogenic, and toxic effects. The most well-known observation about most polymers is their ability to trigger platelet activation upon contact with blood, thereby dictating toxicology assessments before application. Furthermore, knowledge of new modified hydrogel materials that exhibit biocompatibility and biodegradability is essential in order to understand the beneficial properties of these materials [40, 41].

Steam Cell Morphogenesis

Fifteen years ago, scientists began trying in the laboratory to control and regulate the natural regeneration of tissues, with the hope that it could one day help repair defects or even regenerate an organ. The three components in a triad are scaffolds, cells, and signaling biomolecules [42]. Collagen biopolymers compose the Extracellular Matrix (ECM). These porous scaffolds, which resemble the extracellular matrix, can also be used in other polymer organization types, such as gels, foams, and membranes. Enrichment of scaffolds with signaling biomolecules can induce cell *de novo* secretion of extracellular matrix and promote regeneration. Transdifferentiation, also known as plasticity, is the ability of some adult stem cell types to differentiate into multiple cell types. Hematopoietic Stem Cells (HSCs) exemplify this category of cells, capable of differentiating into various cell types, including neuronal, skeletal muscle, and hepatic cells.

Mesenchymal Stem Cells (MSCs) differentiate into osteoblasts, chondrocytes, adipocytes, and various myocytes, and are typically regarded as multipotential; nevertheless, some researchers contend that distinct subpopulations exist with restricted differentiation capabilities. At the molecular level, differentiation is a programmed process, and the microenvironment that influences it is also critical. Despite this, the effects of mechanical signals on stem cells have been directly studied in a few studies. MSC-based tissue engineering still needs further development [43, 44].

Wound Healing

Natural polymers with properties like accessibility, non-toxicity, and efficacy against bacterial infections play a major role in wound dressing applications. Natural polymers are preferable to synthetic polymers due to their therapeutic and antibacterial properties. On the other hand, carrageenan, a natural polysaccharide obtained from edible red seaweeds, is known and studied for wound dressing due to its biocompatibility, blood coagulation, and immunological activity [45]. Chitosan is important in promoting wound healing by preventing bleeding, promoting the aggregation of platelets and erythrocytes, and inhibiting plasminogen activator secretion, which extends the duration of hemostasis. Medicated wound coatings are important for the exchange of necrotic and impaired cell components, which are essential in processes involved in restoring the function of the skin barrier, reconstituting tissue attachments, and maintaining homeostasis in the body. The goal of wound healing is to heal quickly while remaining non-toxic and still antiseptic. Wound healing applications need specific material selection, and biopolymers have been a great choice for their properties that support or initiate typical epidermal and dermal wound healing processes [46].

Skin Tissue Engineering and Regenerative Medicine

Tissue engineering is a multidisciplinary field that aims to create functional structures capable of restoring, repairing, replacing, or maintaining damaged living tissues or organs. Hydrogels maintaining similar mechanical and physicochemical properties have also been proven suitable for biomedical uses because of their tunable properties that align with the necessary properties of the ECM. In addition, natural gum-based hydrogels, through cell-binding treatments, can regulate a variety of cellular activities and may even trigger an immune response in the body. Polysaccharide-based hydrogels are biocompatible with tissues; hence, this hydrogel is relevant in the tissue engineering field [47, 48]. Yongzhen *et al.* conducted *in situ* crosslinking to fabricate XG hydrogels with higher elasticity and toughness than physical XG hydrogels. Crosslinked hydrogels have a porous, interconnected structure, allowing for controlled release, which promotes their application as injectable scaffolds in tissue engineering. Rita *et al.* synthesized Glycosaminoglycan-based physical hydrogel delivery systems with dual functionality, serving both as drug delivery systems and as scaffolds for new bone formation. GG crosslinked with calcium is suitable for tissue engineering scaffolds because it is similar to native glycosaminoglycan materials of the extracellular matrix. A new generation of engineered tissues based on scaffolds with an informational role has been developed, where only materials containing growth factor sequences will be used, thereby offering improved qualities over other non-informational polymers regarding their ability to promote initial cell adhesion, proliferation, and, finally, the differentiation process. Growth factors have been developed as a means of modulating the host healing response at the site of injury to consequently enhance tissue formation, as well as modulating and enhancing *in vitro* tissue development to produce an increased quantity of bio-functionally improved engineered tissues [49]. Natural polymers like polysaccharides, proteins, and other macromolecules perform various functions in their native environments. Nature itself has an optimal set of tools; the current paradigm for biomimetic systems is to use natural biopolymer materials to create a wealth of rich structural and functional complexity at the mesoscale. Cell encapsulation is seen as a potent therapeutic strategy, as it physically dissociates a cell mass from an external milieu while preserving normal cellular physiology within an intended semipermeable constraint [50]. Natural polymers have gained significant attention for medical and reconstructive applications, such as biodegradable sutures, wound dressings, and tissue-engineering scaffolds for regenerative medicine. Tissue engineering combines medicine, biology, and materials science, focusing on creating new tissues and organs for reconstructive purposes by repairing or enhancing tissue functions. Selecting appropriate polymers is critical for developing enhanced tissue regeneration materials, as they affect biological responses. Due to their biodegradability, mechanical characteristics, high porosity, surface-to-volume ratio, and small pore size, natural polymeric materials are used to engineer and regenerate hard and soft tissues. Fibres, micro- and nanoparticles, and porous microparticulate polymeric carriers have been investigated as tissue scaffold materials. Due to their biodegradability and biocompatibility, chitosan, cellulose, and cyclodextrins are employed in tissue regeneration. Scaffold production techniques have improved; however, mimicking the natural extracellular matrix remains difficult.

Cell Encapsulation

Encapsulation technology, which involves enclosing living cells in polymer membranes to protect them from immune system attacks, has evolved significantly since its inception in 1933 by Bisceglie *et al.*, who observed tumor cells surviving in pigs' abdominal cavities. In 1950, Algire *et al.* introduced the infusion chamber concept, emphasizing biocompatibility and the stable properties of polymers for therapeutic cell grafting. Today, encapsulation is used in the treatment of various diseases, including hemophilia B, anemia, dwarfism, kidney and liver failure, pituitary disorders, CNS deficiencies, and diabetes. There are two main types of encapsulation geometries: macro- and microcapsules. Macrocapsules have a low surface-area-to-volume ratio, requiring higher concentrations of nutrients to maintain an adequate diffusion gradient, which limits their use in therapy due to low cell density. In contrast, microcapsules allow rapid exchange of therapeutic molecules and have shown promise in replicating insulin and glucose release, advancing to clinical applications in recent years. Polysaccharides, particularly alginate, are commonly used in encapsulation due to their soft, flexible, mechanically stable, and minimally immunogenic properties. Alginate was first used to encapsulate pancreatic islet cells for the treatment of diabetes and has since been employed for various other applications, including endocrine cell encapsulation, gene therapy, bioartificial organs, and hepatocyte protection. Agarose, another polymer, is used for both macro- and microencapsulation, with applications in preventing islet xenograft rejection and encapsulating genetically altered cells. Chitosan has also been used for encapsulation in various therapies, including Parkinson's disease treatment, drug delivery, wound healing, and tissue regeneration. Cellulose, typically employed in inert diffusion chambers, is used for encapsulating cells like pancreatic cancer cells, insulin-producing lines, and hybridoma cells, providing immunoprotective benefits for research and clinical use [51, 52].

RECENT ADVANCES AND INNOVATIONS IN THE FIELD AND FUTURE OUTLOOK

Researchers are increasingly interested in biopolymers due to their biodegradability, non-toxicity, and biocompatibility. Natural biomaterials, like chitosan, are highly recommended for tissue engineering and drug delivery applications due to their unique properties. Chitosan is used in wound-healing hydrogels, as well as in anticancer, anti-inflammatory, and antioxidant applications [53]. Biodegradable polymer materials used in medicine may be exposed to pressure, flow, temperature, stresses and strains, and electric fields, depending on their placement and purpose. Materials must withstand these impulses and adapt to changing conditions. These factors are the toughest to grasp and fix. Recently, multifunctional biodegradable polymer materials have advanced exponentially. Research should focus on chemical changes and hybrid polymer biocomposites that rebuild bone and soft tissues [54]. Technologies integrating biotechnology, nanotechnology, AI, and sustainable manufacturing practices are revolutionizing the sourcing, production, and application of natural polymers. These advancements can address global challenges like plastic pollution, resource depletion, and climate change, and open new opportunities for innovation in industries like packaging and medicine. Polysaccharides and bio-polyesters are key components of natural materials, and advancements in extraction technologies can significantly transform the chemical industry, urban spaces, and buildings [55]. Advancements in the extraction of natural polymers might be one of the significant factors in changing not only the chemical industry but also city spaces and buildings. Along with traditional chemical technologies, unique extraction technologies have evolved over the last decade.As a result, certain living organisms significantly increase yield and shorten the overall extraction process, while achieving a lower final cost for the obtained polymers [56].

Recent Preclinical/ Clinical Advancements in Natural Polymers

Some key examples focusing on popular natural polymers are as follows:-

Chitosan (derived from crustacean shells/ fungi)

- **Preclinical/ Clinical Application: Wound Healing and Drug Delivery.**
  - **Examples:** Chitosan and its derivatives are extensively studied for wound dressings, especially for diabetic wounds, due to their inherent **antimicrobial, antioxidant, and tissue regeneration effects**. They are used in hydrogels, sponges, and nanoparticles to deliver drugs, promoting faster and more effective healing [57].

Hyaluronic Acid (HA) (present naturally in connective tissue)

- **Preclinical/ Clinical Application: Tissue Engineering and Joint/Ocular Delivery.**
  - **Examples:** HA is a key component in **regenerative medicine scaffolds** and injectable hydrogels. Recent work includes resilient, self-healing HA/chitosan hydrogels for **flexible/ wearable strain sensors** and targeted delivery of therapeutics for conditions like stroke and diabetic wound healing [58].

Alginate (Obtained from Seaweed)

- **Preclinical Application: Controlled Drug Release and Tissue Engineering.**
  - **Examples:** Alginate hydrogels are a hot topic for the **encapsulation and controlled release** of drugs (*e.g.*, anti-inflammatory agents) and cells, often in combination with other polymers like chitosan. Recent studies include the

use of alginate-based microrobots for **targeted intravascular drug delivery** under magnetic drive [59].

Collagen and Gelatin (obtained from animal tissue)

- **Preclinical/Clinical Application: Scaffolds for Tissue Repair.**
  - **Examples:** As the primary component of the extracellular matrix, collagen and its hydrolyzed form, gelatin, are staples in creating **structural scaffolds** for bone repair, cartilage, skin, and nerve regeneration, helping to guide cell migration and tissue formation. These natural materials are valued because they offer **biocompatibility, biodegradability, and a structure** that closely mimics the body's own environment, making them ideal for the next generation of therapeutics [60].

FUTURE OF NATURAL POLYMERS IN BIOMEDICAL APPLICATIONS

Natural Polymers in Biomedical Applications

● Natural polymers are highly sought after in biomedical applications due to their biodegradability and biocompatibility.

● These materials interact well with cells and tissues without causing inflammation or immune responses, making them suitable for niche markets.

● Despite their advantages, natural polymers are underutilized in medical applications due to labor-intensive, less efficient processing techniques, natural variability, batch-to-batch inconsistencies, and seasonal supply.

● New techniques like emulsion and droplet microfluidics and solventless processing methods have been developed but have not yet penetrated many applications, especially at the commercial stage.

● Scaling up a new biopolymer product for biomedical applications faces challenges due to regulatory red tape [57].

Natural polymers are promising for developing functional and creative materials in many industries. However, the principles are inseparable since most materials may be produced with mild solvents (typically water) and simple production methods [58].

● The focus is on interdisciplinary and inter-sectorial research actions.

● Innovations include the development of efficient polymer extraction and purification methods, standardized material production, and the enhancement of the applicability of natural polymers in biological and medical environments.

• Technological innovations include the preparation of explants with a specific profile for biopolymer structures.

• Efforts have been made to develop drug delivery systems based on natural biomass polymers, including lignin, cellulose, starch, chitosan, and pectin.

• Natural polymers like alginate, hyaluronic acid, gelatin, chitosan, and cellulose have been increasingly investigated for biomedical applications because of their biocompatibility, biodegradability, and non-toxicity.

• Natural polymers have been investigated as bioink for 3D printing techniques, offering potential for creating complex structures for soft tissue engineering and personalized food design [59].

Innovative advancements in treating diseases and injuries prevalent in the elderly are emerging through the development of new biomaterials, which are materials compatible with the human body. Coined in 1969, the field of biomaterials is transdisciplinary, focusing on creating materials that interact with biological systems to diagnose, treat, and enhance bodily functions. Successful biomaterial implementation requires collaboration across materials science, life sciences, chemistry, physics, medicine, and engineering to improve human quality of life [60]. The design of a biomaterial is to improve the quality of human life. Progress in the design of polymeric materials has allowed polymer researchers and physicians to make tremendous contributions to the medical field by developing materials comprising surgical sutures, drug-delivery systems, wound dressings, and tissue engineering scaffolds. Also, biohybrid materials can be produced by building up systems that bear functionalities from diverse origins [61].

Numerous treatments and ideas for treating acute and chronic wounds have emerged in healthcare [62]. The rising number of patients with comorbidities and chronic disorders, which can change, delay, or prevent wound healing, has created new challenges in wound care. Academic researchers have swiftly found promising answers, and several sophisticated wound-healing materials have been developed, but translating them to the market is difficult and unlikely without industry specialists. Wound healing applications will help academic and industrial researchers design, evaluate, validate, and sell polymer wound care solutions [63]. The chapter discusses current wound management challenges, the latest products, polymer materials, approval pathways, wound-healing models, and novel technologies that may soon reach customers. This thorough review should emphasize networking and interactions between academia and the healthcare industry. Innovation, manufacturing, regulatory insights, and financial resources are needed to produce wound care products quickly and affordably for patients [64].

The physicochemical properties of polymers can be enhanced through the addition of various inorganic or organic substances, resulting in composites and nanocomposites. These materials are widely used in applications such as superconductors, catalysts, and insulators due to their improved performance [65]. Nanoparticles are particularly valuable in designing composites that enhance mechanical performance, thermal conductivity, and other functional properties, including catalytic action and magnetism, especially in the biomedical sector. Incorporating drugs into nanoscopic biodegradable polymer vehicles allows for controlled and targeted drug delivery, thereby reducing side effects. This has led to the emergence of "nano-medicine," which holds promise for innovative treatments for various diseases. Some of the relevant patents are listed in Table **4**.

Table 4. Patents related to natural polymers and their applications.

S.N.	Title of Patent	Patent Number	Date of Patent	Assignee	Inventors
1	Use of short chain fatty acids for the treatment and prevention of diseases and disorders	US11759442B2	2023-09-19	Temple University of the Commonwealth System of Higher Education	Ira C. Spector, Mark A. Feitelson, Alla Arzumanyan
2	Methods for adhering tissue surfaces and materials and biomedical uses thereof	US20230091258A1	2023-03-23	Ecole Superieur De Physique Et De Chimie Industrielles De Paris, Centre National de la Recherche Scientifique CNRS, Institut National de la Sante et de la Recherche Medicale INSERM, Universite Sorbonne Paris Nord Paris 13, Sorbonne Universite, Universite Paris Cite	Ludwik Leibler, Anne Meddahi-Pellé, Didier Letourneur Alba, Marcellan-Parisot

(Table 4) cont.....

S.N.	Title of Patent	Patent Number	Date of Patent	Assignee	Inventors
3	Photo-crosslinked hydrogel material and preparation, composition, and application thereof photo-crosslinked hydrogel	US20200262802A1	2021-09-14	Zhongshan Guanghe Medical Technology Co Ltd	Linyong Zhu, Yujie Hua, Qiuning Lin, Yiqing Zhang, Chunyan Bao, Xuepeng Zhong
4	Photo-coupled synergistically crosslinked hydrogel material and its composition, preparation method, use, product, and preparation kit	US20200262939A1	2021-06-25	Zhongshan Guanghe Medical Technology Co Ltd	Linyong Zhu, Yujie Hua, Qiuning Lin, Yiqing Zhang, Chunyan Bao, Xuepeng Zhong
5	Synthesis and application of MOFs/natural polymers composite beads adsorbent	US10537873B2	2020-01-21	Nanjing Huachuang Institute Of Environmental Technology Co Ltd	Weiben Yang, Zhen Yang, Ning Zhuo, Xia Zhou, Jiachun Shen, Xuntong Zhang, Xuzeng Wang

CONCLUSION

This chapter has explored the fascinating world of natural polymers, from their historical roots in early human civilization to their modern applications across diverse industries. These polymers, sourced from renewable resources such as plants, animals, and microbes, provide a sustainable alternative to synthetic materials. Their inherent biocompatibility, biodegradability, and often lower cost make them attractive for use in textiles, food products, pharmaceuticals, cosmetics, and biomedical applications. The chapter further delved into specific examples, such as cellulose and starch from plants, as well as collagen and other proteins from animals, showcasing their unique properties and diverse uses. While natural polymers offer numerous advantages, they also have limitations, including potential microbial contamination, batch-to-batch variability, and the need for controlled processing. Despite these challenges, ongoing advancements in natural polymer research are addressing these issues and expanding their potential. The chapter concluded by emphasizing the growing importance of natural polymers in creating advanced materials for applications ranging from drug delivery and tissue engineering to biofabrication and wound healing. As we move towards a more sustainable future, natural polymers will undoubtedly play a critical role in developing eco-friendly and biocompatible solutions for a wide range of societal needs. The continued exploration and refinement of these remarkable materials promise to unlock even greater potential in the years to come.

REFERENCES

[1] Butte Kishor D, Rathod Sudha S. Natural polymers–A comprehensive review. Int J Res Pharm Biomed Sci 2012; 3(4): 1597-613.

[2] Chifiriuc M, Grumezescu A, Grumezescu V, Bezirtzoglou E, Lazar V, Bolocan A. Biomedical applications of natural polymers for drug delivery. Curr Org Chem 2014; 18(2): 152-64. [http://dx.doi.org/10.2174/13852728180214012910452 5]

[3] Puertas-Bartolomé M, Mora-Boza A, García-Fernández L. Emerging biofabrication techniques: A review on natural polymers for biomedical applications. Polymers (Basel) 2021; 13(8): 1209. [http://dx.doi.org/10.3390/polym13081209] [PMID: 33918049]

[4] Aravamudhan A, Ramos DM, Nada AA, Kumbar SG. Natural polymers: polysaccharides and their derivatives for biomedical applications. InNatural and synthetic biomedical polymers 2014; 67-89.

[5] Jacob John M, Thomas S. Natural polymers: an overview. 2012.

[6] Thomas S, Visakh P, Mathew AP. Advances in natural polymers. Advanced Structured Materials 2013; 255: 312-34.

[7] Rajeswari S, Prasanthi T, Sudha N, Swain RP, Panda S, Goka V. Natural polymers: A recent review. World J Pharm Pharm Sci 2017; 6: 472-94. [http://dx.doi.org/10.20959/wjpps20178-9762]

[8] Paradowska-Stolarz A, Wieckiewicz M, Owczarek A, Wezgowiec J. Natural polymers for the maintenance of oral health: Review of recent advances and perspectives. Int J Mol Sci 2021; 22(19): 10337. [http://dx.doi.org/10.3390/ijms221910337] [PMID: 34638678]

[9] Sionkowska A. Collagen blended with natural polymers: Recent advances and trends. Prog Polym Sci 2021; 122: 101452. [http://dx.doi.org/10.1016/j.progpolymsci.2021.101452]

[10] Olatunji O, editor. Natural polymers: industry techniques and applications. Springer; 2015.

[11] Silva ACQ, Silvestre AJD, Vilela C, Freire CSR. Natural polymers-based materials: A contribution to a greener future. Molecules 2021; 27(1): 94. [http://dx.doi.org/10.3390/molecules27010094] [PMID: 35011326]

[12] Shanker U, Rani M, Hussain CM, Eds. Green functionalized nanomaterials for environmental applications. 2021.

[13] Nayak AK, Hasnain MS, Aminabhavi TM. Drug delivery using interpenetrating polymeric networks of natural polymers: A recent update. Journal of Drug Delivery Science and Technology. 202; 66:102915. [http://dx.doi.org/10.1016/j.jddst.2021.102915]

[14] Anwunobi AP, Emeje MO. Recent applications of natural polymers in nanodrug delivery. J Nanomedic Nanotechnol S 2011; 4(002) [http://dx.doi.org/10.4172/2157-7439.S4-002]

[15] Muthukumaran P, Suresh Babu P, Karthikeyan S, Kamaraj M, Aravind J. Tailored natural polymers: a useful eco-friendly sustainable tool for the mitigation of emerging pollutants: a review. Int J Environ Sci Technol 2021; 18(8): 2491-510. [http://dx.doi.org/10.1007/s13762-020-03048-6]

[16] Gowariker VR, Viswanathan NV, Shreedhar J. Polymer Science. New Delhi: New Age International 2005; pp. 1-15.

[17] Pandey R, Khuller G. Polymer based drug delivery systems for mycobacterial infections. Curr Drug Deliv 2004; 1(3): 195-201. [http://dx.doi.org/10.2174/1567201043334669] [PMID: 16305383]

[18] Chamarthy SP, Pinal R. Plasticizer concentration and the performance of a diffusion-controlled polymeric drug delivery system. Colloids Surf A Physicochem Eng Asp 2008; 331(1-2): 25-30. [http://dx.doi.org/10.1016/j.colsurfa.2008.05.047]

[19] Alonso-Sande M, Teijeiro-Osorio D, Remuñán-López C, Alonso MJ. Glucomannan, a promising polysaccharide for biopharmaceutical purposes. Eur J Pharm Biopharm 2009; 72(2): 453-62. [http://dx.doi.org/10.1016/j.ejpb.2008.02.005] [PMID: 18511246]

[20] Guo J, Skinner GW, Harcum WW, Barnum PE. Pharmaceutical applications of naturally occurring watersoluble polymers. PSTT 1998; 1: 254-61.

[21] Girish K. Jani, Dhiren P. Shah, Vipul D. Prajapati, Vineet C. Jain, Gums and mucilages: versatile excipients for pharmaceutical formulations. Asian J Pharm Sci 2009; 4(5): 309-32.

[22] Shirwaikar A, Shirwaikar A, Prabhu SL, Kumar GA. Herbal excipients in novel drug delivery systems. Indian J Pharm Sci 2008; 70(4): 415-22. [http://dx.doi.org/10.4103/0250-474X.44587] [PMID: 20046764]

[23] Nishiyama Y, Langan P, Chanzy H. Crystal structure and hydrogen-bonding system in cellulose Iβ from synchrotron X-ray and neutron fiber diffraction. J Am Chem Soc 2002; 124(31): 9074-82. [http://dx.doi.org/10.1021/ja0257319] [PMID: 12149011]

[24] Scheller HV, Jensen JK, Sørensen SO, Harholt J, Geshi N. Biosynthesis of pectin. Physiol Plant 2007; 129(2): 283-95. [http://dx.doi.org/10.1111/j.1399-3054.2006.00834.x]

[25] Dumitriu S, Ed. Hon, D.N.-S. Cellulose and its derivatives: Structures, Reactions and Medical Uses.Polysaccharides in medicinal applications. New York, NY, USA: Marcel Dekker, Inc 1996; pp. 87-106.

[26] Kamaruzzaman NF, Tan LP, Hamdan RH, *et al.* Antimicrobial polymers: The potential replacement of existing antibiotics? Int J Mol Sci 2019; 20(11): 2747. [http://dx.doi.org/10.3390/ijms20112747] [PMID: 31167476]

[27] Rusu LC, Ardelean LC, Jitariu AA, Miu CA, Streian CG. An insight into the structural diversity and clinical applicability of polyurethanes in biomedicine. Polymers (Basel) 2020; 12(5): 1197. [http://dx.doi.org/10.3390/polym12051197] [PMID: 32456335]

[28] Lebeaux D, Ghigo JM, Beloin C. Biofilm-related infections: bridging the gap between clinical management and fundamental aspects of recalcitrance toward antibiotics. Microbiol Mol Biol Rev 2014; 78(3): 510-43. [http://dx.doi.org/10.1128/MMBR.00013-14] [PMID: 25184564]

[29] Sun D, Babar Shahzad M, Li M, Wang G, Xu D. Antimicrobial materials with medical applications. Mater Technol 2015; 30(sup6): B90-5. [http://dx.doi.org/10.1179/1753555714Y.0000000239]

[30] Dash M, Chiellini F, Ottenbrite RM, Chiellini E. Chitosan—A versatile semi-synthetic polymer in biomedical applications. Prog Polym Sci 2011; 36(8): 981-1014. [http://dx.doi.org/10.1016/j.progpolymsci.2011.02.001]

[31] Kung ML, Lin PY, Peng SW, *et al.* Biomimetic polymer-based Ag nanocomposites as a antimicrobial platform. Appl Mater Today 2016; 4: 31-9. [http://dx.doi.org/10.1016/j.apmt.2016.05.003]

[32] Kumar A, Han SS. PVA-based hydrogels for tissue engineering: A review. Int J Polym Mater 2017; 66(4): 159-82. [http://dx.doi.org/10.1080/00914037.2016.1190930]

[33] Budama-Kilinc Y, Cakir-Koc R, Aslan B, Özkan B, Mutlu H, Üstün E. Hydrogels in Regenerative Medicine.Biomaterials in Regenerative Medicine. London, UK: IntechOpen 2018; pp. 277-301. [http://dx.doi.org/10.5772/intechopen.70409]

[34] Peppas N, Bures P, Leobandung W, Ichikawa H. Hydrogels in pharmaceutical formulations. Eur J Pharm Biopharm 2000; 50(1): 27-46. [http://dx.doi.org/10.1016/S0939-6411(00)00090-4] [PMID: 10840191]

[35] Jonker AM, Löwik DWPM, van Hest JCM. Peptide- and protein-based hydrogels. Chem Mater 2012; 24(5): 759-73. [http://dx.doi.org/10.1021/cm202640w]

[36] Lau HK, Kiick KL. Opportunities for multicomponent hybrid hydrogels in biomedical applications. Biomacromolecules 2015; 16(1): 28-42. [http://dx.doi.org/10.1021/bm501361c] [PMID: 25426888]

[37] Sur S, Rathore A, Dave V, Reddy KR, Chouhan RS, Sadhu V. Recent developments in functionalized polymer nanoparticles for efficient drug delivery system. Nano-Structures & Nano-Objects 2019; 20: 100397. [http://dx.doi.org/10.1016/j.nanoso.2019.100397]

[38] Tong X, Pan W, Su T, Zhang M, Dong W, Qi X. Recent advances in natural polymer-based drug delivery systems. React Funct Polym 2020; 148: 104501. [http://dx.doi.org/10.1016/j.reactfunctpolym.2020.104501]

[39] Tiyaboonchai W. Chitosan Nanoparticles: A Promising System for Drug Delivery. Naresuan Univ J 2003; 11: 51-66.

[40] Kumari A, Yadav SK, Yadav SC. Biodegradable polymeric nanoparticles based drug delivery systems. Colloids Surf B Biointerfaces 2010; 75(1): 1-18. [http://dx.doi.org/10.1016/j.colsurfb.2009.09.001] [PMID: 19782542]

[41] Tibbitt MW, Dahlman JE, Langer R. Emerging frontiers in drug delivery. J Am Chem Soc 2016; 138(3): 704-17. [http://dx.doi.org/10.1021/jacs.5b09974] [PMID: 26741786]

[42] Mukherjee S, Vinugopal JR, Ravichandran R, Ramalingam M, Raghunath M, Ramakrishna S. Nanofiber technology for controlling stem cell functions and tissue engineering. Micro Nanotechnol Eng Stem Cells Tissues 2013; 2: 27-51. [http://dx.doi.org/10.1002/9781118574775.ch2]

[43] Beneke CE, Viljoen AM, Hamman JH. Polymeric plant-derived excipients in drug delivery. Molecules 2009; 14(7): 2602-20. [http://dx.doi.org/10.3390/molecules14072602] [PMID: 19633627]

[44] Malafaya PB, Silva GA, Reis RL. Natural–origin polymers as carriers and scaffolds for biomolecules and cell delivery in tissue engineering applications. Adv Drug Deliv Rev 2007; 59(4-5): 207-33. [http://dx.doi.org/10.1016/j.addr.2007.03.012] [PMID: 17482309]

[45] Jana S, Gandhi A, Sen KK, Basu Sk. Natural polymers and their applications in drug delivery. J Pharm Sci Technol 2011; 1(1): 16-27.

[46] Shanmugam S, Manavalan R, Venkappayya D, Sundaramoorthy K. Natural polymers and their applications. Nat Prod Radiance 2005; 4(6): 478-81.

[47] Katarzyna L, Lewandowicz G. Polymer biodegradation and biodegradable polymers: a review. Pol J Environ Stud 2010; 19(5): 255-66.

[48] Pantani R, Turng LS. Manufacturing of advanced biodegradable polymeric components. J Appl Polym Sci 2015; 132(48): app.42889. [http://dx.doi.org/10.1002/app.42889]

[49] Kim IY, Seo SJ, Moon HS, *et al.* Chitosan and its derivatives for tissue engineering applications.

Biotechnol Adv 2008; 26(1): 1-21.
[http://dx.doi.org/10.1016/j.biotechadv.2007.07.009] [PMID: 17884325]

[50] Venkatesan J, Kim SK. Chitosan composites for bone tissue engineering--an overview. Mar Drugs 2010; 8(8): 2252-66.
[http://dx.doi.org/10.3390/md8082252] [PMID: 20948907]

[51] Jia X, Kiick KL. Hybrid multicomponent hydrogels for tissue engineering. Macromol Biosci 2009; 9(2): 140-56.
[http://dx.doi.org/10.1002/mabi.200800284] [PMID: 19107720]

[52] Przekora A. A concise review on tissue engineered artificial skin grafts for chronic wound treatment: Can we reconstruct functional skin tissue *in vitro*? Cells 2020; 9(7): 1622.
[http://dx.doi.org/10.3390/cells9071622] [PMID: 32640572]

[53] Dovedytis M, Liu ZJ, Bartlett S. Hyaluronic acid and its biomedical applications: A review. Engineered Regeneration 2020; 1: 102-13.
[http://dx.doi.org/10.1016/j.engreg.2020.10.001]

[54] Natalia M. Salwowska, Katarzyna A Bebenek, Dominika A, Zaz dło & Dominika LWcisło-Dziadecka, "Physiochemical properties and application of hyaluronic acid: asystematic review". J Cosmet Dermatol 15: 520-6.

[55] Shen Q, Guo Y, Wang K, Zhang C, Ma Y. Chunhui Zhang andYanli Ma, "A Review of chondroitin sulfate's preparation, properties, functions, and applications". Molecules 2023; 28(20): 7093.
[http://dx.doi.org/10.3390/molecules28207093] [PMID: 37894574]

[56] Divya M, Vijayakumar S, Chen J. A short review on chondroitin sulphate and its based nanomaterials for bone repair and bone remodelling applications. Journal of Composites Science 2023; 8(1): 6.
[http://dx.doi.org/10.3390/jcs8010006]

[57] Rasti H, Parivar K, Baharara J, Iranshahi M, Namvar F. Chitin from the mollusc chiton: Extraction, characterization and chitosan preparation. Iran J Pharm Res 2017; 16(1): 366-79.
[PMID: 28496490]

[58] Younes I, Rinaudo M. Chitin and chitosan preparation from marine sources. Structure, properties and applications. Mar Drugs 2015; 13(3): 1133-74.
[http://dx.doi.org/10.3390/md13031133] [PMID: 25738328]

[59] Guo X, Wang Y, Qin Y, Shen P, Peng Q. Structures, properties and application of alginic acid: A review. Int J Biol Macromol 2020; 162(1): 618-28.
[http://dx.doi.org/10.1016/j.ijbiomac.2020.06.180] [PMID: 32590090]

[60] Ea P, Pavlatou EA. Advanced applications of biomaterials based on alginic acid. American Journal of Biomedical Science & Research 2020; 9(1): 47-53.
[http://dx.doi.org/10.34297/AJBSR.2020.09.001350]

[61] Kamel S, Ali N, Jahangir K, Shah SM, El-Gendy AA. Pharmaceutical significance of cellulose: A review. Express Polym Lett 2008; 2(11): 758-78.
[http://dx.doi.org/10.3144/expresspolymlett.2008.90]

[62] Seddiqi H, Oliaei E, Honarkar H, *et al.* Cellulose and its derivatives: towards biomedical applications. Cellulose 2021; 28(4): 1893-931.
[http://dx.doi.org/10.1007/s10570-020-03674-w]

[63] Bhatia S, Bhatia S. Natural polymers vs synthetic polymer. Natural polymer drug delivery systems: nanoparticles, plants, and algae. 2016:95-118.
[http://dx.doi.org/10.1007/978-3-319-41129-3_3]

[64] Arif U, Haider S, Haider A, Khan N, Alghyamah AA, Jamila N, Khan MI, Almasry WA, Kang IK. Biocompatible polymers and their potential biomedical applications: A review. Current pharmaceutical design. 2019; 1;25(34):3608-19.
[http://dx.doi.org/10.2174/1381612825999191011105148]

[65] Aboulrous AA, Mahmoud T, Alsabagh AM, Abdou MI. Application of natural polymers in engineering. Natural polymers: Industry techniques and applications. 2016:185-218. [http://dx.doi.org/10.1007/978-3-319-26414-1_7]

[66] Aravamudhan A, Ramos DM, Nada AA, Kumbar SG. Natural polymers: polysaccharides and their derivatives for biomedical applications. InNatural and synthetic biomedical polymers 2014; 1: 67-89.

[67] Puertas-Bartolomé M, Mora-Boza A, García-Fernández L. Emerging biofabrication techniques: A review on natural polymers for biomedical applications 2021. [http://dx.doi.org/10.3390/polym13081209]

[68] Pillai O, Panchagnula R. Polymers in drug delivery. Curr Opin Chem Biol 2001; 5(4): 447-51. [http://dx.doi.org/10.1016/S1367-5931(00)00227-1] [PMID: 11470609]

[69] Berthiaume F, Maguire TJ, Yarmush ML. Tissue engineering and regenerative medicine: history, progress, and challenges. Annu Rev Chem Biomol Eng 2011; 2(1): 403-30. [http://dx.doi.org/10.1146/annurev-chembioeng-061010-114257] [PMID: 22432625]

[70] Pina S, Ribeiro VP, Marques CF, *et al.* Scaffolding strategies for tissue engineering and regenerative medicine applications. Materials (Basel) 2019; 12(11): 1824. [http://dx.doi.org/10.3390/ma12111824] [PMID: 31195642]

[71] Malafaya PB, Silva GA, Reis RL. Natural–origin polymers as carriers and scaffolds for biomolecules and cell delivery in tissue engineering applications. Adv Drug Deliv Rev 2007; 59(4-5): 207-33. [http://dx.doi.org/10.1016/j.addr.2007.03.012] [PMID: 17482309]

[72] Kothale D, Verma U, Dewangan N, Jana P, Jain A, Jain D. Alginate as promising natural polymer for pharmaceutical, food, and biomedical applications. Curr Drug Deliv 2020; 17(9): 755-75. [http://dx.doi.org/10.2174/1567201817666200810110226] [PMID: 32778024]

[73] Ahmad Raus R, Wan Nawawi WMF, Nasaruddin RR. Alginate and alginate composites for biomedical applications. Asian Journal of Pharmaceutical Sciences 2021; 16(3): 280-306. [http://dx.doi.org/10.1016/j.ajps.2020.10.001] [PMID: 34276819]

[74] Lavanya DK, Kulkarni PK, Dixit M, Raavi PK, Krishna LN. Sources of cellulose and their applications—A review. International Journal of Drug Formulation and Research 2011; 2(6): 19-38.

[75] Seddiqi H, Oliaei E, Honarkar H, *et al.* Cellulose and its derivatives: towards biomedical applications. Cellulose 2021; 28(4): 1893-931. [http://dx.doi.org/10.1007/s10570-020-03674-w]

[76] Antanitta. S V, Khonde R, Kandasubramanian B. Cellulose and derivatives serving as natural, versatile and biocompatible polymers in biomedical applications. Int J Polym Mater 2024; 13: 1-5. [http://dx.doi.org/10.1080/00914037.2024.2376247]

[77] Bouhlouli M, Pourhadi M, Karami F, Talebi Z, Ranjbari J, Khojasteh A. Applications of bacterial cellulose as a natural polymer in tissue engineering. ASAIO Journal. 2021; 1;67(7):709-20. [http://dx.doi.org/10.1097/MAT.0000000000001356]

[78] Avila Rodríguez MI, Rodríguez Barroso LG, Sánchez ML. Collagen: A review on its sources and potential cosmetic applications. J Cosmet Dermatol 2018; 17(1): 20-6. [http://dx.doi.org/10.1111/jocd.12450] [PMID: 29144022]

[79] Geanaliu-Nicolae RE, Andronescu E. Blended natural support materials—collagen based hydrogels used in biomedicine. Materials (Basel) 2020; 13(24): 5641. [http://dx.doi.org/10.3390/ma13245641] [PMID: 33321865]

[80] Muthukumar T, Sreekumar G, Sastry TP, Chamundeeswari M. Collagen as a potential biomaterial in biomedical applications. Rev Adv Mater Sci 2018; 53(1): 29-39. [http://dx.doi.org/10.1515/rams-2018-0002]

[81] Guerra NB, Sant'Ana Pegorin G, Boratto MH, de Barros NR, de Oliveira Graeff CF, Herculano RD. Biomedical applications of natural rubber latex from the rubber tree Hevea brasiliensis. Mater Sci Eng

C 2021; 126: 112126.
[http://dx.doi.org/10.1016/j.msec.2021.112126] [PMID: 34082943]

[82] Andrade KL, Ramlow H, Floriano JF, Acosta ED, Faita FL, Machado RAF. Latex and natural rubber: recent advances for biomedical applications. Polímeros 2022; 32(2): e2022015.
[http://dx.doi.org/10.1590/0104-1428.20210114]

[83] Srivastava P, Malviya R. Sources of pectin, extraction and its applications in pharmaceutical industry– An overview. Indian J Nat Prod Resour 2011; 2(1): 10-8.

[84] Sultana N. Biological properties and biomedical applications of pectin and pectin-based composites: A review. Molecules 2023; 28(24): 7974.
[http://dx.doi.org/10.3390/molecules28247974] [PMID: 38138464]

[85] Mishra RK, Banthia AK, Majeed AB. Pectin based formulations for biomedical applications: a review. Asian J Pharm Clin Res 2012; 5(4): 1-7.

[86] Zia KM, Tabasum S, Nasif M, *et al.* A review on synthesis, properties and applications of natural polymer based carrageenan blends and composites. Int J Biol Macromol 2017; 96: 282-301.
[http://dx.doi.org/10.1016/j.ijbiomac.2016.11.095] [PMID: 27914965]

[87] Das IJ, Bal T. Exploring carrageenan: From seaweed to biomedicine—A comprehensive review. Int J Biol Macromol 2024; 268(Pt 2): 131822.
[http://dx.doi.org/10.1016/j.ijbiomac.2024.131822] [PMID: 38677668]

[88] Pacheco-Quito EM, Ruiz-Caro R, Veiga MD. Carrageenan: drug delivery systems and other biomedical applications. Mar Drugs 2020; 18(11): 583.
[http://dx.doi.org/10.3390/md18110583] [PMID: 33238488]

CHAPTER 4

Plant-Derived Polymers and Their Contribution to the Management of Inflammatory Bowel Disease.

Sakshi Gupta[1], **Nidhi Agrawal**[1], **Mohammad Akbar Siddiqui**[1], **Meenakshi Jaiswal**[1] and **S.K. Lanjhiyana**[1,*]

[1] *Department of Pharmacy, Guru Ghasidas Vishwavidyalaya, Bilaspur 495009, Chhattisgarh, India*

Abstract: Inflammatory Bowel Disease (IBD) is a chronic inflammation of the small and large intestines that results from host-microbial interactions in genetically susceptible individuals. It includes Crohn's disease and ulcerative colitis, causing symptoms like diarrhoea, pain, bloody stools, and vomiting. IBD is characterised by a complex interaction of genetic, environmental, and microbial factors. It needs novel therapeutic strategies that overcome conventional anti-inflammatory and immunosuppressive treatments. Plant-derived polymers, including pectin, inulin, cyclodextrin, guar gum, cellulose, carrageenan, and alginate, have the capacity to regulate IBD. These polysaccharides are distinguished by their biodegradability, biocompatibility, and distinctive physicochemical properties, allowing them to function as efficient drug transporters while possessing intrinsic anti-inflammatory and immunomodulatory effects. Pectin and inulin have prebiotic properties, fortifying the Gastrointestinal (GI) barrier and diminishing intestinal permeability. Cyclodextrins enhance the solubility and stability of medicinal medicines, whilst guar gum and cellulose facilitate targeted drug delivery. Carrageenan and alginate are utilised in advanced encapsulation methods for targeted medication delivery. Advanced extraction methods and biotechnological improvements have further refined these polymers for medicinal use. Incorporating these natural chemicals into IBD treatment protocols shows potential for enhancing patient results, reducing unwanted effects, and promoting a more sustainable, comprehensive strategy for managing this severe disease.

Keywords: Alginate, Carrageenan, Cellulose, Cyclodextrin, Guar gum, Inflammatory bowel disease, Inulin, Pectin, Plant-derived polymer.

* **Corresponding author S.K. Lanjhiyana:** Department of Pharmacy, Guru Ghasidas Vishwavidyalaya, Bilaspur 495009, Chhattisgarh, India; E-mail: sklanjh1975@gmail.com

Meenakshi Jaiswal & S.K. Lanjhiyana (Eds.)

INTRODUCTION

IBD has markedly risen across Europe and North America over the past 25 years, with a twofold increase in incident cases in the UK during the previous 20 years. The condition, conventionally categorized as Crohn's disease and ulcerative colitis, is a complicated 'continuum' disease with a comparable etiology encompassing genetic, environmental, and microbial influences [1]. Treatment is predominantl empirical, requiring current input to ensure optimal long-term outcomes for patients. The etiology of elevated illness incidence remains unclear; however, hypotheses about diminished microbial exposure during early life, the westernization of nutrition, and the hygiene theory may contribute to this phenomenon [2]. IBD is a persistent inflammatory condition of the GI system, marked by abnormal immune response and changes in the gut flora. The diagnosis of IBD and its subtypes requires the evaluation of clinical symptoms and clinical methods. Molecular markers, including serological, histological, and faecal signs, can aid in differential diagnosis. Treatment techniques often encompass pharmaceutical measures to manage inflammation and, in extreme instances, surgical procedures. Probiotics, live microorganisms, drug-loaded natural polysaccharide systems, and genetically modified probiotics are potential approaches to the treatment of IBD [3]. The inflammation sites of Crohn's disease and ulcerative colitis are illustrated in Fig. (**1**).

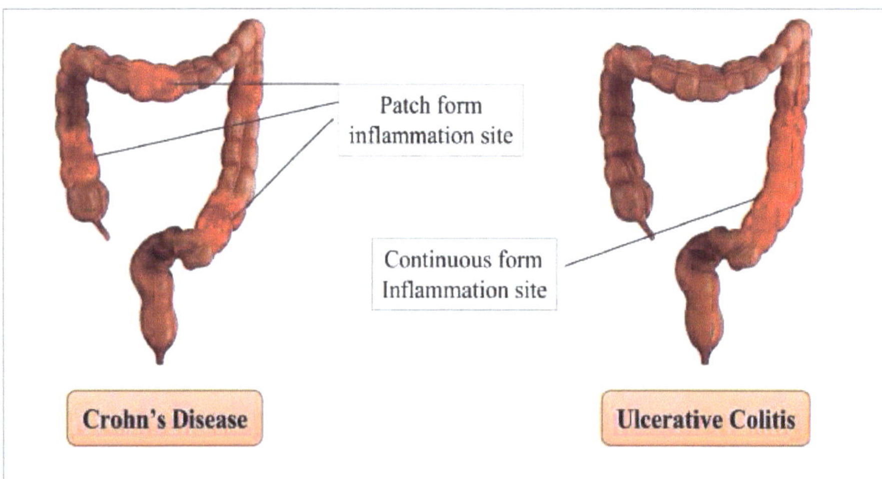

Fig. (1). Schematic illustration of Crohn's disease and ulcerative colitis.

Polysaccharides are a class of pharmacologically active compounds with anti-inflammatory, immunomodulatory, glycolipid, and anticancer properties. They are well known for their safety and can serve as substrates for certain gut microbiomes to enhance the spread of beneficial bacteria. The International Scientific Association of Probiotics and Prebiotics (ISAPP) defines prebiotics as substances preferentially employed by host bacteria and confer health benefits [4]. The health-enhancing properties of polysaccharides derived from the same source but exhibiting varying structural types are frequently associated with the composition, diversity, enterotypes, or metabolites of the gut microbiome. Understanding the probable processes of dietary polysaccharide-gut microbiome-host interactions and the correlation between polysaccharide structure and prebiotic activity will contribute to the advancement and improvement of plant-derived polysaccharides in the food sector. They are essential in the management of IBD due to their anti-inflammatory and immunoregulatory properties. They modulate inflammatory cytokines, the intestinal microbiota, and the immune system, and can attach to the ulcerated surface of the colon [5]. Polysaccharides can function as drug carriers, exhibiting effective controlled-release properties, high affinity, and biodegradability. They can efficiently mitigate and manage IBD through several mechanisms, rendering them appropriate for immediate intervention and the continuous release of therapeutic agents. This chapter offers a summary of the classifications and therapeutic mechanisms of polysaccharides [6].

Basic Introduction to Plant-derived Polymers

Pectin

Pectin is a heteropolysaccharide consisting of a linear polymer of Galacturonic Acid (GalA), referred to as Homogalacturonan (HG). It is categorized as High-Methoxyl Pectin (HMP) and Low-methoxyl Pectin (LMP). HMP originates from the extraction of juice by-products, whereas LMP is generated by acid, alkaline, or enzymatic de-esterification processes. Sunflower Heads (SH) serve as an alternative source of natural LMP, potentially containing up to 20% of this polysaccharide. LMP possesses a net negative charge due to the free carboxyl groups of the GalA residues, which engage with positively charged amino acids, facilitating its penetration through the mucus layer of the intestinal wall. The extraction of pectin requires the use of strong acids and is both time- and energy-intensive. Ultrasound-Assisted Extraction (UAE) has been examined for its benefits, such as reduced energy expenses and enhanced yield and quality [7, 8]. The chemical structure of pectin is illustrated in Fig. (**2**).

Inulin

Inulin, discovered by German scientist Rose in 1804, is a fructose-containing polymer found in the roots of Inula helenium, a perennial plant native to temperate parts of Europe, Asia, and Africa. It is classified as a fructan and functions as a storage polymer in several members of the Compositae family. Inulin consists mostly of linear fructose units linked by a β-(2-6) glycosidic bond and is derived from chicory, a naturally occurring polydisperse carbohydrate. Inulin, a multifaceted compound with many health and scientific benefits, is found in more than 3000 vegetables and plants. It is acquired from asparagus, leek, onion, banana, wheat, and garlic [9]. Inulin-type fructans are derived from sucrose and are extensively utilized in processed meals as substitutes for fat or sugar, or to enhance beneficial attributes. It provides just 25-35% of the energy offered by digestible carbs and has a sweetness level around 10% that of sucrose [10]. The chemical structure of inulin comprises linear (2→1)-linked -d-fructosyl units connected to the fructosyl component of sucrose. The Degree of Polymerization (DP) and branching influence functioning, with plants exhibiting a comparatively low DP (maximum < 200) and bacteria demonstrating a significantly high DP (ranging from 10,000 to over 100,000). Inulin manufacture consists of two stages: the extraction and initial purification of raw syrup, followed by additional refinement to yield commercial goods with a purity of above 99.5% in the second phase of processing. Advanced technologies such as supercritical Carbon Dioxide (CO_2), ultrasound, simultaneous ultrasonic/microwave, and Pulsed Electric Field (PEF) are employed in the extraction process to achieve higher yields of purified finished products while minimizing energy usage [11]. The chemical structure of inulin is illustrated in Fig. (**3**).

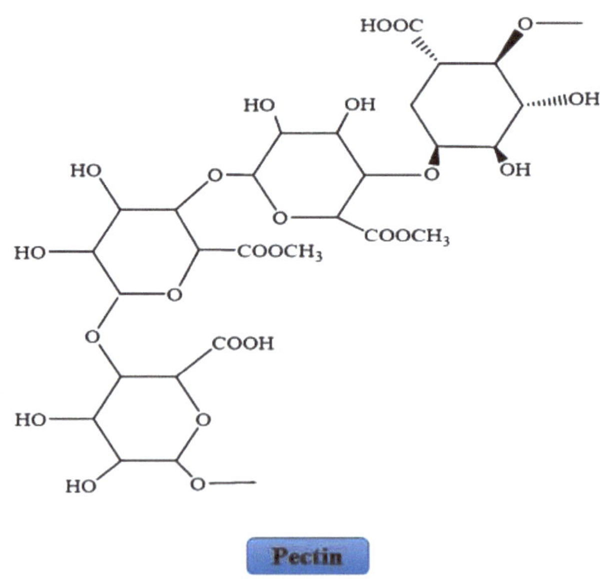

Fig. (2). Chemical structure of pectin.

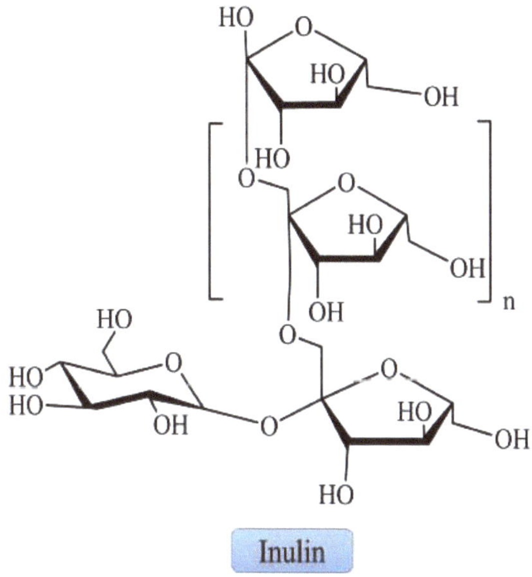

Fig. (3). Chemical structure of Inulin.

Cyclodextrin

The first documented description of cyclodextrins was published in 1891 by the French scientist A. Villiers, who extracted a crystalline compound produced during the bacterial digestion of starch. Austrian scientist Franz Schardinger investigated several microorganisms responsible for food degradation, particularly in starch, and identified two crystalline substances, A and B, in potato starch. These compounds were subsequently designated as Schardinger's cyclodextrins in his tribute. Three principals natural cyclodextrins were identified and described during the discovery phase. They were identified as oligosaccharides; nonetheless, their molecular weight and precise chemical structure remained undetermined. Advancements in analytical instruments and biotechnology resulted in the development of cyclodextrins, which are utilized in medicinal formulations. The evolution of cyclodextrins has been influenced by progress in analytical instruments and biotechnology [12, 13]. Cyclodextrins are a kind of starch generated by enzymatic treatment of starch with amylase derived from *Bacillus macerans*. The combination is challenging to purify, and it often contains additional linear and branched dextrins, proteins, and contaminants. Biotechnological advancements in the 1970s resulted in significant enhancements in production, with genetic engineering increasing the activity and specificity of several cyclomaltodextrin glucanotransferases for the synthesis of cyclodextrin. These enzymes and technical advancements facilitated the availability of highly pure cyclodextrin for use as medicinal excipients. The water solubility of cyclodextrin is significantly lower than that of linear dextrins due to robust binding and intramolecular hydrogen bonding [14]. The chemical structure of cyclodextrin is illustrated in Fig. (**4**).

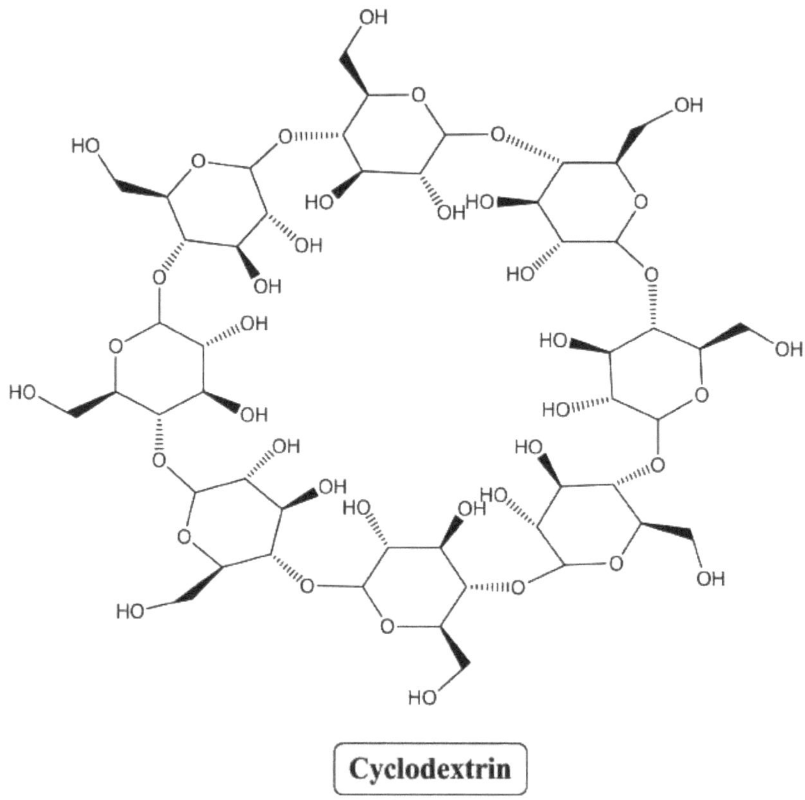

Fig. (4). Chemical structure of cyclodextrin.

Guar Gum

Guar gum is a naturally occurring water-soluble polysaccharide composed of mannose backbones and galactose side chains. Its unique structure and -OH functional groups are responsible for hydrophilicity and high solubility. Guar gum is also used as a dispersant for organic systems and a coagulant for inorganic ones, especially in clay-characterized systems [15]. Guar gum is safe for oral administration, making it suitable for drug delivery applications. Its mucoadhesive properties make it a suitable material for wound healing applications. Guar gum's high hydrophilic nature leads to invasion swelling, making it suitable for disintegrating agents and binding in hydrophilic matrix systems for prolonged release and controlled drug delivery. Due to its versatility, guar gum is widely used in various forms for targeted drug delivery, offering protection from degradation, prolonging pharmacological action, and improving therapeutic effects [16]. The chemical structure of guar gum is illustrated in Fig. (**5**).

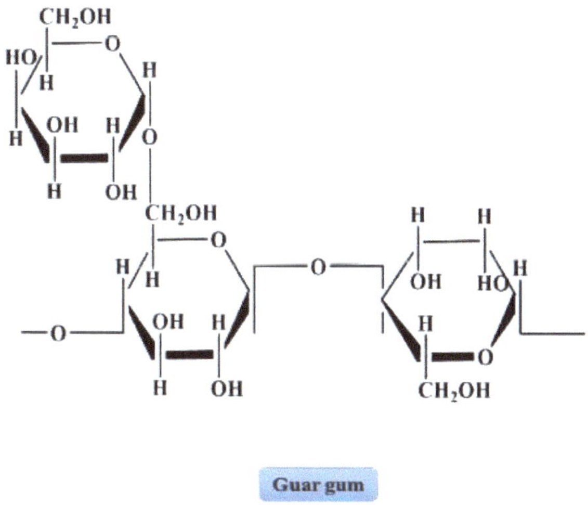

Fig. (5). Chemical structure of guar gum.

Cellulose

Cellulose, a naturally occurring biopolymer, is extensively utilized in many applications owing to its advantages for the green economy. It consists of elongated chains of Anhydro-D-Glucopyranose Units (AGU) covalently linked between the equatorial groups of the C_1 and C_4 carbon atoms. The chemical structure of cellulose has three hydroxyl groups per AGU unit, which engage in intra- and intermolecular hydrogen bonding to create a supramolecular polymer with crystalline domains. Nevertheless, cellulose possesses intrinsic limitations, including inadequate crease resistance, undesirable solubility in solvent media, and an absence of thermoplasticity. Surface functionalization enhances cellulose characteristics by incorporating foreign groups into cellulose molecules [17]. Cellulose can be converted into several derivatives through processes including etherification, esterification, depolymerization, and radical grafting. These compounds are appropriate for the administration of human and veterinary medications owing to their distinctive characteristics, including increased water-retention capacity and biocompatibility [18]. The chemical structure of cellulose is illustrated in Fig. (**6**).

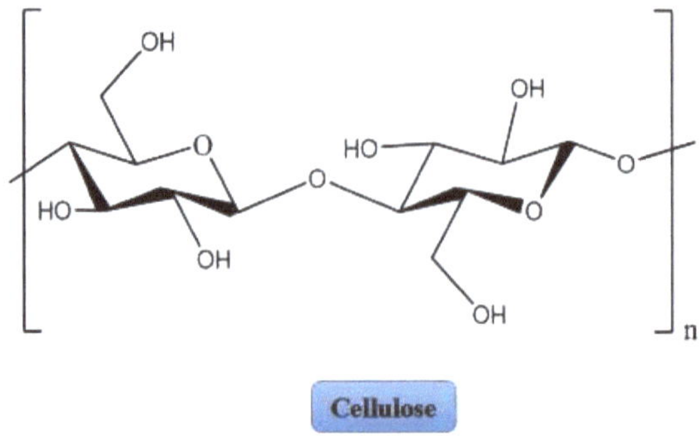

Fig. (6). Chemical structure of cellulose.

Carrageenan

Carrageenan is a group of sulfated polysaccharides found in the cell walls of red seaweed. It serves as a thickening agent, emulsifier, and stabilizer, devoid of nutritional value. It is used as a food additive in processed foods, pet foods, cosmetics, textiles, and the pharmaceutical sector [19]. Carrageenan can be categorized by molecular mass, degree of sulfation, and the position and distribution of the sulfate group. The principal varieties of carrageenan are ι (iota), κ (kappa), and lambda, which vary based on the frequency of unit sulfation (1, 2, or 3 sulfate groups). Carrageenan is included in several processed foods, such as ice cream, soymilk, meats, and nutritional supplements. Carrageenan enhances yield in processed chicken, ham, and red meat products by retaining water and binding meat fluids to minimize loss. It is utilized as a browning inhibitor for the regulation of fresh fruit processing [20]. The chemical structure of carrageenan is illustrated in Fig. (7).

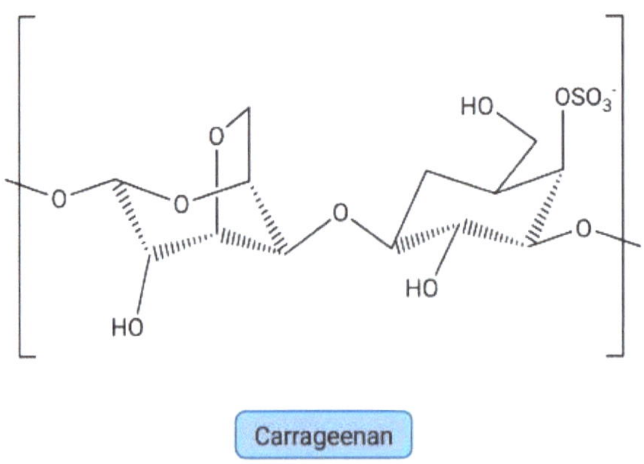

Fig. (7). Chemical structure of carrageenan.

Alginate

The Alginate (AG) polymer has benefits such as biodegradability, low toxicity, chemical versatility, cross-linking ability, and pH sensitivity. They are the favoured polymer substrate for drug delivery researchers because of their intrinsic modifiability. AG is a linear anionic polysaccharide composed of alpha-1,4-L-Gulonuronic Acid (G) and beta-1,4-D-Mannuronic Acid (M) segments. The configuration and extent of polymerization of AG are contingent upon the ratio of M residues to G residues. The mechanical characteristics of AG gel can be enhanced by augmenting the length and molecular weight of G-blocks. AG is derived from the cell walls of brown algae or bacterial sources, and its production can yield a more precise chemical structure and physical characteristics. Recent advancements in bacterial biosynthesis and modification may enable tailored properties and applications in the biomedical sector [21, 22]. Summary of the source and pharmaceutical applications of various plant-based polymers is elaborated in Table **1**. The chemical structure of AG is illustrated in Fig. (**8**).

Table 1. Summary of the source and pharmaceutical applications of various plant-based polymers.

S. No.	Plant-based Polymer	Source	Pharmaceutical Applications	References
1.	Pectin [23]	Citrus fruits like oranges, lemons, grapefruit, and apples.	Drug delivery, wound healing, cholesterol reduction, tissue engineering, contact lenses, artificial corneas, and anticancer activities.	Freitas *et al.* (2021)
2.	Inulin [24]	Asparagus, Jerusalem artichoke, agave, wheat, onion, bananas, garlic, and chicory.	Aids weight loss, improves food composition, regulates the GI tract, has antidiabetic activity, promotes prebiotics and beneficial bacteria while preventing constipation, diarrhea, and colon cancer.	Du *et al.* (2023)
3.	Cyclodextrin [25]	Potatoes, corn, cassava starches, and maize.	Used as solubilizers, mask unpleasant tastes, reduce tissue irritation, convert liquid drugs to solids, and achieve controlled drug release.	Jacob *et al.* (2018)
4.	Guar Gum [26]	From the seeds of the Cyamopsis tetragonoloba plant	Its gel-forming nature can lower cholesterol and glucose levels, and its resistance to cholera- and diarrhea-causing pathogens makes it effective in relieving chronic functional bowel diseases, *etc.*	George *et al.*, (2018)
5.	Cellulose [27]	Cell walls of wood and plants	It has inherent characteristics that can be tailored for tissue engineering, drug delivery, and wound dressing systems.	Seddiqi *et al.* (2021)

(Table 1) cont.....

S. No.	Plant-based Polymer	Source	Pharmaceutical Applications	References
6.	Carrageenan [19]	From red edible seaweeds (marine plant)	Hydrogel-forming ability, has shown good bioactive properties for controlling viral infections, bacterial infections, and pathophysiological processes despite their safety, effectiveness, and biocompatibility.	Quito *et al.* (2020)
7.	Alginate [28]	Brown seaweed (also called kelp), also produced by certain bacteria.	Gel-forming capabilities, moist healing environment, and functions as a carrier for drugs or cells during targeted delivery processes, reinforcing agent during tissue regeneration and providing a suitable cell microenvironment, scaffolding capabilities, *etc.*	Raus *et al.* (2021)

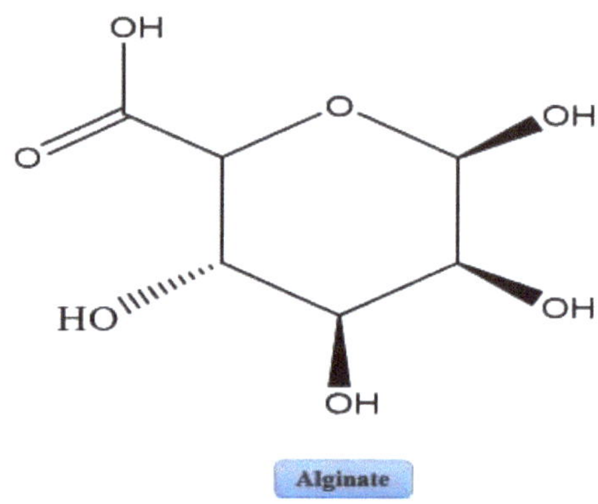

Fig. (8). Chemical structure of alginate.

ROLE OF PLANT-DERIVED POLYMERS IN THE MANAGEMENT OF IBD

Pectin in IBD

Pectin, a dietary fibre with a unique structure, can affect the GI immune barrier by directly linking with immune cells or affecting the intestinal microbiota. Their effects involve deepening the mucus layer, strengthening epithelial integrity, and activating dendritic cell and macrophage reactions. Pectins can stimulate the beneficial microbiome and enhance the GI immune barrier through short-chain fatty acids. Further human studies are needed to understand pectin's potential role in managing and preventing inflammatory conditions [29]. Almagro *et al.* (2023) evaluated the structural properties and activity of sunflower pectin, suggesting its potential as a preventive treatment for IBD. *In vivo* experiments demonstrated that ultrasonic extraction produced the most efficacious pectin, exhibiting increased viscosity that conferred superior protection against IBD. The research further identified a reduction in intestinal permeability and reduced production of pro-inflammatory cytokines and chemokines associated with tissue injury [30]. Dang *et al.* (2023), in their study, found that pectin enhances gut health in pigs by facilitating tryptophan metabolism. It reduced Actinobacteria, increased Proteobacteria, and decreased *Streptococcus*. Pectin also enhanced the proliferation of indole-derivative-producing bacteria, hence fostering gut health. It also elevated levels of AhR, IL-22, and p-Stat3, which are involved in the synthesis of antimicrobial compounds. This indicates that dietary pectin supplementation may enhance gut integrity and immune function [31].

Inulin in IBD

Inulin is a potential nutraceutical for the treatment of GI illnesses, particularly IBD, owing to its convenience, cost-effectiveness, and low toxicity. It can serve as a dietary supplement to preserve health and regulate issues. Inulin's prebiotic effects diminish mucosal inflammation in IBD and inhibit the proliferation of endogenous bacteria while obstructing adhesion and invasion. This prebiotic strategy is advantageous for vulnerable patients and individuals with chronic GI conditions [32]. Soltani *et al.* (2023) developed an enhanced single-layer coating technique for budesonide (BUD) pellets utilizing inulin and eudragit RS. The formulation, comprising 9% inulin and 91% eudragit RS, inhibited premature drug release in the stomach and enabled regulated drug release along the intestine. The coated pellets demonstrated enhanced therapeutic efficacy in the treatment of colitis compared with untreated pellets, indicating that the coating technology successfully protected the drug [33].

Niu *et al.* (2024) found that in a colitis animal model, inulin has been shown to reduce symptoms by changing the gut microbiota profile, specifically the abundance of *Blautia* and *Faecalibacterium*. The study investigated the impact of inulin and its combination with two probiotics on colitis in a Dextran Sulfate Sodium (DSS)- induced mouse model. According to the results, inulin can enhance the intestinal barrier, alter the relative abundance of *Blautia* and *Faecalibacterium*, and modulate pro- and anti-inflammatory cytokines. All of these results point to inulin as a possible functional food therapy strategy for the treatment of colitis [34].

Cyclodextrin (CDs) in IBD

CDs are employed to enhance current therapies, increasing their efficacy, stability, and safety. They serve as multifunctional excipients, improving solubility, mitigating drug-drug and drug-additive interactions, masking undesirable odours and flavours, and diminishing adverse effects. They are available in several pharmaceutical formulations and can be utilized to develop sophisticated drug delivery systems. CDs are optimal for the formation of anti-inflammatory pharmaceuticals and bioactive substances, and can complex larger molecules such as proteins [35]. Lazaro *et al.* (2020) developed new formulations of BUD-CD inclusion complexes in poloxamer-based hydrogels to reduce colonic inflammation in rats. *In vivo* results showed these formulations significantly reduced inflammation compared to conventional drugs. The self-assembled micelle-micelle network in the gel structure acts as a drug reservoir, allowing slow and prolonged release of BUD after rectal administration. The best formulation, BUD 2: BUD Hydroxypropyl (HP) β-CDs + Poloxamer (PL) 407 (20%), demonstrated safety and effectiveness [36]. Akkari *et al.* (2016) purposed to enhance the physicochemical features of BUD *via* complexation with HP-cyclodextrin and incorporation of its inclusion complex into PL-based hydrogels. The objective is to create self-assembled stimuli-responsive structures. The physicochemical properties of the integartion of BUD-Hydroxypropyl (HP)--CDs into PL407 or PL407-PL403 systems were examined. The findings indicated that complexation with HP-CDs enhanced the solubility of BUD in simulated colon juices. CDs can form complexes with therapeutic molecules, resulting in enhanced water solubility and a competitive mechanism between PL and the drug for complexation within the hydrophobic cavity of the CDs. The research indicated that the rivalry between the medication and PL for the HP-CDs cavity did not affect the interaction between BUD and PL [37].

Guar gum in IBD

Guar gum, a multifaceted substance characterized by biocompatibility, biodegradability, low toxicity, and immunological properties, has been extensively utilized in biomedical applications owing to its adaptability. It has undergone modification by esterification, carboxymethylation, grafting, etherification, and cross-linking to develop drug delivery systems such as hydrogels, nanoparticles, nanocomposites, and scaffolds. The binding, stabilizing, gelling, mucoadhesive, and enzymatic degrading characteristics of guar gum render it appropriate for oral, buccal, transdermal, intravenous, and gene delivery applications [16]. Jhundoo *et al.* (2021) revealed that acacia and guar gum exhibit considerable anti-inflammatory properties in a mouse model of experimental colitis. Acacia demonstrated a more pronounced impact at a dosage of 300mg/kg, but guar gum exhibited greater viscosity. Both polysaccharides influence the digestion process in the large intestine, resulting in the generation of volatile fatty acids. The results may facilitate the development of customized formulations for oral or rectal delivery, utilizing acacia as a stabilizer, emulsifier, and tablet binder and guar gum as an anti-inflammatory excipient in gel form [38]. Sharma *et al.* (2018) investigated colon-targeted embelin-loaded microparticles both *in vitro* and *in vivo* to elucidate their GI behavior. Microparticles infused with embelin, derived from plant extracts, have anti-inflammatory and antioxidant characteristics. The average particle size in F4 is 14.7 ± 0.9 mm, and *in vitro*, regulated drug release is facilitated by guar gum. Embelin inhibits dinitrobenzene sulfonic acid-induced colitis *in vivo* [39].

Cellulose in IBD

Cellulose, an insoluble fibre found in plant tissues, has a proliferative effect on the colon, mainly in rodent models. Although it can be fermented, its secondary production of short-chain fatty acids is limited. Despite this, cellulose has been shown to significantly modify colonic microbial composition, making it a potential prebiotic [40]. Jagdale *et al.* (2017) developed and optimized a colon-targeted drug delivery using Chitosan (CS) and cellulose acetate phthalate, aiming to avoid first-pass metabolism and treat colon diseases. The optimized batch, F8, was found to have a significant impact on drug release, with the swelling index playing a crucial role. The formulation's swelling property, influenced by CS and cellulose acetate phthalate, could be a potential treatment for colon diseases [41]. The study by Li *et al.* (2022) reported the anti-inflammatory effects of high-substituted Hydroxypropyl Cellulose (HHPC) and low-substituted Hydroxypropyl Cellulose (LHPC) on dextran sodium sulfate-induced colitis in mice. Results showed that HHPC inhibited excessive TNF-α and IL-6 secretion, mitigated colon tissue damage, suppressed spleen edema, preserved thymus index, reduced inflammatory mediators, increased sIgA secretion, and restored intestinal flora balance [42].

Carrageenan in IBD

Carrageenan, a prevalent food ingredient in the Western diet, may provoke intestinal inflammation, either as a result of gastric digestion or interaction with intestinal bacterial flora. Research indicates that decreasing dietary carrageenan can alleviate GI problems. The carrageenan-activated cascade encompasses reactive oxygen species and the innate immune system, including toll-like receptors and B-cell leukemia/lymphoma. The rising incidence of IBD in recent years is associated with heightened use of carrageenan [43]. Various diets, including the Specific Carbohydrate Diet and the Mediterranean diet, may assist in managing chronic IBD by eliminating dairy products and processed foods [44]. Stavarache *et al.* (2021) developed a novel hydrogel particle, coated with CS-sodium Tripolyphosphate (TPP)- k-Carrageenan (kCG), by utilizing ionic gelation and TPP as a crosslinking agent. The particles were analyzed by FT-IR spectrometry and dynamic light scattering, demonstrating the drug's incorporation and interactions. The hydrogel beads exhibited a more refined texture than core-shell beads coated with kCG, signifying the presence of the protective polymer.

The biocompatibility assessment demonstrated favourable viability for CCD 841 CoN cells, accompanied by a modest enhancement in cell growth. The maximum mesalamine encapsulation reached around 40% for beads with a CS/TPP weight ratio of 1:5. The drug-encapsulated CS-TPP-kCG particles represent a viable option for regulated drug delivery systems [45]. Wu *et al.* (2017) examined the capacity of k-carrageenan to improve the inflammatory response in human colonic cells utilizing a *Citrobacter freundii* DBS100-induced intestinal inflammation model. Results indicate that k-carrageenan synergizes with lipopolysaccharide to elicit a heightened inflammatory response, with elevated levels seen in HT-29 cells. The research evaluated the activation of the inflammatory pathway in HT-29 cells. Nonetheless, elevated dosages of k-carrageenan alone induce only a marginal increase. The research indicated that α-carrageenan elevates proinflammatory cytokines TNF, Interleukin (IL)-8, and IL-6 in mice subjected to *Citrobacter freundii* DBS100, implying humoral immune tolerance. The research indicates that α-carrageenan functions as a possible inflammatory agent that exacerbates pre-existing intestinal inflammation [46].

Alginate in IBD

Alginate is a linear, anionic polysaccharide obtained from brown seaweed, recognized for its biodegradability, low toxicity, and chemical flexibility. It produces stable gels in aqueous environments and is applicable for drug delivery and cell immobilization. The alginate matrix can be synthesized *via* physical or chemical crosslinking, with ionic crosslinking forming a three-dimensional network. The predominant cation is Ca^{2+}, which is readily absorbed by humans owing to its role in the skeletal system and physiological processes. Additional crosslinking agents include hydrogen bonds, electrostatic interactions, covalent bonds, and stereocomplexation. Covalent crosslinking yields more robust and stable networks *via* bifunctional crosslinkers such as glutaraldehyde or epichlorohydrin, amide bond production *via* water-soluble carbodiimide chemistry, and photo-crosslinking. This chemical junction is linked to chronic exposure to hazardous chemicals that may be physiologically harmful to humans [47]. Qiu *et al.* (2023) investigated the application of alginate in drug products, particularly emphasizing nanoscale dimensions to enhance drug loading efficacy and facilitate degradation by gut microbes. Dietary fibres, indigestible in the human small intestine, consist of neutral sugars and β-glucan, which exhibit physiological action in the body. The research suggests a codelivery approach utilizing an anti-IL-1β monoclonal antibody and bovine serum albumin as a linker to covalently attach mesalamine to the Nanoscale Dietary Fibres (NDF). Microspheres composed of alginate were developed to encapsulate NDF-Pro/mesalamine and probiotics, ensuring protection from acidic and enzymatic conditions in the stomach and facilitating targeted delivery of mesalamine to the intestinal mucosa. The technique may result in an increased and more consistent drug usage rate [48]. Sun *et al.* (2022) aimed to develop mucus-penetrating AG-CS-NPs for oral delivery of Berberine Hydrochloride (BH) to the site of colonic ulcer lesions. The NPs, with a particle size of 257 nm and a negative charge, showed high mucus-penetrating ability. An *ex vivo* retention study showed high retention of BH-AG-CS NPs at the colon site for over 16 hours. *In vivo* therapeutic effectiveness showed that the NPs could alleviate colonic injury and improve immunologic function [49].

The advantages and limitations of plant-based polymer is illustrated in Table **2**.

Table 2. The advantages and limitations of plant-based polymers.

S. No.	Polymer	Advantages	Limitation
1.	Pectin [50]	Pectin, a soluble fiber, aids digestion, lowers cholesterol, acts as a prebiotic, and is used in the food industry as a gelling agent. It also has potential health benefits, including anticancer properties and potential use in targeted drug and gene delivery.	Pectin supplements may cause gas, bloating, or upset stomach, reduce mineral absorption, and interact with certain drugs. Pectin has limited nutritional value and may cause side effects, medication interactions, and allergic reactions.
2.	Inulin [33]	Inulin is a prebiotic fiber that supports gut health by feeding beneficial gut bacteria, improving bowel regularity, aiding blood sugar control, aiding weight management, reducing inflammation, and enhancing mineral absorption.	Gastrointestinal side effects and variable metabolic effects.
3.	Cyclodextrin [51]	Cyclodextrins enhance drug solubility, bioavailability, stability, and control drug release.	It has potential toxicity, rapid clearance, drug displacement, limited administration routes, and destabilizing effects.
4.	Guar gum [52]	Guar gum is a versatile, cost-effective thickening agent. It aids digestive health, supports weight management, manages blood sugar, and lowers cholesterol.	It can cause digestive discomfort, interfere with drugs, and cause health risks.
5.	Cellulose [17]	Cellulose is a renewable and biodegradable natural polymer. It is well-tolerated by the body, making it suitable for biomedical applications like tissue engineering and drug delivery systems.	It has limitations such as insolubility in water and organic solvents, difficulty in melting, limited antimicrobial properties, and processing challenges, which may require chemical modification.

(Table 2) cont.....

S. No.	Polymer	Advantages	Limitation
6.	Carrageenan [53]	Carrageenan can be used as a fat substitute in dairy and meat products due to its hydrophilic nature. Its antiviral effects, cholesterol-lowering properties, anticancer effects, and biocompatibility make it a sustainable, eco-friendly alternative.	Health concerns, such as inflammation and gastrointestinal issues, need further research.
7.	Alginate [21]	Alginate is an affordable, easy-to-use, and biocompatible material suitable for dental impressions. Its setting time can be adjusted for flexibility and is comfortable for patients.	It has limitations such as poor stability, low mechanical strength, and a one-time use nature. It may not reproduce fine details as accurately as other materials and may be messy during mixing and handling.

In summary, we can say that plant-derived polymers play various roles in the management of IBD. The specific role of polymers in the management of IBD is mentioned in Table **3**.

Table 3. Specific role of plant-based polymers in the management of IBD.

S. No.	Plant-derived Polymers	Specific Role in IBD	References
1.	Pectin	Modulates the production of Short-chain Fatty Acids (SCFAs); reduces inflammation; strengthens the intestinal barrier; promotes beneficial gut bacteria, *etc.*	[54, 55]
2.	Inulin	Increases the expression of MUC2 in intestinal epithelial cells (reduces inflammation); increases SCFAs in caecal content, enhances growth of indigenous lactobacilli, *etc.*	[56, 57]
3.	Cyclodextrin	Reduces irritation; modulates the effect of TNF-α inhibitors; promotes gut microbiota balance, *etc.*	[58, 59]
4.	Guar gum	Provides relief from constipation and diarrhoea, softens stool; reduces ulceration; enriches actinobacteria, *etc.*	[60, 61]
5.	Cellulose	Refulates gut health; interacts with the intestinal lining; reduces intestinal permeability; suppresses the activation of immune cells like T-cells and macrophages; restores gut microbiota balance, *etc.*	[62, 63]
6.	Carrageenan	Reduces the release of pro-inflammatory cytokines like TNF-alpha, IL-6, and IL-1β; reduces permeability; improves gut mucosal integrity; suppresses inflammatory responses, *etc.*	[64, 65]
7.	Alginate	Reduces acid reflux; reduces the activation of inflammatory pathways in the gut; contributes to the production of SCFAs; functions as a protective barrier on the mucosal surface, *etc.*	[66, 67]

CONCLUSION

IBD is an escalating disorder in Europe and North America, requiring novel treatment approaches. Plant-derived polymers, including pectin, inulin, cyclodextrin, guar gum, cellulose, carrageenan, and alginate, have shown to be effective in the management of IBD, owing to their anti-inflammatory, immunomodulatory, and prebiotic characteristics. These polymers can regulate the gut microbiota, strengthen the immunological barrier, and function as effective drug carriers with controlled-release properties. They can augment intestinal integrity, diminish inflammation, promote medication solubility and stability, and facilitate targeted drug delivery and tissue protection. These polymers provide a versatile platform for developing novel treatment approaches, reducing adverse effects and improving therapeutic outcomes. Additional clinical research is required to enhance their applicability and comprehensively elucidate their processes.

REFERENCES

[1] Ashton JJ, Beattie RM. Inflammatory bowel disease: recent developments. Archives of Disease in Childhood 2024; (5): 370-6.
[http://dx.doi.org/10.1136/archdischild-2023-325668]

[2] Stojanov S, Berlec A. Smart bionanomaterials for treatment and diagnosis of inflammatory bowel disease. Nanotechnology Reviews 2024; (1):
[http://dx.doi.org/10.1515/ntrev-2024-0057]

[3] Yeshi K, Jamtsho T, Wangchuk P. Current treatments, emerging therapeutics, and natural remedies for inflammatory bowel disease. Molecules 2024; (16):
[http://dx.doi.org/10.3390/molecules29163954]

[4] Yang W, Zhao P, Li X, Guo L, Gao W. The potential roles of natural plant polysaccharides in inflammatory bowel disease: A review. Carbohydrate Polymers 2022.
[http://dx.doi.org/10.1016/j.carbpol.2021.118821]

[5] Wang X, Li X, Zhang L, *et al.* Recent progress in plant-derived polysaccharides with prebiotic potential for intestinal health by targeting gut microbiota: a review. Critical Reviews in Food Science and Nutrition 2024; (33): 12242-71.
[http://dx.doi.org/10.1080/10408398.2023.2248631]

[6] Li Q, Li L, Li Q, Wang J, Nie S, Xie M. Influence of natural polysaccharides on intestinal microbiota in inflammatory bowel diseases: An overview. Foods 2022; (8):
[http://dx.doi.org/10.3390/foods11081084]

[7] Martin B. The effects of different dietary fiber pectin structures on the gastrointestinal immune barrier: impact *via* gut microbiota and direct effects on immune cells. Experimental and Molecular Medicine 2020; 1-3.
[http://dx.doi.org/10.1038/s12276-020-0449-2]

[8] Fernandez ML. Pectin. Handbook of Dietary Fiber 2001; 566-84.
[http://dx.doi.org/10.1201/9780203904220.ch30]

[9] Shoaib M, Shehzad A, Omar M, *et al.* Inulin: Properties, health benefits and food applications. Carbohydrate Polymers 2016; 444-54.
[http://dx.doi.org/10.1016/j.carbpol.2016.04.020]

[10] Akram W, Garud N, Joshi R. Role of inulin as prebiotics on inflammatory bowel disease. Drug discoveries & therapeutics. 2019; pp. 1-8.
[http://dx.doi.org/10.5582/ddt.2019.01000]

[11] Du Y, Kusama K, Hama K, *et al.* Protective effects of inulin on stress-recurrent inflammatory bowel disease. International Journal of Molecular Sciences 2024; (5):
[http://dx.doi.org/10.3390/ijms25052494]

[12] Loftsson T, Duchene D. Cyclodextrins and their pharmaceutical applications. International Journal of Pharmaceutics 2007; (1-2): 1-11.
[http://dx.doi.org/10.1016/j.ijpharm.2006.10.044]

[13] Jambhekar SS, Breen P. Cyclodextrins in pharmaceutical formulations I: structure and physicochemical properties, formation of complexes, and types of complex. Drug Discovery Today 2016; (2): 356-62.
[http://dx.doi.org/10.1016/j.drudis.2015.11.017]

[14] Poulson BG, Alsulami QA, Sharfalddin A, *et al.* Cyclodextrins: Structural, chemical, and physical properties, and applications. Polysaccharides 2021; (1): 1-31.
[http://dx.doi.org/10.3390/polysaccharides3010001]

[15] Ellis PR, Wang Q, Rayment P, Ren Y, Sb R. Guar gum: agricultural and botanical aspects, physicochemical and nutritional properties, and its use in the development of functional foods. Handbook of dietary fiber. 2001; pp. 613-57.

[16] Verma D, Sharma SK. Recent advances in guar gum-based drug delivery systems and their administrative routes. International Journal of Biological Macromolecules 2021; 653-71.
[http://dx.doi.org/10.1016/j.ijbiomac.2021.03.087]

[17] Mcmullen RL, Ozkan S, Gillece T. Physicochemical properties of cellulose ethers. Cosmetics 2022; (3):
[http://dx.doi.org/10.3390/cosmetics9030052]

[18] Heinze T. Cellulose: structure and properties. Advances in Polymer Science 2015; 1-52.
[http://dx.doi.org/10.1007/12_2015_319]

[19] Pacheco-Quito E, Ruiz-Caro R, Veiga M. Carrageenan: Drug delivery systems and other biomedical applications. Marine Drugs 2020; (11):
[http://dx.doi.org/10.3390/md18110583]

[20] Liu J, Zhan X, Wan J, Wang Y, Wang C. Review for carrageenan-based pharmaceutical biomaterials: Favourable physical features versus adverse biological effects. Carbohydrate Polymers 2015; 27-36.
[http://dx.doi.org/10.1016/j.carbpol.2014.11.063]

[21] Draget KI, Taylor C. Chemical, physical and biological properties of alginates and their biomedical implications. Food Hydrocolloids 2011; 251-6.
[http://dx.doi.org/10.1016/j.foodhyd.2009.10.007]

[22] Agüero L, Zaldivar-Silva D, Peña L, Dias ML. Alginate microparticles as oral colon drug delivery device: A review. Carbohydrate Polymers 2017; 32-43.
[http://dx.doi.org/10.1016/j.carbpol.2017.03.033]

[23] Freitas CMP, Coimbra JSR, Souza VGL, Sousa RCS. Structure and applications of pectin in food, biomedical, and pharmaceutical industry: A review. Coatings 2021; (8):
[http://dx.doi.org/10.3390/coatings11080922]

[24] Du M, Cheng X, Qian L, Huo A, Chen J, Sun Y. Extraction, physicochemical properties, functional activities and applications of inulin polysaccharide: a review. Plant Foods for Human Nutrition 2023; (2): 243-52.
[http://dx.doi.org/10.1007/s11130-023-01066-6]

[25] Jacob S, Nair AB. Cyclodextrin complexes: Perspective from drug delivery and formulation. Drug

Development Research. 2018; pp. 201-17.
[http://dx.doi.org/10.1002/ddr.21452]

[26] George A, Shah PA, Shrivastav PS. Guar gum: Versatile natural polymer for drug delivery applications. European Polymer Journal 2019; 722-35.
[http://dx.doi.org/10.1016/j.eurpolymj.2018.10.042]

[27] Seddiqi H, Oliaei E, Honarkar H, *et al.* Cellulose and its derivatives: towards biomedical applications. Cellulose 2021; (4): 1893-931.
[http://dx.doi.org/10.1007/s10570-020-03674-w]

[28] Raus RA, Nawawi WM, Nasaruddin RR. Alginate and alginate composites for biomedical applications. Asian Journal of Pharmaceutical Sciences 2021; (3): 280-306.
[http://dx.doi.org/10.1016/j.ajps.2020.10.001]

[29] Chung WSF, Meijerink M, Zeuner B, *et al.* Prebiotic potential of pectin and pectic oligosaccharides to promote anti-inflammatory commensal bacteria in the human colon. FEMS Microbiology Ecology 2017; (11):
[http://dx.doi.org/10.1093/femsec/fix127]

[30] Muñoz-Almagro N, Molina-Tijeras JA, Montilla A, *et al.* Pectin from sunflower by-products obtained by ultrasound: Chemical characterization and *in vivo* evaluation of properties in inflammatory bowel disease. International Journal of Biological Macromolecules 2023.
[http://dx.doi.org/10.1016/j.ijbiomac.2023.125505]

[31] Dang G, Wen X, Zhong R, *et al.* Pectin modulates intestinal immunity in a pig model *via* regulating the gut microbiota-derived tryptophan metabolite-AhR-IL22 pathway. Journal of Animal Science and Biotechnology 2023; (1):
[http://dx.doi.org/10.1186/s40104-023-00838-z]

[32] Afinjuomo F, Abdella S, Youssef SH, Song Y, Garg S. Inulin and its application in drug delivery. Pharmaceuticals 2021; (9):
[http://dx.doi.org/10.3390/ph14090855]

[33] Soltani F, Kamali H, Akhgari A, *et al.* Combination of time-dependent polymer and inulin as a coating for sustained delivery of budesonide pellets aimed for use in IBD treatment. Journal of Drug Delivery Science and Technology 2023.
[http://dx.doi.org/10.1016/j.jddst.2023.104927]

[34] Niu B, Li F, Lv X, *et al.* Unveiling the therapeutic potential and mechanism of inulin in DSS-induced colitis mice. International Journal of Biological Macromolecules 2024.
[http://dx.doi.org/10.1016/j.ijbiomac.2024.135861]

[35] Appleton L, Navarro-Orcajada S, Martinez-Navarro S, *et al.* Cyclodextrins as antiinflammatory agents: basis, drugs and perspectives. Biomolecules 2021; (9):
[http://dx.doi.org/10.3390/biom11091384]

[36] Lázaro CM, De Oliveira CC, Gambero A, *et al.* Evaluation of budesonide–hydroxypropyl--cyclodextrin inclusion complex in thermoreversible gels for ulcerative colitis. Digestive Diseases and Sciences 2020; (11): 3297-304.
[http://dx.doi.org/10.1007/s10620-020-06075-y]

[37] Akkari AC, Campos EV, Keppler AF, *et al.* Budesonide-hydroxypropyl-β-cyclodextrin inclusion complex in binary poloxamer 407/403 system for ulcerative colitis treatment: A physico-chemical study from micelles to hydrogels. Colloids and Surfaces B: Biointerfaces 2016; 138-47.
[http://dx.doi.org/10.1016/j.colsurfb.2015.11.048]

[38] Jhundoo HD, Siefen T, Liang A, *et al.* Anti-inflammatory effects of acacia and guar gum in 5-amino salicylic acid formulations in experimental colitis. International Journal of Pharmaceutics: X 2021.
[http://dx.doi.org/10.1016/j.ijpx.2021.100080]

[39] Sharma A, Kaur N, Sharma S, *et al.* Embelin-loaded guar gum microparticles for the management of

ulcerative colitis. Journal of microencapsulation 2018; (2): 181-91.
[http://dx.doi.org/10.1080/02652048.2018.1452991]

[40] Lavanya DK, Kulkarni PK, Dixit M, Raavi PK, Krishna LN. Sources of cellulose and their applications-A review. International Journal of Drug Formulation and Research 2011; (6): 19-38.

[41] Jagdale S, Chandekar A. Optimization of chitosan and cellulose acetate phthalate controlled delivery of methylprednisolone for treatment of inflammatory bowel disease. Maad Rayan Publishing Company 2017; (2): 203-13.
[http://dx.doi.org/10.15171/apb.2017.025]

[42] Li X, Lv H, Shi F, Song J, Zhang Z. The potential therapeutic effects of hydroxypropyl cellulose on acute murine colitis induced by DSS. Carbohydrate Polymers 2022.
[http://dx.doi.org/10.1016/j.carbpol.2022.119430]

[43] Komisarska P, Pinyosinwat A, Saleem M, Szczuko M. Carrageenan as a potential factor of inflammatory bowel diseases. Nutrients 2024; (9):
[http://dx.doi.org/10.3390/nu16091367]

[44] Borsani B, De Santis R, Perico V, *et al.* The role of carrageenan in inflammatory bowel diseases and allergic reactions: Where do we stand?. Nutrients 2021; (10):
[http://dx.doi.org/10.3390/nu13103402]

[45] Stavarache CE, Ghebaur A, Dinescu S, *et al.* 5-aminosalicylic acid loaded chitosan-carrageenan hydrogel beads with potential application for the treatment of inflammatory bowel disease. Polymers 2021; (15):
[http://dx.doi.org/10.3390/polym13152463]

[46] Wu W, Zhen Z, Niu T, *et al.* Carrageenan enhances lipopolysaccharide-induced interleukin-8 secretion by stimulating the Bcl10-NF-B pathway in HT-29 cells and aggravates freundii induced inflammation in mice. Mediators of Inflammation 2017; (1): 1-16.
[http://dx.doi.org/10.1155/2017/8634865]

[47] Hecht H, Srebnik S. Structural characterization of sodium alginate and calcium alginate. Biomacromolecules 2016; (6): 2160-7.
[http://dx.doi.org/10.1021/acs.biomac.6b00378]

[48] Qiu L, Shen R, Wei L, *et al.* Designing a microbial fermentation-functionalized alginate microsphere for targeted release of 5-ASA using nano dietary fiber carrier for inflammatory bowel disease treatment. Journal of Nanobiotechnology 2023; (1):
[http://dx.doi.org/10.1186/s12951-023-02097-6]

[49] Sun L, Nie X, Lu W, *et al.* Mucus-penetrating alginate-chitosan nanoparticles loaded with berberine hydrochloride for oral delivery to the inflammation site of ulcerative colitis. AAPS PharmSciTech 2022; (6):
[http://dx.doi.org/10.1208/s12249-022-02327-4]

[50] Xiang T, Yang R, Li L, Lin H, Kai G. Research progress and application of pectin: A review. Journal of Food Science 2024; (11): 6985-7007.
[http://dx.doi.org/10.1111/1750-3841.17438]

[51] Tian B, Liu J. The classification and application of cyclodextrin polymers: a review. New Journal of Chemistry 2020; (22): 9137-48.
[http://dx.doi.org/10.1039/c9nj05844c]

[52] Li D, Li J, Wang S. Guar gum in drug delivery. Natural Biopolymers for Drug Delivery 2025; 163-87.
[http://dx.doi.org/10.1016/b978-0-323-95367-2.00008-9]

[53] Kumar S, Bhatt A, Purohit P. Carrageenan modifications: Improving biomedical applications. Journal of Polymers and the Environment 2025; (4): 1667-88.
[http://dx.doi.org/10.1007/s10924-025-03501-y]

[54] Yener S, Akbulut KG, Karakuş R, Erdoğan D, Acartürk F. Development of melatonin loaded pectin

nanoparticles for the treatment of inflammatory bowel disease: *In vitro* and *in vivo* studies. Journal of Drug Delivery Science and Technology 2022.
[http://dx.doi.org/10.1016/j.jddst.2021.102861]

[55] Zhang S, Zhang M, Li W, *et al.* Research progress of natural plant polysaccharides inhibiting inflammatory signaling pathways and regulating intestinal flora and metabolism to protect inflammatory bowel disease. International Journal of Biological Macromolecules 2023.
[http://dx.doi.org/10.1016/j.ijbiomac.2023.126799]

[56] Tawfick MM, Xie H, Zhao C, Shao P, Farag MA. Inulin fructans in diet: Role in gut homeostasis, immunity, health outcomes and potential therapeutics. International Journal of Biological Macromolecules 2022; 948-61.
[http://dx.doi.org/10.1016/j.ijbiomac.2022.03.218]

[57] Roy S, Dhaneshwar S. Role of prebiotics, probiotics, and synbiotics in management of inflammatory bowel disease: Current perspectives. World Journal of Gastroenterology 2023; (14): 2078-100.
[http://dx.doi.org/10.3748/wjg.v29.i14.2078]

[58] Wang W, Li X, Wu H, Shi F, Zhang Z, Lv H. Explore the underlying oral efficacy of α-, β-, γ-Cyclodextrin against the ulcerative colitis using *in vitro* and *in vivo* studies assisted by network pharmacology. Journal of Biomolecular Structure and Dynamics 2024; (10): 4985-5000.
[http://dx.doi.org/10.1080/07391102.2023.2239901]

[59] Appleton L, Navarro-Orcajada S, Martinez-Navarro S, *et al.* Cyclodextrins as antiinflammatory agents: basis, drugs and perspectives. Biomolecules 2021; (9):
[http://dx.doi.org/10.3390/biom11091384]

[60] Nair DVT, Paudel D, Cantorna M, Singh V. Dietary fiber guar gum exacerbates colonic inflammation in multiple experimental models of inflammatory bowel disease. Inflammatory Bowel Diseases 2021; (Supplement_1): S2-3.
[http://dx.doi.org/10.1093/ibd/izaa347.004]

[61] Moutaharrik S, Meroni G, Soggiu A, *et al.* Guar gum as a microbially degradable component for an oral colon delivery system based on a combination strategy: formulation and *in vitro* evaluation. Drug Delivery and Translational Research 2024; (3): 826-38.
[http://dx.doi.org/10.1007/s13346-023-01439-z]

[62] Kim Y, Hwang SW, Kim S, *et al.* Dietary cellulose prevents gut inflammation by modulating lipid metabolism and gut microbiota. Gut Microbes 2020; (4): 944-61.
[http://dx.doi.org/10.1080/19490976.2020.1730149]

[63] Caro D, Alcamo V, Cummings AM, *et al.* Effect of dietary cellulose supplementation on gut barrier function and apoptosis in a murine model of endotoxemia. PLoS One 2019; (12):
[http://dx.doi.org/10.1371/journal.pone.0224838]

[64] Kimilu N, Gładyś-Cieszyńska K, Pieszko M, Mańkowska-Wierzbicka D, Folwarski M. Carrageenan in the diet: Friend or Foe for inflammatory bowel disease?. Nutrients 2024; (11):
[http://dx.doi.org/10.3390/nu16111780]

[65] Liyanage NM, Nagahawatta DP, Jayawardena TU, Jeon Y. The role of seaweed polysaccharides in gastrointestinal health: Protective effect against inflammatory bowel disease. Life 2023; (4):
[http://dx.doi.org/10.3390/life13041026]

[66] Swastha D, Varsha N, Aravind S, *et al.* Alginate-based drug carrier systems to target inflammatory bowel disease: A review. International Journal of Biological Macromolecules 2023.
[http://dx.doi.org/10.1016/j.ijbiomac.2023.125472]

[67] Wang Q, Wang G, Zhou J, Gao L, Cui Y. Colon targeted oral drug delivery system based on alginate-chitosan microspheres loaded with icariin in the treatment of ulcerative colitis. International Journal of Pharmaceutics 2016; (1-2): 176-85.
[http://dx.doi.org/10.1016/j.ijpharm.2016.10.002]

CHAPTER 5

Exploring the Role of Polymers Derived from Animals in the Treatment of Inflammatory Bowel Disease

Rashmi Dewangan[1], **Nidhi Agrawal**[1], **S.K. Lanjhiyana**[1], **Sanjay Kumar Bharti**[1] and **Meenakshi Jaiswal**[1,*]

[1] *Department of Pharmacy, Guru Ghasidas Vishwavidyalaya, Bilaspur 495009, Chhattisgarh, India*

Abstract: Inflammatory Bowel Disease (IBD), encompassing Crohn's Disease (CD) and Ulcerative Colitis (UC), is a chronic inflammatory condition of the gastrointestinal tract. The primary challenge in IBD treatment is the limited bioavailability of therapeutic agents at the inflamed site, necessitating higher systemic doses that can lead to adverse effects. Animal-derived polymers are becoming recognized as efficient carriers for targeted drug administration due to their biocompatibility, biodegradability, and ability to enhance drug retention in the colon. Natural polymers such as gelatin, chitosan, collagen, hyaluronic acid, albumin, and chondroitin sulfate demonstrate potential in improving drug absorption, modulating inflammation, and extending drug release. These biomaterials exhibit mucoadhesive properties, prolong intestine retention, and promote mucosal healing, hence enhancing therapeutic efficiency. Moreover, they can be engineered to encapsulate anti-inflammatory agents and biologics, ensuring localized pharmacological effectiveness while minimizing systemic toxicity. Innovative methods, including enzymatic and biological modifications, have been explored to improve the structural and functional properties of these polymers, hence increasing their effectiveness in drug delivery applications. Notwithstanding these advancements, challenges remain in refining polymer formulations for improved stability, precise release, and controlled degradation. This chapter highlights recent developments in animal-derived polymeric nanocarriers for the treatment of IBD, emphasizing their role in enhancing drug targeting and therapeutic effectiveness. The progression of innovative animal-derived polymers or their derivatives with superior properties remains a crucial area for future research, offering potential improvements in IBD therapy.

Keywords: Animal-derived polymers, Inflammatory bowel disease (IBD), Nano-carriers, Natural polymers, Targeted drug delivery.

[*] **Corresponding author Meenakshi Jaiswal**: Department of Pharmacy, Guru Ghasidas Vishwavidyalaya, Bilaspur 495009, Chhattisgarh, India; E-mail: jaiswalmeenakshiggu@gmail.com

Meenakshi Jaiswal & S.K. Lanjhiyana (Eds.)

INTRODUCTION

Inflammatory Bowel Disease (IBD) encompasses Crohn's Disease (CD) and Ulcerative Colitis (UC), both of which are persistent inflammatory disorders of the gastrointestinal tract [1]. The highest prevalence is observed in North America an Northern Europe, with 9–20 cases per 100,000 individuals per year [2]. UC is more prevalent in adults, while CD is more common in children [3]. The prevalence of IBD is rising in traditionally low-risk areas, including Asia, the Middle East, and South America, presumably attributable to urbanization and westernized lifestyles [4]. Environmental factors, including diet, pollution, and hygiene, affect the emergence of disease in people with a genetic disposition [5]. Before the age of 20, an appendectomy reduces the chance of UC by 69%, but it increases the risk of CD [6]. IBD often presents throughout the first three decades of life, causing chronic recurring inflammation [7]. It causes significant morbidity and mortality and is associated with an increased risk of Colorectal Cancer (CRC) [8]. While CD can affect any part of the gastrointestinal system and is characterized by transmural inflammation that results in strictures and fistulas, UC primarily affects the colon, causing surface mucosal inflammation [9]. Immunological dysregulation, gut microbiota, environmental variables, and genetic vulnerability all contribute to its emergence, although the exact cause is still unknown [10]. Systemic disorders may arise from IBD, which typically manifests as a relapsing-remitting pattern in early adulthood [11]. Intestinal epithelial barrier deficiencies and increased immunological activity are linked to IBD, which causes tissue deterioration over time [12]. CRC is the leading cause of cancer-related mortality, and it is a major risk factor for the disease. An important public health issue that demands improved treatment strategies is the growing incidence of IBD worldwide [13]. Due to the complex physiology and environment of the gastrointestinal system, colorectal medication distribution in IBD faces significant challenges [14]. Drug formulations that are both targeted and resistant to stomach transit are required because the colon's located farther from the stomach [15]. Formulation design is crucial because changes in intestinal fluid volume, transit time, and pH affect the breakdown and absorption of medications. [16] Drug mobility is limited by the increased viscosity of colonic contents, while medications may become inactive or lose their efficacy due to colonic bacterial enzymatic destruction [17]. Additionally, pharmacologically active, inert, or possibly dangerous metabolites may be produced *via* intestinal metabolism. Drug bioavailability may be hampered by inadequate solubility and high dosage requirements, necessitating the use specially designed delivery systems [18]. In order to ensure targeted and effective therapy, colorectal medication administration strategies in IBD include a variety of cutting-edge techniques [19]. For targeted drug release, colon-specific biodegradable methods of delivery include enzyme-sensitive polymers or bacterial fermentation of polysaccharides [20]. Pharmaceuticals are encapsulated in matrix-based methods using biodegradable or pH-sensitive polymers to prevent early release [21]. Although gastrointestinal transit time is the basis for timed-release techniques, drug administration may be impacted by motility variations [22]. By improving drug retention in the intestinal mucosa, bioadhesive techniques improve absorption and efficacy [23]. The uniformity of drug distribution and absorption by colonic macrophages is enhanced by multiparticulate systems like microspheres [24]. Enzyme-mediated drug release, stability, and biocompatibility are all offered by polysaccharide-based delivery systems [25]. For controlled release, pH-sensitive coatings dissolve at colonic pH and shield medications from stomach acid [26]. Although variations in viscosity may affect effectiveness, pressure-controlled formulations use increased intestinal lumen pressure to start drug release [27]. To enhance targeted drug delivery, osmotic and pulsincap systems combine timed-release mechanisms with pH-sensitive coatings [16]. Animal-derived natural polymers, which use colonic bacterial enzymatic breakdown for precise release, are crucial for colon-specific drug delivery in IBD [15]. Compared to synthetic polymers, they are safer because they are non-toxic, biodegradable, and biocompatible [28]. Collagen, gelatin, chitosan, and hyaluronic acid are examples of animal-derived polymers that are valued for their structural similarity to human biomolecules, biocompatibility, and biodegradability [29]. Strict ISO 10993 testing is necessary for safety, as impurities or inadequate purification can cause cytotoxic or inflammatory reactions [30]. Additionally, these polymers may possess antigenic properties, such as α-Gal epitopes, that trigger an immune response [31]. In order to ensure increased purity, improved biocompatibility, and reduced immunogenicity, advanced purification and chemical modification techniques are employed to remove or mask antigenic residues [32]. In addition, they are affordable, easily obtainable, and free of adverse effects [29]. The properties of animal-derived polymers and their application in targeted medication delivery for the management of IBD are covered in this chapter.

THE IMPORTANCE OF ANIMAL-DERIVED POLYMERS IN IBD

Animal-derived polymers enhance stability, bioavailability, and controlled release, and are considered significant for targeted colorectal drug delivery in IBD [30]. Chitosan, hyaluronic acid, collagen, gelatin, and chondroitin are examples of polymers that are used as excipients in formulations such as tablets, hydrogels, microparticles, microspheres, nanoparticles, nanovesicles, and composites (Table **1**) [31]. These biopolymers enhance mucoadhesion, prevent drug degradation, and facilitate targeted delivery to inflamed areas, thereby minimizing systemic side effects (Fig. **1**) [32].

Table 1. Applications of animal-derived polymer for the treatment of IBD.

Animal-derived Polymers	Key Application	Mechanism of Action in IBD	Example of Formulation
Chitosan	Colon-targeted delivery, Mucoadhesion	pH-responsive, Bioadhesive	Budesonide nanoparticles
Gelatin	Controlled drug release	Enzyme-degradable matrix	5-ASA capsules
Collagen	Mucosal healing scaffold	Promotes epithelial repair	Collagen enema
Hyaluronic acid	Anti-inflammatory hydrogel	Reduces cytokine release	HA enemas
Albumin	Nano-carrier for biologics	Sustained protein release	TNF-α inhibitor nanoparticles

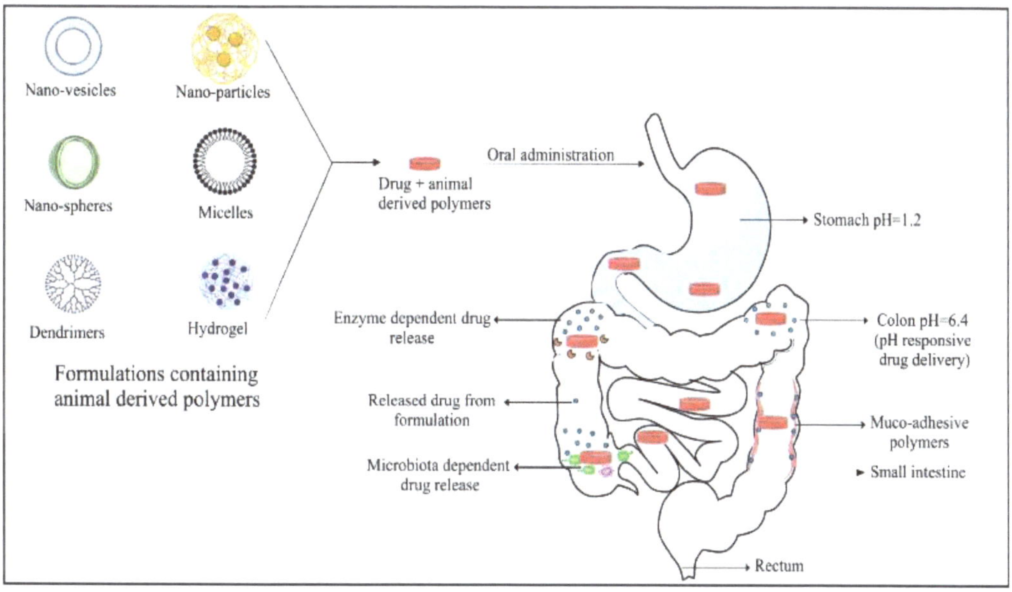

Fig. (1). Animal-derived polymer-containing formulations in colorectal drug delivery for the treatment of IBD.

Chitosan

Chitosan, derived from chitin found in crab shells, insect exoskeletons, and fungal cell walls, is a biodegradable and biocompatible polysaccharide [33]. It consists of β-(1→4) linked glucosamine and N-acetylglucosamine units, with solubility influenced by the degree of deacetylation and pH [34]. Chitosan exhibits protonation in acidic conditions (pKa ~6.5) and is modified by phosphorylation or quaternization to enhance solubility and functionality [35]. It shows destruction through acid hydrolysis, enzymatic cleavage (chitinases, chitosanases), or oxidative mechanisms [36]. Crosslinked chitosan enhances drug entrapment and enables controlled release in drug delivery systems [37]. pH-sensitive drug release is made possible by chitosan-based formulations, which protect drugs in the stomach and deliver their contents into the colon [38]. Glycosidic linkages are hydrolyzed by colonic bacteria, allowing site-specific drug delivery [15]. Aldehyde-crosslinked chitosan is insoluble under acidic conditions but swells at intestinal pH, enabling controlled drug release. [35] Chitosan oligosaccharides reduce oxidative damage and inflammation by modifying NF-κB signaling [39]. By improving medication targeting and therapeutic efficacy, chitosan-based formulations show potential for the treatment of IBD [40].

In 2015, Castangia *et al.* developed chitosan-coated nanovesicles to enhance drug delivery for Inflammatory Bowel Disease (IBD) by providing mucoadhesion, stability, and targeted release in the colon. The coating protects quercetin from gastric breakdown, enabling controlled release at neutral pH by enzymatic degradation. Chitosan improves drug retention *via* mucoadhesion, colon targeting, and therapeutic efficacy, compared to uncoated vesicles, as evidenced in TNBS-induced colitis mice. Moreover, its enzymatic degradability and prebiotic properties enhance gut health and mitigate symptoms of IBD, including diarrhea [41].

Chitosan–poly(methyl acrylate) nanoparticles loaded with diclofenac sodium were formulated using a unique multiplestep, spinning-disk processing technique for colon-targeted drug delivery. A protective nanocore formed by chitosan inhibits drug release immediately from the formulation in the upper GIT. In inflamed colonic tissues, its protonation at colonic pH promotes cellular absorption and localized drug release by improving bioadhesion to the anionic-charged mucosal layer. Within 8-hours, the improved formulation achieved over 90% release in simulated colonic fluid, pH- and enzyme-controlled release, and significant drug entrapment (88%), as evidenced by cellular uptake experiments that showed improved drug absorption in Caco-2 cells [42].

Chitosan-based composites formulated as colon-targeted resveratrol depots for the treatment of IBD. Ionic cross-linking was used to incorporate resveratrol-loaded nanoparticles into chitosan hydrogels after they were modified for encapsulation efficiency. Due to the organized chitosan network, the composite hydrogels demonstrated lower resveratrol release rates (29–34% after 48 hours) than nanoparticles alone (79–81%). Thermal and morphological evaluations demonstrated the formulations' ability to sustain long-term colonic drug administration by ensuring stability and scaffold porosity [43].

In 2010, Dubey *et al.* designed enzyme-responsive drug delivery microspheres based on chitosan to specifically transport 5-aminosalicylic acid and camylofine dihydrochloride to the colon to address UC. After enzyme induction, the enteric-coated microspheres demonstrated increased drug release (70–72%) in the presence of 3% rat caecal matter, improving to 92–95%. Effective colonic targeting has been demonstrated by *in vivo* tests (76.55% drug release in 9 h) [44].

Chitosan plays a role in IBD treatment as a biocompatible and biodegradable carrier for targeted siRNA delivery. In a chitosan/alginate hydrogel system, nanoparticles loaded with CD98 siRNA and functionalized with single-chain CD98 antibodies efficiently target colonic cells that overexpress CD98. These nanoparticles improve mucus penetration, promote endosomal escape, and inhibit CD98 expression, thereby diminishing colitis severity in preclinical models. This targeted methodology diminishes systemic adverse effects, indicating a feasible strategy for IBD management [45].

Gelatin

Bovine bone gelatin peptides show anti-inflammatory properties by inhibiting pro-inflammatory cytokines (TNF-α, IL-6, IL-1β, MCP-1) and altering the gut microbiota composition in dextran sodium sulfate-induced colitis models. Bovine bone gelatin peptides restore intestinal barrier integrity by downregulating TLR-4/NF-κB signaling and increasing tight junction proteins (ZO-1, occludin). Additionally, bovine bone gelatin peptides reduce inflammatory bacteria (*Peptococcus, Bifidobacterium, Saccharibacteria*) while increasing beneficial microbiota (*Akkermansia, Parasutterella*). According to these findings, bovine bone gelatin peptides may be a useful dietary or remedial component for IBD [46].

Recombinant IL-10 was delivered *via* gelatin microspheres to enhance its therapeutic efficacy in IL-10-deficient mice with colitis. Colonic inflammation was significantly reduced by rectal diffusion of the Gelatin-IL-10 microsphere, which decreased the expression of CD40 and IL-12 mRNA in Mac-1-positive cells. Unlike polylactic acid microspheres, gelatin microspheres preserved the biological activity of IL-10, enabling prolonged release and customized anti-inflammatory effects. This approach highlights the potential of gelatin-based medication delivery for IBD treatment [47].

Treating IBD requires the use of type B gelatin, as it serves as a biocompatible vehicle for orally delivering siRNA. TNF-α siRNA was encapsulated in type B gelatin nanoparticles and then trapped in poly-ε-caprolactone microspheres in a nanoparticles-in-microspheres oral system. In a DSS-induced animal model, this strategy reduces the severity of colitis and downregulates TNF-α by preventing siRNA from degrading, facilitating controlled release in the inflammatory colon, and improving cellular absorption [48].

Curcumin-encapsulated carboxymethyl chitosan microspheres were incorporated into a pH-sensitive hydrogel made of hyaluronic acid and gelatin for the purpose of treating colitis. Gelatin enhances the structural integrity of the hydrogel and controls medication release, whereas hyaluronic acid promotes intestinal healing and reduces inflammation. The formulation reduced pro-inflammatory cytokines (IL-6, TNF-α), extended curcumin release, maintained elevated colonic concentrations for over 24 hours, and effectively treated colitis in DSS-induced mice. This strategy improves the bioavailability of curcumin and provides a practical means of controlled medication delivery in IBD [49].

Gelatin-based nanoparticles facilitate the targeted delivery of 5-aminosalicylic acid to the inflamed colon, offering a compelling strategy for ulcerative colitis. By preventing 5-aminosalicylic acid from degrading in the stomach, Eudragit-S10--coated gelatin nanoparticles enable tailored release and enhanced bioavailability. By suppressing markers including TNF-α, IL-1β, and COX-2, these nanoparticles significantly reduce inflammation while restoring intestinal histoarchitecture. The study highlights how gelatin nanoparticles are more therapeutically efficient than free 5-aminosalicylic acid at reducing the symptoms of colitis [50].

Collagen

One of the main structural components of the extracellular matrix, which is present in skin, bone, cartilage, tendons, ligaments, and blood vessels, is collagen, a naturally occurring protein that is common in animals [51]. Chemically, it consists of three polypeptide chains with repeating Gly-X-Y sequences that create a triple-helix structure supported by interchain hydrogen bonding (where X and Y are usually proline and hydroxyproline) [52]. Collagen is a fibrous, water-insoluble protein that exhibits unique swelling properties owing to its amino and carboxyl groups, which provide polyelectrolyte characteristics [57]. The degree of crosslinking, pH, temperature, and the presence of hydrophilic monomers-all of which are critical for drug loading and release-have an impact on the swelling capacity [54]. Collagen is an excellent candidate for oral formulations of medications, particularly for IBD, due to its biocompatibility and its ability to undergo functional group changes. [55] In IBD, excessive collagen degradation by Matrix Metalloproteinases (MMPs), especially MMP-1, causes mucosal ulceration and compromises the intestinal barrier [56]. Because of their pliable swelling properties, collagen-based hydrogels can serve as regulated drug delivery vehicles, enhancing drug retention and release at inflammatory sites and promoting mucosal healing and targeted treatment for IBD [57]. Collagen peptides derived from cod skin demonstrated notable anti-inflammatory properties *in vitro* by decreasing pro-inflammatory cytokines, diminishing oxidative stress, and regulating NF-κB/MAPK signaling pathways. In a DSS-induced UC model, collagen peptides mitigated colonic damage, reinstated intestinal barrier function by enhancing tight junction proteins (ZO-1, Occludin, Claudin-1), and regulated gut microbiota by augmenting probiotics and diminishing pathogenic microorganisms [58].

In another study, researchers found that collagen, an essential extracellular matrix protein that facilitate tissue regeneration, was integrated with fucoidan to form an *in situ* hydrogel exhibiting a sol-gel transition, thereby ensuring prolonged 12-hour release of fucoidan. In a DSS-induced colitis model, this formulation markedly diminished clinical scores and rectal bleeding compared with the conventional treatment, mesalamine, as well as with individual treatments with either fucoidan or collagen alone [59].

Collagen and its hydrolysate are crucial in the treatment of IBD by promoting mucosal healing and reducing inflammation. In a DSS-induced colitis model, both collagen and collagen hydrolysate significantly reduced rectal bleeding and downregulated key inflammatory markers (VEGF, TNF-α, IL-1β, IL-6) more effectively than mesalamine. Enhanced mucosal regeneration was found in histological examination, underscoring that collagen serves a dual function in tissue repair and inflammatory regulation [60].

In an additional experiment, researchers found that prolyl endopeptidase, MMP8, MMP9, and collagen degradation in IBD produce tripeptide Proline-Glycin--Proline (PGP), which in turn promotes neutrophil chemotaxis *via* CXCR2. Intestinal tissues from DSS-induced colitis mice and IBD patients showed elevated PGP levels. Peripheral blood polymorphonuclear cells in IBD were shown to produce more PGP from collagen in *ex vivo* investigations. Its significance in sustaining inflammation in IBD was highlighted when neutrophil infiltration was decreased by neutralizing it [61].

The potential of collagen as a treatment is highlighted by mucosal ulceration resulting from excessive collagen breakdown driven by matrix metalloproteinases in UC. Mesalamine was added to a pH/temperature-sensitive collagen hydrogel, which demonstrated a prolonged 12-hour release and significantly reduced mucosal damage and rectal bleeding in a DSS-induced colitis model in comparison to mesalamine suspension. For effective localized control of UC, this synergistic approach combines their anti-inflammatory qualities with the regenerative potential of collagen [62].

Fish collagen peptide Naticol®Gut reduces colonic inflammation in DSS-induced colitis by promoting an antioxidant and anti-inflammatory macrophage phenotype *via* mannose receptor recognition. Intestinal eubiosis is restored, CD8 T-cell activation is reduced, and CD4 T-cells are guided toward a Th2 response. Similar to this, Naticol®Gut rewires monocytes in IBD patients, highlighting its potential as a functional food for gut health [63].

Hyaluronic Acid

A significant glycosaminoglycan found in the extracellular matrix of connective tissues like skin, heart valves, umbilical cords, and synovial fluid, hyaluronic acid was first isolated from the vitreous body of cows in 1934 [64]. Hyaluronic acid is a linear, non-sulfated, biodegradable mucopolysaccharide consisting of repeated units of N-acetylglucosamine and D-glucuronic acid interconnected by β-1,4- and β-1,3-glycosidic linkages [65]. Because of its remarkable flexibility and water-retention capacity, it may absorb thousands of times its own weight in water, which alters its viscoelastic and rheological properties [66]. The molar mass of hyaluronic acid polymers ranges from 100 kDa to 8 MDa, and their lengths range from 10 nm to 25 μm [64]. By acting as a scaffold for proteoglycans and encouraging hyaluronic acid–protein interactions, it plays an essential role in the extracellular matrix [67]. Hyaluronic acid is not produced in the Golgi apparatus like other glycosaminoglycans [68]. Viscosity-dependent shear-thinning properties are seen in its aqueous solutions [66]. By interacting with immune cells and modifying cytokine responses, hyaluronic acid regulates inflammation, tissue repair, and the integrity of the epithelial barrier in IBD [66, 69]. Hyaluronic acid-based drug delivery systems use their mucoadhesive properties and enzymatic breakdown in the colon to enable targeted and sustained release in colorectal applications [70].

Amphiphilic conjugates of hyaluronic acid were used to formulate budesonide-loaded hyaluronic acid nanoparticles, which showed a significant affinity for CD44 receptors, which are overexpressed in inflammatory colonic tissues, and a negative charge. In rats with acetic acid-induced colitis, these nanoparticles improved the therapeutic efficacy of budesonide by enabling both passive and active targeting. Budesonide-loaded hyaluronic acid nanoparticles significantly reduced inflammation, TNF-α levels, and MPO activity as compared to free budesonide, which promoted tissue repair. The effectiveness of using hyaluronic acid-based nanoparticles as a targeted drug delivery strategy to treat IBD is confirmed by this study [71].

Using galactosylated bovine serum albumin, researchers developed a polyphenol-based nanodelivery system (GBP-HA NPs) that transports tannic acid and epigallocatechin gallate while encasing them in a "nanoarmor" of hyaluronic acid and ε-polylysine. While hyaluronic acid provides protection against gastric breakdown and selectively targets inflammatory colonic areas through CD44 binding, bovine serum albumin enhances the stability and bioavailability of polyphenols. By modulating the Keap1-Nrf2, NF-κB, and Caspase-1-dependent pyroptosis pathways, GBP-HA demonstrated notable anti-inflammatory and antioxidant activity in addition to targeting macrophages and reducing UC symptoms [72].

By conjugating poly(N-isopropylacrylamide) to hyaluronic acid, researchers created a sprayable topical treatment for IBD that improves mucoadhesion and adhesiveness to injured gut mucosa through temperature-induced phase transition. The formulation produces a thin protective layer within 5 minutes at physiological temperature. In an *ex vivo* IBD model, prednisolone was encapsulated to optimize treatment efficacy and drastically restore mucosal tissue. Repair of the mucosal barrier is confirmed by histological examination and elevated mRNA levels of ZO-1 and Muc-2 [73].

In models of moderate and severe colitis, a rectal formulation containing hyaluronic acid and 5-aminosalicylic acid demonstrated improved therapeutic efficacy. By exhibiting mucoprotective, anti-inflammatory, and bioadhesive characteristics, hyaluronic acid, a non-sulfated glycosaminoglycan, impedes the retention of 5-aminosalicylic acid at inflammatory sites. More effectively than 5-aminosalicylic acid alone, the combination decreased inflammation markers (MPO, TNF-α, IL-6, and IL-1β), demonstrating a synergistic impact. By improving mucosal healing and drug uptake, this formulation offers a possible alternative to corticosteroids for severe IBD cases [74].

A thermoresponsive hydrogel technology based on methylcellulose and hyaluronic acid was investigated by researchers for the rectal delivery of biologics in IBD. The therapeutic potential of the hydrogel is enhanced by hyaluronic acid, which is well known for its mucoadhesive and mucosal-healing properties. As a model biologic, bovine serum albumin showed transintestinal permeability and prolonged release, especially when combined with an absorption enhancer. The hydrogel demonstrated appropriate rheological characteristics for rectal application, indicating potential as a safe but effective biologics delivery strategy in IBD [75].

Aprodu A *et al.* formulated an oral creatine-modified selenium-based hyaluronic acid nanogel for the treatment of IBD, emphasizing the role of hyaluronic acid in targeting IBD lesions *via* CD44 interaction and electrostatic adsorption. By effectively removing ROS and restoring mitochondrial energy metabolism, the prepared nanogel reduces the symptoms of IBD, including immunological response, gut microbiota imbalance, and mitochondrial dysfunction. This treatment combines the removal of ROS with the stimulation of energy metabolism, offering a dual-targeted approach to successful IBD therapy [76].

Albumin

Albumin, a naturally occurring globular protein, is sourced from human serum, bovine serum, and egg white (ovalbumin) [77]. It consists of a single polypeptide chain (~66–69 kDa) with three α-helical domains stabilized by disulfide bonds [78]. Its hydrophobic pockets enhance its significant drug-binding capacity, making it an effective drug carrier [79]. Formulations incorporating albumin improve therapeutic efficacy, reduce systemic toxicity, and improve medication targeting in IBD [80]. Certain intestinal conditions, such as a neutral to slightly alkaline pH (6.8–7.4), the presence of colonic bacteria, and inflammation linked to conditions like IBD, influence the release of medications from albumin-based polymers in the colon [77]. Albumin-based carriers demonstrate pH sensitivity, remaining stable in the acidic conditions of the stomach (pH 1.5–3.5) and the small intestine (pH 5.5–6.8), but deteriorating at the elevated pH of the colon [81]. Additionally, polymer degradation is facilitated by microbial enzymes, such as proteases and azoreductases, which initiate the release of drugs [82]. In inflamed colonic tissue, increased proteolytic enzyme activity, reactive oxygen species, and inflammatory cytokines promote drug release, enabling targeted therapy [83].

An innovative medication delivery method targeting inflammation, utilizing albumin-based nanoparticles, was formulated for the treatment of IBD. At the inflammatory mucosa, these nanoparticles interact with positively charged proteins after being coated with heparin to boost their negative charge. Budesonide and granulocyte macrophage colony-stimulating factor-loaded dual-drug nanoparticles showed improved anti-inflammatory effects and specific targeting of the inflamed gut in a mouse model of colitis. With IBD, this strategy presents a viable way to improve treatment results while reducing systemic side effects [84].

In order to treat UC, human serum albumin nanoparticles loaded with 5-aminosalicylic acid were developed for targeted delivery to inflammatory areas of the colon. Upon specific interaction with Myeloperoxidase (MPO), these nanoparticles, with an average size of 190 nm, showed strong localization in the inflamed colon. *In vivo* studies showed significant therapeutic effects at a much lower dose of 5-aminosalicylic acid compared to conventional formulations, suggesting that human serum albumin nanoparticles are a promising carrier for site-specific delivery in IBD [85].

Researchers developed a ROS-responsive human serum albumin-based nanomedicine to enhance the therapeutic efficacy of tofacitinib for UC. The formulation selectively targeted inflamed colons, reducing pro-inflammatory cytokines and inhibiting T-cell migration. It showed anti-inflammatory effects by promoting M2 macrophage polarization during wound healing. *In vitro* and *in vivo* studies demonstrated improved drug delivery, offering a promising approach to UC treatment with fewer side effects [86].

Chondroitin

Chondroitin sulfate is a glycosaminoglycan found in the extracellular matrix, bone, cartilage, epidermis, nerve tissue, and blood vessels of humans, other animals (such as pigs, cattle, and chickens), sharks, invertebrates, and some bacteria [87, 88]. It consists of alternating units of D-glucuronic acid and N-acetyl-D-galactosamine, exhibiting diverse sulfation patterns that influence its charge and molecular weight (50–100 kDa) [89]. Chondroitin sulfate demonstrated considerable water solubility, which can be modified using swellable polymers or enteric coatings for drug delivery [90]. Its biodegradability, biocompatibility, and affinity for CD44 receptors enable targeted drug accumulation in the colon, making it an effective carrier for colorectal drug delivery [91].

A novel oral drug delivery system has been developed by encapsulating epigallocatechin gallate with Poly(N-vinylpyrrolidone) (PVP) and conjugating chondroitin sulfate for targeted delivery in UC. Chondroitin sulfate improves gastrointestinal stability, facilitates CD44-mediated active targeting, and concentrates epigallocatechin in the inflamed colon. The system exhibited anti-inflammatory properties, reinstated the intestinal barrier, and altered gut microbiota in DSS-induced UC mice, underscoring its potential for polyphenol-based IBD treatment [92].

Researchers designed colon-targeted aceclofenac matrix tablets utilizing chondroitin sulfate as a microbially degradable polymeric carrier. Colloidal silica was crucial for regulating drug release, maintaining stability in gastric and intestinal fluids while undergoing enzymatic degradation in colonic fluid, which initiated the fast release of aceclofenac. FT-IR and DSC validated the compatibility of the medicines with the polymer, whereas dissolving studies demonstrated that chondroitin sulfate efficiently modulated drug release in the colon. The results emphasize chondroitin sulfate as an effective vehicle for the administration of customized medications [90].

A chondroitin sulfate-glycyl-prednisolone combination was produced using carbodiimide coupling, resulting in nanogels with prednisolone concentrations of

5.5% and 21.1% (w/w). The negatively charged nanoparticles demonstrated pH-sensitive, sustained release of prednisolone, with the nanogel exhibiting a decreased release rate and improved transport to the lower intestines. In a TNBS-induced colitis rat model, the nanogel demonstrated greater therapeutic efficacy compared to prednisolone alone. Chondroitin sulfate played a vital role in nanogel synthesis, drug retention, and targeted administration, underscoring its promise in ulcerative colitis therapy [93].

Rosmarinic acid was conjugated with chondroitin sulfate A to enhance water solubility and targeting for the treatment of UC. The rosmarinic acid-chondroitin sulfate A, nanoconjugate self-assembled into nanoassemblies around 247.3 nm in size, demonstrating antioxidant and anti-inflammatory properties. It significantly reduced intestinal inflammation, pro-inflammatory cytokine expression, and disease severity in mice with DSS-induced colitis. Chondroitin sulfate A improved the absorption and therapeutic efficacy of rosmarinic acid, making rosmarinic acid-chondroitin sulfate A nanoconjugate a potent treatment for UC [94].

Amrutkar JR *et al.* developed colon-targeted matrix tablets employing cross-linked chitosan and chondroitin sulfate as a polyelectrolyte complex carrier. Chondroitin sulfate facilitated colon-targeted drug delivery by electrostatic interactions with cross-linked chitosan, as shown by FTIR, DSC, and XRD analyses. The disintegration rate depended on polysaccharide concentration and cross-linking duration. The findings demonstrated that chondroitin sulfate promotes the localized release of indomethacin in the colon [95].

ETHICAL CONSIDERATIONS IN OBTAINING ANIMAL-DERIVED POLYMERS

The procurement of animal-derived polymers, such as gelatin, collagen, chitosan, and hyaluronic acid, raises substantial ethical concerns about animal welfare, sustainability, and cultural sensitivity [28]. Animals should be treated with consideration, emphasizing the utilization of by-products rather than their sacrifice just for extraction [100]. Transparency and traceability of the source are essential for guaranteeing ethical procurement. Religious and cultural beliefs must be respected, particularly when sourcing products from pigs or cattle. To alleviate environmental harm, emphasis must be placed on sustainable and environmentally benign extraction techniques and the development of non-animal alternatives [101]. Adherence to international and national ethical norms, including CPCSEA (India), EU Directives, and IAEC recommendations, ensures responsible sourcing in pharmaceutical applications [102].

Safety Considerations in Sourcing Animal-derived Polymers

Safety issues for acquiring animal-derived polymers are crucial to ensure their suitability for pharmaceutical applications. Raw materials must be obtained from healthy, certified animals with full traceability to prevent contamination and ensure ethical sourcing [103]. A primary concern is the transmission of diseases such as Bovine Spongiform Encephalopathy (BSE) and other zoonotic infections; thus, sourcing must comply with WHO and EMA guidelines for TSE/BSE-free products [104]. Aseptic processing, sterilization, and regular bioburden evaluation are essential to guarantee sterility and microbiological safety. Adherence to ethical and regulatory standards, including compliance with FDA, EU, and ISO 22442 rules, is essential [105]. It is essential to ensure the removal of residual chemicals, heavy metals, and crosslinking agents that may cause toxicity. Assessment of biocompatibility and immunogenicity, in compliance with ISO 10993, confirms safety for biomedical applications [106]. Thorough documentation, certificate of analysis, and GMP compliance are crucial to ensure transparency and quality assurance in the sourcing and processing of animal-derived polymers [107].

CONCLUSION

Polymers derived from animals, including chitosan, gelatin, collagen, hyaluronic acid, albumin, and chondroitin sulfate, have significant potential for targeted treatment of IBD. These biopolymers enhance medication stability, bioavailability, and controlled release through pH-sensitive and enzyme-responsive mechanisms. Their biocompatibility and ability to regulate inflammation make them effective in reducing systemic side effects while promoting mucosal healing. Innovative delivery methods improve therapeutic effectiveness, such as nanoparticles, hydrogels, and microspheres. These polymers offer novel ways to improve IBD treatment through tailored medication delivery because of their biodegradability and safety profile.

DISCLOSURE (ARTIFICIAL INTELLIGENCE)

AI-based tools were used only to refine the language of this manuscript and enhance clarity and readability, while all scientific interpretations and intellectual contributions remain entirely those of the authors.

REFERENCES

[1] Rubin DC, Shaker A, Levin MS. Chronic intestinal inflammation: inflammatory bowel disease and colitis-associated colon cancer. Front Immunol 2012; 3: 107. [http://dx.doi.org/10.3389/fimmu.2012.00107] [PMID: 22586430]

[2] Shivashankar R, Tremaine WJ, Harmsen WS, Loftus EV Jr. Incidence and prevalence of Crohn's

disease and ulcerative colitis in olmsted county, minnesota from 1970 through 2010. Clin Gastroenterol Hepatol 2017; 15(6): 857-63. [http://dx.doi.org/10.1016/j.cgh.2016.10.039] [PMID: 27856364]

[3] Rosen MJ, Dhawan A, Saeed SA. Inflammatory Bowel Disease in Children and Adolescents. JAMA Pediatr 2015; 169(11): 1053-60. [http://dx.doi.org/10.1001/jamapediatrics.2015.1982] [PMID: 26414706]

[4] Selvaratnam S, Gullino S, Shim L, *et al.* Epidemiology of inflammatory bowel disease in South America: A systematic review. World J Gastroenterol 2019; 25(47): 6866-75. [http://dx.doi.org/10.3748/wjg.v25.i47.6866] [PMID: 31885427]

[5] Virolainen SJ, VonHandorf A, Viel KCMF, Weirauch MT, Kottyan LC. Gene–environment interactions and their impact on human health. Genes Immun 2022; 24(1): 1-11. [http://dx.doi.org/10.1038/s41435-022-00192-6] [PMID: 36585519]

[6] Arjomand Fard N, Armstrong H, Perry T, Wine E. Appendix and ulcerative colitis: A key to explaining the pathogenesis and directing novel therapies? Inflamm Bowel Dis 2023; 29(1): 151-60. [http://dx.doi.org/10.1093/ibd/izac106] [PMID: 35749298]

[7] Hendrickson BA, Gokhale R, Cho JH. Clinical aspects and pathophysiology of inflammatory bowel disease. Clin Microbiol Rev 2002; 15(1): 79-94. [http://dx.doi.org/10.1128/CMR.15.1.79-94.2002] [PMID: 11781268]

[8] Sawicki T, Ruszkowska M, Danielewicz A, Niedźwiedzka E, Arłukowicz T, Przybyłowicz KE. A review of colorectal cancer in terms of epidemiology, risk factors, development, symptoms and diagnosis. Cancers (Basel) 2021; 13(9): 2025. [http://dx.doi.org/10.3390/cancers13092025] [PMID: 33922197]

[9] O'Neill L. Crohn's disease gene is given the NOD. Trends Immunol 2001; 22(8): 418-9. [http://dx.doi.org/10.1016/S1471-4906(01)02002-6] [PMID: 11473823]

[10] Maciel-Fiuza MF, Muller GC, Campos DMS, *et al.* Role of gut microbiota in infectious and inflammatory diseases. Front Microbiol 2023; 14: 1098386. [http://dx.doi.org/10.3389/fmicb.2023.1098386] [PMID: 37051522]

[11] Sun Y, Li L, Xie R, Wang B, Jiang K, Cao H. Stress triggers flare of inflammatory bowel disease in children and adults. Front Pediatr 2019; 7: 432. [http://dx.doi.org/10.3389/fped.2019.00432] [PMID: 31709203]

[12] Lee SH, Kwon J, Cho ML. Immunological pathogenesis of inflammatory bowel disease. Intest Res 2018; 16(1): 26-42. [http://dx.doi.org/10.5217/ir.2018.16.1.26] [PMID: 29422795]

[13] Marabotto E, Kayali S, Buccilli S, *et al.* Colorectal cancer in inflammatory bowel diseases: epidemiology and prevention: a review. Cancers (Basel) 2022; 14(17): 4254. [http://dx.doi.org/10.3390/cancers14174254] [PMID: 36077786]

[14] Mattar MC, Lough D, Pishvaian MJ, Charabaty A. Current management of inflammatory bowel disease and colorectal cancer. Gastrointest Cancer Res 2011; 4(2): 53-61. [PMID: 21673876]

[15] McCoubrey LE, Favaron A, Awad A, Orlu M, Gaisford S, Basit AW. Colonic drug delivery: Formulating the next generation of colon-targeted therapeutics. J Control Release 2023; 353: 1107-26. [http://dx.doi.org/10.1016/j.jconrel.2022.12.029] [PMID: 36528195]

[16] Amidon S, Brown JE, Dave VS. Colon-targeted oral drug delivery systems: design trends and approaches. AAPS PharmSciTech 2015; 16(4): 731-41. [http://dx.doi.org/10.1208/s12249-015-0350-9] [PMID: 26070545]

[17] Sun C, Chen L, Shen Z. Mechanisms of gastrointestinal microflora on drug metabolism in clinical practice. Saudi Pharm J 2019; 27(8): 1146-56. [http://dx.doi.org/10.1016/j.jsps.2019.09.011] [PMID: 31885474]

[18] Bhalani DV, Nutan B, Kumar A, Singh Chandel AK. Bioavailability enhancement techniques for poorly aqueous soluble drugs and therapeutics. Biomedicines 2022; 10(9): 2055. [http://dx.doi.org/10.3390/biomedicines10092055] [PMID: 36140156]

[19] Cai Z, Wang S, Li J. Treatment of inflammatory bowel disease: A comprehensive review. Front Med (Lausanne) 2021; 8: 765474. [http://dx.doi.org/10.3389/fmed.2021.765474] [PMID: 34988090]

[20] Chaudhary PK, Kim S. An insight into GPCR and G-proteins as cancer drivers. Cells 2021; 10(12): 3288. [http://dx.doi.org/10.3390/cells10123288] [PMID: 34943797]

[21] Borandeh S, van Bochove B, Teotia A, Seppälä J. Polymeric drug delivery systems by additive manufacturing. Adv Drug Deliv Rev 2021; 173: 349-73. [http://dx.doi.org/10.1016/j.addr.2021.03.022] [PMID: 33831477]

[22] Varum FJO, Merchant HA, Basit AW. Oral modified-release formulations in motion: The relationship between gastrointestinal transit and drug absorption. Int J Pharm 2010; 395(1-2): 26-36. [http://dx.doi.org/10.1016/j.ijpharm.2010.04.046] [PMID: 20546855]

[23] Gómez-Guillén MC, Montero MP. Enhancement of oral bioavailability of natural compounds and probiotics by mucoadhesive tailored biopolymer-based nanoparticles: A review. Food Hydrocoll 2021; 118: 106772. [http://dx.doi.org/10.1016/j.foodhyd.2021.106772]

[24] Navarro-Ruíz E, Álvarez-Álvarez C, Peña MÁ, Torrado-Salmerón C, Dahma Z, de la Torre-Iglesias PM. Multiparticulate systems of meloxicam for colonic administration in cancer or autoimmune diseases. Pharmaceutics 2022; 14(7): 1504. [http://dx.doi.org/10.3390/pharmaceutics14071504] [PMID: 35890399]

[25] Visan AI, Cristescu R. Polysaccharide-based coatings as drug delivery systems. Pharmaceutics 2023; 15(9): 2227. [http://dx.doi.org/10.3390/pharmaceutics15092227] [PMID: 37765196]

[26] Liu L, Yao W, Rao Y, Lu X, Gao J. pH-Responsive carriers for oral drug delivery: challenges and opportunities of current platforms. Drug Deliv 2017; 24(1): 569-81. [http://dx.doi.org/10.1080/10717544.2017.1279238] [PMID: 28195032]

[27] Philip A, Philip B. Colon targeted drug delivery systems: a review on primary and novel approaches. Oman Med J 2010; 25(2): 70-8. [http://dx.doi.org/10.5001/omj.2010.24] [PMID: 22125706]

[28] Satchanska G, Davidova S, Petrov PD. Natural and synthetic polymers for biomedical and environmental applications. Polymers (Basel) 2024; 16(8): 1159. [http://dx.doi.org/10.3390/polym16081159] [PMID: 38675078]

[29] Hu T, Fang J, Shen Y, *et al.* Advances of naturally derived biomedical polymers in tissue engineering. Front Chem 2024; 12: 1469183. [http://dx.doi.org/10.3389/fchem.2024.1469183] [PMID: 39635576]

[30] Rosa V, Silikas N, Yu B, *et al.* Guidance on the assessment of biocompatibility of biomaterials: Fundamentals and testing considerations. Dent Mater 2024; 40(11): 1773-85. [http://dx.doi.org/10.1016/j.dental.2024.07.020] [PMID: 39129079]

[31] Weiss AM, Hossainy S, Rowan SJ, Hubbell JA, Esser-Kahn AP. Immunostimulatory polymers as adjuvants, immunotherapies, and delivery systems. Macromolecules 2022; 55(16): 6913-37. [http://dx.doi.org/10.1021/acs.macromol.2c00854] [PMID: 36034324]

[32] Carvalho DN, Gonçalves C, Sousa RO, Reis RL, Oliveira JM, Silva TH. Extraction and purification of biopolymers from marine origin sources envisaging their use for biotechnological applications. Mar Biotechnol (NY) 2024; 26(6): 1079-119. [http://dx.doi.org/10.1007/s10126-024-10361-5] [PMID: 39254780]

[33] Jacob EM, Borah A, Pillai SC, Kumar DS. Inflammatory bowel disease: The emergence of new trends in lifestyle and nanomedicine as the modern tool for pharmacotherapy. Nanomaterials (Basel) 2020; 10(12): 2460.
[http://dx.doi.org/10.3390/nano10122460] [PMID: 33316984]

[34] Teruel AH, Gonzalez-Alvarez I, Bermejo M, *et al.* New insights of oral colonic drug delivery systems for inflammatory bowel disease therapy. Int J Mol Sci 2020; 21(18): 6502.
[http://dx.doi.org/10.3390/ijms21186502] [PMID: 32899548]

[35] Jain S, Jain A, Jain R, Chauhan NS. Potential of natural polymeric materials in pharmaceutics. Pharmacol Res - Nat Prod [Internet] 2024.
[http://dx.doi.org/10.1016/j.prenap.2024.100014]

[36] Dubashynskaya NV, Petrova VA, Skorik YA. Biopolymer drug delivery systems for oromucosal application: Recent trends in pharmaceutical R&D. Int J Mol Sci 2024; 25(10): 5359.
[http://dx.doi.org/10.3390/ijms25105359] [PMID: 38791397]

[37] Veranič P, Erman A, Kerec-Kos M. Interactions of biopolymer chitosan with plasma membrane in biomedical applications. Colloids Surf B Biointerfaces 2012; 75-91.
[http://dx.doi.org/10.1016/B978-0-12-396534-9.00003-9]

[38] Aranaz I, Alcántara AR, Civera MC, *et al.* Chitosan: An overview of its properties and applications. Polymers (Basel) 2021; 13(19): 3256.
[http://dx.doi.org/10.3390/polym13193256] [PMID: 34641071]

[39] Yadav M, Kaushik B, Rao GK, Srivastava CM, Vaya D. Advances and challenges in the use of chitosan and its derivatives in biomedical fields: A review. Carbohydrate Polymer Technologies and Applications 2023; 5: 100323.
[http://dx.doi.org/10.1016/j.carpta.2023.100323]

[40] Kaczmarek MB, Struszczyk-Swita K, Li X, Szczęsna-Antczak M, Daroch M. Enzymatic modifications of chitin, chitosan, and chitooligosaccharides. Front Bioeng Biotechnol 2019; 7: 243.
[http://dx.doi.org/10.3389/fbioe.2019.00243] [PMID: 31612131]

[41] Jafernik K, Ładniak A, Blicharska E, *et al.* Chitosan-based nanoparticles as effective drug delivery systems—A review. Molecules 2023; 28(4): 1963.
[http://dx.doi.org/10.3390/molecules28041963] [PMID: 36838951]

[42] Du H, Liu M, Yang X, Zhai G. The design of pH-sensitive chitosan-based formulations for gastrointestinal delivery. Drug Discov Today 2015; 20(8): 1004-11.
[http://dx.doi.org/10.1016/j.drudis.2015.03.002] [PMID: 25769687]

[43] Liu M, Li Z, Li J, *et al.* Chitosan oligosaccharide alleviates DON-induced liver injury *via* suppressing ferroptosis in mice. Ecotoxicol Environ Saf 2025; 290: 117530.
[http://dx.doi.org/10.1016/j.ecoenv.2024.117530] [PMID: 39674026]

[44] Liu X, Dong Y, Wang C, Guo Z. Application of chitosan as nano carrier in the treatment of inflammatory bowel disease. Int J Biol Macromol 2024; 278(Pt 4): 134899.
[http://dx.doi.org/10.1016/j.ijbiomac.2024.134899] [PMID: 39187100]

[45] Castangia I, Nácher A, Caddeo C, *et al.* Therapeutic efficacy of quercetin enzyme-responsive nanovesicles for the treatment of experimental colitis in rats. Acta Biomater 2015; 13: 216-27.
[http://dx.doi.org/10.1016/j.actbio.2014.11.017] [PMID: 25463498]

[46] Huanbutta K, Sriamornsak P, Luangtana-anan M, *et al.* Application of multiple stepwise spinning disk processing for the synthesis of poly(methyl acrylates) coated chitosan–diclofenac sodium nanoparticles for colonic drug delivery. Eur J Pharm Sci 2013; 50(3-4): 303-11.
[http://dx.doi.org/10.1016/j.ejps.2013.07.010] [PMID: 23896171]

[47] Iglesias N, Galbis E, Díaz-Blanco MJ, Lucas R, Benito E, de-Paz MV. Nanostructured chitosan-based biomaterials for sustained and colon-specific resveratrol release. Int J Mol Sci 2019; 20(2): 398.
[http://dx.doi.org/10.3390/ijms20020398] [PMID: 30669264]

[48] Dubey R, Dubey R, Omrey P, Vyas SP, Jain SK. Development and characterization of colon specific drug delivery system bearing 5-ASA and camylofine dihydrochloride for the treatment of ulcerative colitis. J Drug Target 2010; 18(8): 589-601.
[http://dx.doi.org/10.3109/10611860903572933] [PMID: 20088681]

[49] Xiao B, Laroui H, Viennois E, *et al.* Nanoparticles with surface antibody against CD98 and carrying CD98 small interfering RNA reduce colitis in mice. Gastroenterology 2014; 146(5): 1289-1300.e19, 19.
[http://dx.doi.org/10.1053/j.gastro.2014.01.056] [PMID: 24503126]

[50] Xing L, Fu L, Cao S, Yin Y, Wei L, Zhang W. The anti-inflammatory effect of bovine bone-gelati--derived peptides in LPS-induced RAW264.7 macrophages cells and dextran sulfate sodium-induced C57BL/6 Mice. Nutrients 2022; 14(7): 1479.
[http://dx.doi.org/10.3390/nu14071479] [PMID: 35406093]

[51] Nakase H, Okazaki K, Tabata Y, *et al.* New cytokine delivery system using gelatin microspheres containing interleukin-10 for experimental inflammatory bowel disease. J Pharmacol Exp Ther 2002; 301(1): 59-65.
[http://dx.doi.org/10.1124/jpet.301.1.59] [PMID: 11907157]

[52] Kriegel C, Amiji M. Oral TNF-α gene silencing using a polymeric microsphere-based delivery system for the treatment of inflammatory bowel disease. J Control Release 2011; 150(1): 77-86.
[http://dx.doi.org/10.1016/j.jconrel.2010.10.002] [PMID: 20959130]

[53] Zhang S, Kang L, Hu S, *et al.* Carboxymethyl chitosan microspheres loaded hyaluronic acid/gelatin hydrogels for controlled drug delivery and the treatment of inflammatory bowel disease. Int J Biol Macromol 2021; 167: 1598-612.
[http://dx.doi.org/10.1016/j.ijbiomac.2020.11.117] [PMID: 33220374]

[54] Ahmad A, Ansari MM, Mishra RK, *et al.* Enteric-coated gelatin nanoparticles mediated oral delivery of 5-aminosalicylic acid alleviates severity of DSS-induced ulcerative colitis. Mater Sci Eng C 2021; 119: 111582.
[http://dx.doi.org/10.1016/j.msec.2020.111582] [PMID: 33321628]

[55] Amirrah IN, Lokanathan Y, Zulkiflee I, Wee MFMR, Motta A, Fauzi MB. A comprehensive review on collagen type I development of biomaterials for tissue engineering: From biosynthesis to bioscaffold. Biomedicines 2022; 10(9): 2307.
[http://dx.doi.org/10.3390/biomedicines10092307] [PMID: 36140407]

[56] Dubey NK, Deng WP. Polymeric gels for cartilage tissue engineering. Polymeric Gels. Elsevier 2018; pp. 505-25. Internet
[http://dx.doi.org/10.1016/B978-0-08-102179-8.00020-X]

[57] Bakar AJA, Azam NSM, Sevakumaran V, *et al.* Effectiveness of collagen and gatifloxacin in improving the healing and antibacterial activities of gellan gum hydrogel films as dressing materials. Int J Biol Macromol 2023; 245: 125494.
[http://dx.doi.org/10.1016/j.ijbiomac.2023.125494] [PMID: 37348586]

[58] Sarrigiannidis SO, Rey JM, Dobre O, González-García C, Dalby MJ, Salmeron-Sanchez M. A tough act to follow: collagen hydrogel modifications to improve mechanical and growth factor loading capabilities. Mater Today Bio 2021; 10: 100098.
[http://dx.doi.org/10.1016/j.mtbio.2021.100098] [PMID: 33763641]

[59] Zhang W, Michalowski CB, Beloqui A. Oral delivery of biologics in inflammatory bowel disease treatment. Front Bioeng Biotechnol 2021; 9: 675194.
[http://dx.doi.org/10.3389/fbioe.2021.675194] [PMID: 34150733]

[60] O'Sullivan S, Gilmer JF, Medina C. Matrix Metalloproteinases in Inflammatory Bowel Disease: An Update. Oral HB, editor. Mediators Inflamm 2015; 8(1)
[http://dx.doi.org/10.1155/2015/964131]

[61] Lu P, Ruan D, Huang M, *et al.* Harnessing the potential of hydrogels for advanced therapeutic applications: current achievements and future directions. Signal Transduct Target Ther 2024; 9(1): 166.
[http://dx.doi.org/10.1038/s41392-024-01852-x] [PMID: 38945949]

[62] Xin XY, Zhou J, Liu GG, Zhang MY, Li XZ, Wang Y. Anti-inflammatory activity of collagen peptide *in vitro* and its effect on improving ulcerative colitis. NPJ Sci Food [Internet] 2025; 9(1)

[63] Kuppusamy S, Sathesh Kumar K, Devadasan V, Kuppusamy S. Formulation of a thermo-sensitive hydro-gel for ulcerative colitis treatment. Bioinformation 2022; 18(10): 925-37.
[http://dx.doi.org/10.6026/97320630018925] [PMID: 37654823]

[64] Ramadass SK, Jabaris SL, Perumal RK, HairulIslam VI, Gopinath A, Madhan B. Type I collagen and its daughter peptides for targeting mucosal healing in ulcerative colitis: A new treatment strategy. Eur J Pharm Sci 2016; 91: 216-24.
[http://dx.doi.org/10.1016/j.ejps.2016.05.015] [PMID: 27185300]

[65] Koelink PJ, Overbeek SA, Braber S, *et al.* Collagen degradation and neutrophilic infiltration: a vicious circle in inflammatory bowel disease. Gut 2014; 63(4): 578-87.
[http://dx.doi.org/10.1136/gutjnl-2012-303252] [PMID: 23525573]

[66] Ramadass SK, Perumal S, Jabaris SL, Madhan B. Preparation and evaluation of mesalamine collagen *in situ* rectal gel: A novel therapeutic approach for treating ulcerative colitis. Eur J Pharm Sci 2013; 48(1-2): 104-10.
[http://dx.doi.org/10.1016/j.ejps.2012.10.015] [PMID: 23137838]

[67] Rahabi M, Salon M, Bruno-Bonnet C, *et al.* Bioactive fish collagen peptides weaken intestinal inflammation by orienting colonic macrophages phenotype through mannose receptor activation. Eur J Nutr 2022; 61(4): 2051-66.
[http://dx.doi.org/10.1007/s00394-021-02787-7] [PMID: 34999930]

[68] Valachová K, Hassan ME, Šoltés L. Hyaluronan: Sources, structure, features and applications. Molecules 2024; 29(3): 739.
[http://dx.doi.org/10.3390/molecules29030739] [PMID: 38338483]

[69] de Oliveira JD, Carvalho LS, Gomes AMV, Queiroz LR, Magalhães BS, Parachin NS. Genetic basis for hyper production of hyaluronic acid in natural and engineered microorganisms. Microb Cell Fact 2016; 15(1): 119.
[http://dx.doi.org/10.1186/s12934-016-0517-4] [PMID: 27370777]

[70] Dovedytis M, Liu ZJ, Bartlett S. Hyaluronic acid and its biomedical applications: A review. Eng Regen [Internet] 2020; 1: 102-3.
[http://dx.doi.org/10.1016/j.engreg.2020.10.001]

[71] Dicker KT, Gurski LA, Pradhan-Bhatt S, Witt RL, Farach-Carson MC, Jia X. Hyaluronan: A simple polysaccharide with diverse biological functions. Acta Biomater 2014; 10(4): 1558-70.
[http://dx.doi.org/10.1016/j.actbio.2013.12.019] [PMID: 24361428]

[72] Inubushi T, Nag P, Sasaki JI, Shiraishi Y, Yamashiro T. The significant role of glycosaminoglycans in tooth development. Glycobiology 2024; 34(5): cwae024.
[http://dx.doi.org/10.1093/glycob/cwae024] [PMID: 38438145]

[73] Petrey AC, de la Motte CA. Hyaluronan in inflammatory bowel disease: Cross-linking inflammation and coagulation. Matrix Biol 2019; 78-79: 314-23.
[http://dx.doi.org/10.1016/j.matbio.2018.03.011] [PMID: 29574062]

[74] Kaur L, Bala R, Kanojia N, Nagpal M, Dhingra GA. Formulation development and optimization of fast dissolving tablets of aceclofenac using natural superdisintegrant. ISRN Pharm 2014; 2014: 1-10.
[http://dx.doi.org/10.1155/2014/242504] [PMID: 24944837]

[75] Vafaei SY, Abdolghaffari AH, Mahjub R, Eslami SM, Esmaeili M, Abdollahi M, *et al.* Budesonide-Loaded Hyaluronic Acid Nanoparticles for Targeted Delivery to the Inflamed Intestinal Mucosa in a

Rodent Model of Colitis. Ahad A, editor Biomed Res Int [Internet] 2022; 27(1) [http://dx.doi.org/10.1155/2022/7776092]

[76] Zhao X, Zhang Y, Wang P, *et al.* Layer by layer self-assembled hyaluronic acid nanoarmor for the treatment of ulcerative colitis. J Nanobiotechnology 2024; 22(1): 633. [http://dx.doi.org/10.1186/s12951-024-02933-3] [PMID: 39420343]

[77] Mairal A, Mehrotra S, Kumar A, Maiwal R, Marsal J, Kumar A. Hyaluronic acid-conjugated thermoresponsive polymer-based bioformulation enhanced wound healing and gut barrier repair of a TNBS-induced colitis injury *ex vivo* model in a dynamic perfusion device. ACS Appl Mater Interfaces 2024; 16(5): 5382-400. [http://dx.doi.org/10.1021/acsami.3c14113] [PMID: 38266010]

[78] Jhundoo HD, Siefen T, Liang A, *et al.* Hyaluronic acid increases anti-inflammatory efficacy of rectal 5-amino salicylic acid administration in a murine colitis model. Biomol Ther (Seoul) 2021; 29(5): 536-44. [http://dx.doi.org/10.4062/biomolther.2020.227] [PMID: 34059563]

[79] Aprodu A, Mantaj J, Raimi-Abraham B, Vllasaliu D. Evaluation of a methylcellulose and hyaluronic acid hydrogel as a vehicle for rectal delivery of biologics. Pharmaceutics 2019; 11(3): 127. [http://dx.doi.org/10.3390/pharmaceutics11030127] [PMID: 30893796]

[80] Huai M, Pei M, Chen J, *et al.* Oral creatine-modified selenium-based hyaluronic acid nanogel mediated mitochondrial energy recovery to drive the treatment of inflammatory bowel disease. J Nanobiotechnology 2024; 22(1): 740. [http://dx.doi.org/10.1186/s12951-024-03007-0] [PMID: 39609811]

[81] Hutapea TPH, Madurani KA, Syahputra MY, Hudha MN, Asriana AN. Suprapto, et al. Albumin: Source, preparation, determination, applications, and prospects. J Sci Adv Mater Devices [Internet] 2023; 8(2): 100549.

[82] Mishra V, Heath RJ. Structural and biochemical features of human serum albumin essential for eukaryotic cell culture. Int J Mol Sci 2021; 22(16): 8411. [http://dx.doi.org/10.3390/ijms22168411] [PMID: 34445120]

[83] Larsen MT, Kuhlmann M, Hvam ML, Howard KA. Albumin-based drug delivery: Harnessing nature to cure disease. Mol Cell Ther 2016; 4(1): 3. [http://dx.doi.org/10.1186/s40591-016-0048-8] [PMID: 26925240]

[84] Gao J, Li J, Luo Z, Wang H, Ma Z. Nanoparticle-based drug delivery systems for inflammatory bowel disease treatment. Drug Des Devel Ther 2024; 18: 2921-49. [http://dx.doi.org/10.2147/DDDT.S461977] [PMID: 39055164]

[85] Raghuwanshi VS, Yu B, Browne C, Garnier G. Reversible pH responsive bovine serum albumin hydrogel sponge nanolayer. Front Bioeng Biotechnol 2020; 8: 573. [http://dx.doi.org/10.3389/fbioe.2020.00573] [PMID: 32582681]

[86] Kragh-Hansen U. Possible mechanisms by which enzymatic degradation of human serum albumin can lead to bioactive peptides and biomarkers. Front Mol Biosci 2018; 5: 63. [http://dx.doi.org/10.3389/fmolb.2018.00063] [PMID: 30038906]

[87] Watanabe K, Kinoshita H, Okamoto T, Sugiura K, Kawashima S, Kimura T. Antioxidant properties of albumin and diseases related to obstetrics and gynecology. Antioxidants 2025; 14(1): 55. [http://dx.doi.org/10.3390/antiox14010055] [PMID: 39857389]

[88] Zhang S, Cho WJ, Jin A, Korzenik J, Lennerz J, Traverso C. Albumin-based nanoparticles for drug combination in inflammatory bowel disease. Gastroenterology 2021; 160(3): S46. [http://dx.doi.org/10.1053/j.gastro.2021.01.129] [PMID: 33022277]

[89] Iwao Y, Tomiguchi I, Domura A, *et al.* Inflamed site-specific drug delivery system based on the interaction of human serum albumin nanoparticles with myeloperoxidase in a murine model of experimental colitis. Eur J Pharm Biopharm 2018; 125: 141-7.

[http://dx.doi.org/10.1016/j.ejpb.2018.01.016] [PMID: 29407223]

[90] Li B, Liu X, Long Q, *et al.* Inflammation responsive tofacitinib loaded albumin nanomedicine for targeted synergistic therapy in ulcerative colitis. Nano Res 2023; 16(7): 9873-84. [http://dx.doi.org/10.1007/s12274-023-5743-6]

[91] Mneimneh AT, Mehanna MM. Chondroitin Sulphate: An emerging therapeutic multidimensional proteoglycan in colon cancer. Int J Biol Macromol 2024; 254(Pt 1): 127672. [http://dx.doi.org/10.1016/j.ijbiomac.2023.127672] [PMID: 38287564]

[92] Shen Q, Guo Y, Wang K, Zhang C, Ma Y. A review of chondroitin sulfate's preparation, properties, functions, and applications. Molecules 2023; 28(20): 7093. [http://dx.doi.org/10.3390/molecules28207093] [PMID: 37894574]

[93] Miller T, Goude MC, McDevitt TC, Temenoff JS. Molecular engineering of glycosaminoglycan chemistry for biomolecule delivery. Acta Biomater 2014; 10(4): 1705-19. [http://dx.doi.org/10.1016/j.actbio.2013.09.039] [PMID: 24121191]

[94] Ramasamy T, Subbaih Khandasamy U, Shanmugam S, Ruttala H. Formulation and evaluation of chondroitin sulphate tablets of aceclofenac for colon targeted drug delivery. Iran J Pharm Res IJPR [Internet] 2012; 11(2): 465-79.

[95] Azimijou N, Karimi-Soflou R, Karkhaneh A. CD44 targeted-chondroitin sulfate nanoparticles: Fine-tuning hydrophobic groups to enhance *in vitro* pH-responsiveness and *in vivo* efficacy for advanced breast cancer treatment. Biomaterials Advances 2024; 158: 213776. [http://dx.doi.org/10.1016/j.bioadv.2024.213776] [PMID: 38244368]

[96] Chen Y, Shui M, Yuan Q, *et al.* Oral chondroitin sulfate functionalized natural polyphenol for targeted therapy of ulcerative colitis. Mater Des 2024; 238: 112645. [http://dx.doi.org/10.1016/j.matdes.2024.112645]

[97] Onishi H, Ikeuchi-Takahashi Y, Kawano K, Hattori Y. Preparation of chondroitin sulfate-glycy--prednisolone conjugate nanogel and its efficacy in rats with ulcerative colitis. Biol Pharm Bull 2019; 42(7): 1155-63. [http://dx.doi.org/10.1248/bpb.b19-00020] [PMID: 31257292]

[98] Long M, Li J, Yang M, *et al.* Rosmarinic acid-chondroitin sulfate nanoconjugate for targeted treatment of ulcerative colitis. Int J Biol Macromol 2025; 306(Pt 3): 141008. [http://dx.doi.org/10.1016/j.ijbiomac.2025.141008] [PMID: 39971022]

[99] Amrutkar JR, Gattani SG. Chitosan-chondroitin sulfate based matrix tablets for colon specific delivery of indomethacin. AAPS PharmSciTech 2009; 10(2): 670-7. [http://dx.doi.org/10.1208/s12249-009-9253-y] [PMID: 19459052]

[100] Ferdowsian HR, Beck N. Ethical and Scientific Considerations Regarding Animal Testing and Research. MacCallum CJ, editor PLoS One [Internet] 2011; 6(9): e24059. [http://dx.doi.org/10.1371/journal.pone.0024059]

[101] Varzakas T, Antoniadou M. A holistic approach for ethics and sustainability in the food chain: the gateway to oral and systemic health. Foods 2024; 13(8): 1224. [http://dx.doi.org/10.3390/foods13081224] [PMID: 38672896]

[102] Pereira S, Veeraraghavan P, Ghosh S, Gandhi M. Animal experimentation and ethics in India: the CPCSEA makes a difference. Altern Lab Anim 2004; 32(1_suppl) (Suppl. 1B): 411-5. [http://dx.doi.org/10.1177/026119290403201s67] [PMID: 23581110]

[103] Wang JR, Oh E, Aronow B, Bernstein WK. The unseen animal behind medicine: exploring considerations of animal-derived medications and anaesthetics in today's landscape. BJA Open 2025; 13: 100360. [http://dx.doi.org/10.1016/j.bjao.2024.100360] [PMID: 39802095]

[104] Koutsoumanis K, Allende A, Bolton D, *et al.* BSE risk posed by ruminant collagen and gelatine derived from bones. EFSA J 2024; 22(7): e8883.

[PMID: 39015303]

[105] Marsit NM, Saadawi S, Alennabi K. Challenges of growth-based microbiological methods in sterility assurance of pharmaceutical product manufacturing. Discov Pharm Sci [Internet] 2025; 1(1): 13. [http://dx.doi.org/10.1007/s44395-025-00020-6]

[106] Singh VK, Gunasekaran P, Kumari M, Krishnan D, Ramachandran VK. Animal sourced biopolymer for mitigating xenobiotics and hazardous materials. Physical Sciences Reviews 2024; 9(4): 1731-46. [http://dx.doi.org/10.1515/psr-2022-0221]

[107] Khodaei D, Álvarez C, Mullen AM. Biodegradable packaging materials from animal processing co-products and wastes: An overview. Polymers (Basel) 2021; 13(15): 2561. [http://dx.doi.org/10.3390/polym13152561] [PMID: 34372163]

CHAPTER 6

Microbial-Derived Polymers: Revolutionizing Inflammatory Bowel Disease Treatment

Rashmi Dewangan[1] and **Nikita Verma**[2,*]

[1] *Department of Pharmacy, Guru Ghasidas Vishwavidyalaya, Bilaspur 495009, Chhattisgarh, India*

[2] *MATS School of Pharmacy, MATS University, Raipur 493441, Chhattisgarh, India*

Abstract: Inflammatory Bowel Disease (IBD), comprising Crohn's disease and ulcerative colitis, is a persistent gastrointestinal disorder marked by immune dysregulation and imbalances in gut flora. Conventional therapy modalities, including corticosteroids, immunosuppressants, and monoclonal antibodies, frequently result in side effects and inconsistent patient responses. Recent advancements in biomaterials have underscored the potential of microbial-derived polymers as novel therapeutic carriers for the management of IBD. Polymers isolated from microbes are sourced from bacterial, fungal, and algal origins. Bacterial polysaccharides, such as xanthan gum, dextran, pullulan, curdlan, and bacterial cellulose, provide superior biocompatibility, muco-adhesive characteristics, and controlled drug release potential. Polymers derived from fungi, such as xanthan-like polymers, chitosan, and β-glucan, have bioadhesive and antibacterial properties that facilitate mucosal healing. Algal polysaccharides such as alginate and carrageenan facilitate pH-sensitive drug release, ensuring precise delivery to the inflamed intestinal mucosa. Microbial-derived polymers function as multifaceted carriers in IBD drug delivery, developing advanced formulations including hydrogels, nanoparticles, dendrimers, nanofibers, nanosuspensions, microspheres, and vesicles. Hydrogels enable prolonged drug release, preserving moisture and enhancing mucosal regeneration. Nanoparticles and microspheres improve drug stability and bioavailability, facilitating accurate targeting of inflamed regions. Dendrimers and nanofibers have substantial drug-loading capacities, facilitating sustained and controlled therapeutic effects, whereas nanosuspensions enhance solubility and absorption. This chapter discusses microbial-derived polymers, their optimal characteristics for colorectal drug delivery, classifications based on charge, various biological sources, and the multifunctional roles of these polymers as therapeutic carriers. By utilizing these advanced drug delivery technologies, microbial polymers are enabling more effective and targeted treatments for IBD, resulting in diminished side effects and enhanced patient compliance.

[*] **Corresponding author Nikita Verma** MATS School of Pharmacy, MATS University, Raipur 493441, Chhattisgarh, India; E-mail: nikitaverma510@gmail.com

Meenakshi Jaiswal & S.K. Lanjhiyana (Eds.)

Keywords: Alginates, Beta-glucan, Exopolysaccharides, IBD, Microbial-derived polymers.

INTRODUCTION

The mucosal immune system maintains a balanced response between pro- and anti-inflammatory micellar responses in a healthy gut [1]. This allows for appropriate defence against pathogens while also preventing an overwhelming immune response against a large number of harmless food antigens and commensal microbes [2]. Due to the hyperactivation of immune effector cells that produce high quantities of pro-inflammatory cytokines such as TNF-α, IL-6, and IFN-γ, the immunological response in IBD is turned towards pro-inflammation [3]. Nuclear Factor kappa B (NF-κB), a transcription factor, is essential for the regulation and modulation of the mucosal immune system [4]. NF-κB is widely expressed in all cell types and triggers several pro-inflammatory genes, including pro-inflammatory cytokines [5]. Increased NF-κB p65 expression in biopsied tissue from IBD patients, especially those with Crohn's disease, indicates that NF-κB is significantly overactivated in IBD [6]. IBD is a serious public health issue on a global scale [7]. Current therapeutic techniques, such as immunosuppressants, biological therapies, and anti-inflammatory drugs, are often ineffective and have detrimental effects on health [8]. The use of natural compounds to target key pathogenic pathways in IBD is therefore of great interest [9]. Seaweed contains a wide range of structurally varied biologically active compounds. Intestinal epithelium cells, reactive oxygen, nitrogen, cytokines, chemokines, adhesion molecules, and nuclear factor NF-kB [10, 11]. This is why it is necessary to consider a personalised medicine delivery method for IBD. The novel tailored drug-delivery approach can deliver medication directly to the site of inflammation based on the pathological characteristics associated with IBD, improving medication accumulation and reducing adverse effects [11]. A better knowledge of the mechanisms underlying the effects of polysaccharides from different algal species, each with a distinct structure and molecular weight, on intestinal microbes, as well as immunological and epithelial cells, will aid in the development of pharmaceuticals and nutritional supplements [12]. Faecal transplantation, medication therapy, and surgery are all part of the treatment for IBD [13]. However, because many patients have post-operative recurrence, which lowers their quality of life and causes more intestinal damage, surgery does not cure the problem [14]. Mesenchymal Stem Cells (MSCs) have recently attracted a lot of attention due to their immunomodulatory and tissue-healing capabilities, which makes cell-based therapies a promising treatment option for IBD. MSCs release a variety of bioactive compounds that can influence immune responses and hasten tissue regeneration, including growth factors and anti-inflammatory cytokines [15]. Understanding the effects of these interactions on human health is still necessary, though. For instance, individuals with inflammatory bowel illness have been shown to express TLR4 more than normal [16]. Sulfated polysaccharides, found in seaweed, have demonstrated an anti-inflammatory effect on the illness. Using an enzymatic process, LMW-ulvan, a new low molecular weight sulfate Ulva polysaccharide, was produced. [17] The availability of treatments with a variety of modes of action, such as anti-integrins that block leukocyte trafficking or anti-tumor necrosis factor and anti-interleukin [18]. These studies generally showed that active targeting is a promising strategy for improving drug accumulation and uptake in IBD inflammatory tissues, even though more research is needed to evaluate the efficacy and stability of various targeted ligands and formulations in IBD models [19].

Microbial-derived polymers have numerous advantages over synthetic polymers for the treatment of IBD, owing to their biocompatibility, biodegradability, and biological functioning [20, 21]. In contrast to synthetic polymers, which frequently necessitate surface modification to enhance biocompatibility or cellular contact, microbial polymers inherently possess bioadhesive and immunomodulatory characteristics, hence facilitating mucosal healing and medication retention at inflamed intestinal sites [22]. They are biologically derived, non-toxic, and able to replicate the natural extracellular milieu, facilitating epithelium regeneration [23]. Additionally, microbial polymers like dextran, xanthan gum, gellan gum, pullulan, and bacterial cellulose exhibit mucoadhesive and pH-sensitive properties, facilitating targeted and prolonged release of drugs in the colon, thus reducing systemic adverse effects [24]. Synthetic polymers, by contrast, can provide hazardous breakdown products and lack biological recognition, hence constraining their therapeutic efficacy in chronic inflammatory disorders such as IBD [20]. Microbial-derived polymers integrate natural bioactivity, environmentally sustainable manufacturing, and patient safety, rendering them exceptional prospects for colon-targeted delivery of drugs and mucosal tissue healing in IBD treatment [25]. This chapter will examine microbial-derived polymers, their categorization, and their function in the management of IBD.

MICROBIAL-DERIVED POLYMERS

Microbial-derived polymers can be produced by various microorganisms, including bacteria, actinomycetes, yeast, archaea, and fungi [19]. Every biopolymer has distinct characteristics and can be modified for the colon-targeted drug delivery in the treatment of IBD [20].

Ideal Characteristics of Microbial-derived Polymers for IBD Treatment

Biocompatibility and Biodegradability

The microbial-derived polymer must be non-toxic and decompose into safe by-products to prevent adverse effects on the sensitive gut environment and ensure compatibility with intestinal bacteria [21].

pH-responsive

Microbial-derived polymer must maintain stability at the acidic pH of the stomach while degrading or releasing the drug at the neutral to slightly alkaline pH of the colon (pH 6–7.5), ensuring targeted delivery [22].

Enzyme-responsive Behaviour

The polymer must exhibit sensitivity to certain enzymes generated by colonic bacteria, such as β-glucuronidase and azoreductase, to enable targeted drug release in the colon [23].

Mucus-Penetrating Ability

The polymer must possess adequate hydrophilicity and particle size to traverse the dense mucus barrier of the gut walls without being entrapped [24].

Stability During GI Transit

To ensure stability throughout gastrointestinal transit, the polymer must endure the acidic milieu, proteolytic enzymes, and mechanical stresses in the upper gastrointestinal tract before arriving intact in the colon [25].

Controlled and Sustained Release

The polymer must facilitate regulated and prolonged drug release at the site of inflammation, thereby decreasing dosage frequency and minimizing systemic adverse effects [26].

Anti-inflammatory and Prebiotic Properties

The polymer may assist in diminishing inflammation or regulating the gut microbiota to foster a healthy bacterial equilibrium, therefore facilitating disease management [27].

Adhesion and Retention inside the Colon

The polymer must adhere to the intestinal mucosa to localize the drugs to the site of inflammation, hence improving therapeutic efficacy [28].

Ease of Functionalization

The polymer must facilitate chemical modifications to conjugate with therapeutic drugs, diagnostic agents, or ligands for the targeted delivery of therapeutics to inflamed areas [29].

Scalable and Economical Production

Polymers generated from microbes must be easily scalable, reproducible, and cost-effective to formulate, while ensuring consistent quality for clinical applications [30].

Classification of Microbial-derived Polymers

Microbial-derived polymers can be classified on the basis of the charges they carry, their structure, and their biological origin [31].

According to the charge they carry, they can be classified into three categories (Fig. **1**).

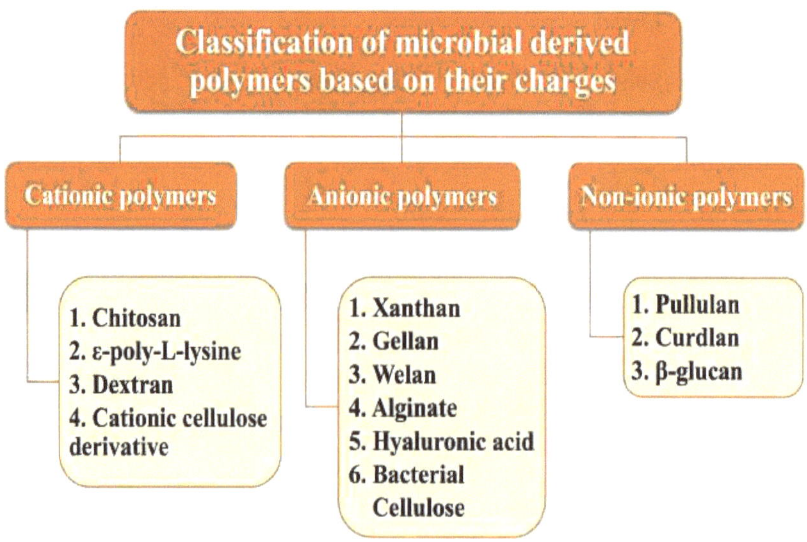

Fig. (1). Classification of microbial-derived polymers based on their charges.

Cationic Polymers

These biopolymers have a net positive charge, which allows them to interact well with drug molecules and biological macromolecules that have a negative charge [32]. Examples include chitosan, ε-poly-L-lysine, dextran, derivatives of PGA, pullulan derivatives, cationic cellulose derivatives, *etc.* [19].

Anionic Biopolymers

These biopolymers exhibit a net negative charge, enabling interactions with positively charged molecules. Illustrations include the following: xanthan, gellan, welan gum, alginate, hyaluronic acid, and bacterial cellulose [31].

Non-Ionic Biopolymers

These biopolymers are neutral and devoid of substantial cationic or anionic charges. They are widely used for their stabilizing and structural attributes. Few non-ionic polymers include pullulan, curdlan, and β-glucan [33].

On the basis of biological origin, they are classified into three classes (Fig. **2**);

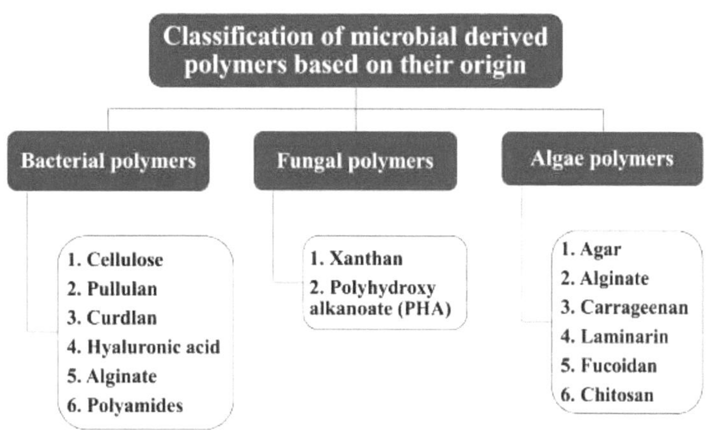

Fig. (2). Classification of microbial-derived polymers based on their source of extraction.

Bacteria-derived Polymers

Bacteria synthesize diverse biopolymers, such as polysaccharides, polyamides, polyesters, and polyphosphates, each serving unique structural and functional purposes [34]. Polysaccharides, glycosidically linked to sugar or sugar acids, may be intracellular, as exemplified by glycogen and levan, or secreted as capsular polysaccharides, including polysialic acid, pneumococcal polysaccharides, and

Staphylococcus capsular polysaccharides [35]. Additionally, they may produce exopolysaccharides that support the biofilm matrix in sessile bacterial culture, including cellulose, pullulan, curdlan, hyaluronic acid, and alginate [36]. Polyamides, shown by PGA, are formed by peptide linkage between amino acids, whereas poly-hydroxyalkanoates like polyesters are composed of ester linkage between hydroxyl-fatty acids [37]. Furthermore, inorganic phosphates are linked by anhydride bonds to form polyphosphates. These biopolymers perform multiple roles, such as energy storage, structural reinforcement, and augmentation of bacterial virulence [38].

Fungal-derived Polymers

Fungal polysaccharides, including chitosan and β-glucans, possess mucoadhesive properties, provide controlled drug release, and exhibit immunomodulatory effects, rendering them appropriate for the delivery of anti-inflammatory drugs to inflamed intestinal regions [39]. Exopolysaccharides, such as xanthan-like polymers, confer stability and elevated viscosity, facilitating the development of colon-targeted drug delivery systems [40]. Lipid-based fungal polymers, including PHAs, can function as biocompatible carriers for encapsulating and delivering therapeutic agents to inflamed mucosa, thereby minimizing systemic side effects [41].

Algae-derived Polymers

Polymers derived from algae are very advantageous in the treatment of IBD owing to their biocompatibility, gel-forming capabilities, and targeted drug release characteristics [42]. Alginate-based systems, comprising sodium alginate, calcium alginate, and alginate hydrogels, are extensively utilized for pH-sensitive and colon-specific drug delivery, facilitating the efficient release of drugs in the intestinal milieu [43]. Anionic polysaccharides, including carrageenan and agar, improve formulation stability and facilitate prolonged drug release [44]. Hybrid polymers, such as alginate-chitosan composites, enhance mucoadhesion and facilitate regulated drug release, whilst neutral polysaccharides like laminarin demonstrate anti-inflammatory effects, hence aiding in the management of IBD (Fig. **3**) [45]. These polymers facilitate the development of targeted formulations, including hydrogels, microspheres, and nanocarriers, for targeted and effective IBD treatment [10].

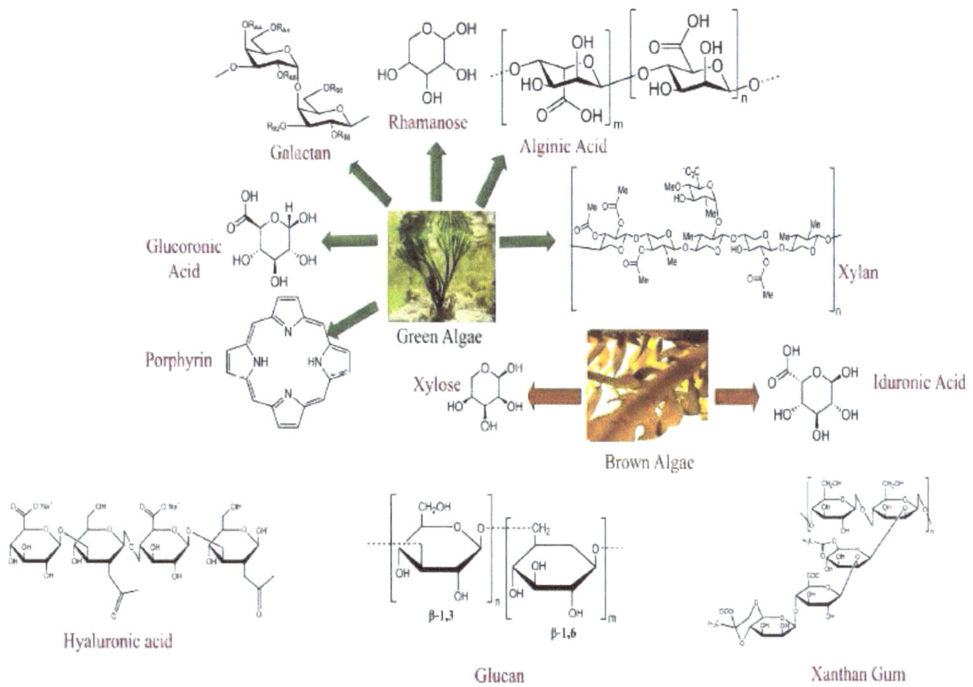

Fig. (3). Microbial-derived polymer for treatment of IBD.

ROLE OF MICROBIAL-DERIVED POLYMERS IN IBD

Polymers derived from microbes are increasingly utilized for targeting the colon in the treatment of IBD, including ulcerative colitis and Crohn's disease [64]. They function as nanocarriers to improve permeability, penetration, and bioavailability, or as microcarriers for localized and sustained drug release, employing pH-responsive and time-dependent mechanisms for efficient delivery (Fig. **4**) [65, 66].

Alginate

Alginate, an anionic polysaccharide consisting of β-D-mannuronic acid and α L-guluronic acid connected by 1,4-glycosidic linkages, is predominantly derived from brown seaweeds (*e.g.*, Laminaria, Macrocystis) and bacteria such as Pseudomonas and Azotobacter [67]. Its distinctive characteristics, including pH sensitivity, biodegradability, and the capacity to undergo a sol-gel transition under the influence of bivalent metal cations such as Ca^{2+}, render it optimal for drug delivery applications [68]. Alginate-based solutions in IBD facilitate targeted drug release, improved biocompatibility, and regulated encapsulation, resulting in higher therapeutic efficacy [69]. Applications encompass nanoparticle formulations to enhance bioavailability, microparticles for localized release, and *in situ* gels for targeted delivery within the gastrointestinal system [70].

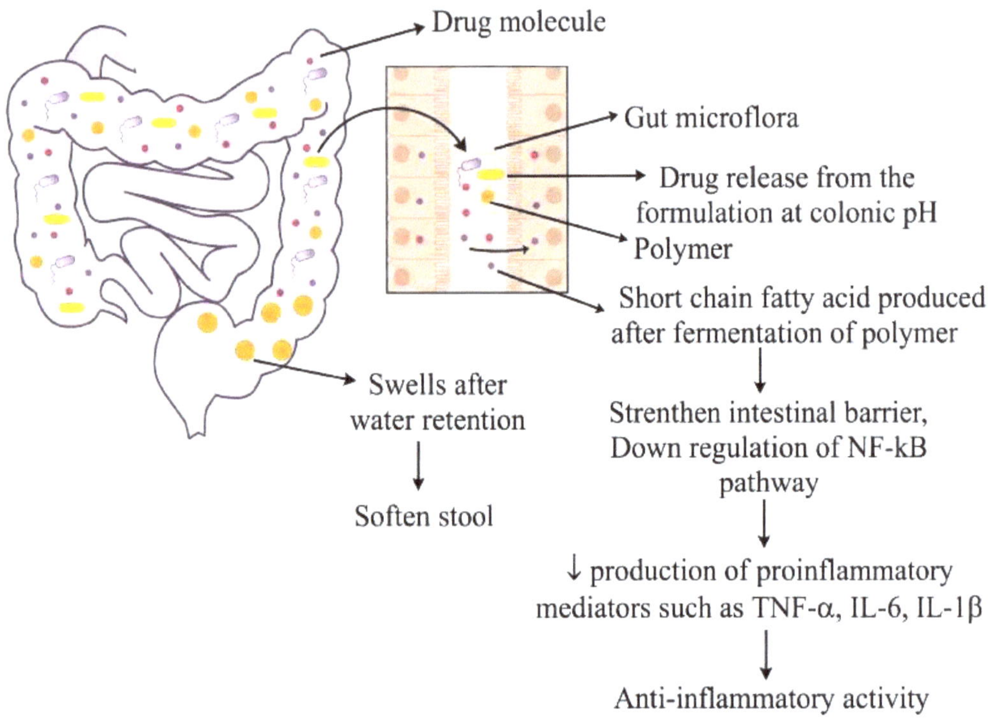

Fig. (4). Mechanism of action of various polymers for the treatment of IBD.

Infliximab (IFX) was encapsulated in chitosan/carboxymethyl chitosan and alginate-based nano-in-microparticles for oral administration in IBD. These polymers safeguard IFX against gastrointestinal degradation and facilitate targeted delivery to the inflamed intestine. *In vivo* experiments demonstrated that the nanocarriers significantly mitigated colitis by diminishing inflammation and retaining the functionality of the gastrointestinal mucosal membrane. This polymeric delivery method improves IFX stability and therapeutic effectiveness in IBD [71].

In 2023, X. Zhang *et al.* formulated a novel nanotherapeutic, LBL-CO@MPDA, for the treatment of IBD by employing a layer-by-layer assembly of chitosan/alginate polyelectrolytes on mesoporous Polydopamine Nanoparticles (MPDA) loaded with a CO prodrug [72]. The anionic polymer covering promotes targeted deposition in inflammatory colon lesions through electrostatic interactions. In the oxidative colonic microenvironment, the system releases carbon monoxide in a responsive manner, scavenging reactive oxygen species and modifying immune responses [73]. Carbon monoxide emission activates heme oxygenase-1, facilitating macrophage M2 polarization and inhibiting inflammatory pathways (p38 MAPK, NF-κB). This method reinstates gut barrier integrity and homeostasis by mitigating oxidative stress, immunological dysfunction, and microbial imbalance [72].

Xu *et al.* formulated a sodium alginate-based hydrogel encapsulating lutein nanoparticles to efficiently provide lutein to the inflamed colon and address DSS-induced colitis. The hydrogel augmented the production of ZO-1, claudin-1, and occludin-like intestinal tight junction proteins, inhibited the NF-κB pathway, and reduced inflammatory factors (TNF-α, iNOS, NLRP3, and IL-1β), thereby preserving intestinal barrier integrity. It also altered the gut microbiota by decreasing *Desulfovibrionaceae* and increasing *Erysipelotrichaceae* and *Rikenellaceae*. In comparison to lutein crystals, the hydrogel demonstrated enhanced anti-inflammatory properties, underscoring the promise of sodium alginate as a slow-release vehicle for IBD treatment (Table **1**) [74].

Table 1. Microbial-derived polymers used in IBD.

Sr. No.	Microbial-derived Polymers	Source	Experimental Assay	References
1.	Fucoidan	Brown Algae *Cladosiphon okamuranus, Tokida* and *Kjellmaniella crassifolia*	Reduces chronic colitis in the colon of dextran sodium sulfate-treated mice, which has been shown to inhibit IL-6 production in CMT-93 cells and decrease NF-kB nuclear translocation.	[46]
2.	β-glucan	*Laminaria hyperborea* and *Laminaria digitate*	Decrease the expression of Th17-associated cytokines (IL-17a, IL-17F, and IL-22), as well as receptor IL-23R, and IL-6, with no alteration to the T regulatory cell (TREG)–related targets.	[47]
3.	Oligosaccharide	*Ulva*	Induce the proliferation of RAW264.7 macrophages.	[48]
4.	Polysaccharide	*Ulva lactuca*	Protective effect on DSS-induced acute colitis in mice, and ULP-SeNPs inhibited the activation of macrophages by suppressing the nuclear translocation of NF-κB.	[49]
5.	Alginate	*Enterococcus fecium; Staphylococcus succinus*	Enhancement of the bioavailability of the probiotic strains.	[50]

(Table 1) cont.....

Sr. No.	Microbial-derived Polymers	Source	Experimental Assay	References
6.	Fucoidan	*Laminaria japonica*	Reduces H_2O_2-induced paracellular permeability. Up-regulates the expression of claudin-1, claudin-2, and occludin.	[51]
7.	Polysaccharides	*Gracilaria lemaneiformis*	Improves DSS-induced colitis symptoms, alters intestinal microbes, increases SCFA production, and downregulates CCL25/CCR9 and TGF-β1 levels.	[52]
8.	Polysaccharides	*Blidingia minima*	Repairs colon dysfunction and colonic morphology, improves the expression of tight junction proteins, and decreases pro-inflammatory cytokine levels.	[53]
9.	Sulfate ulva polysaccharide	*Ulva pertusa*	Decreases colon shortening and colonic tissue damage.	[17]
10.	Fucoidan	*Ecklonia cava*	Inhibits ROS and NO production.	[54]
11.	Crude polysaccharide	*Sargassum thungbergii*	Increases intestinal beneficial bacteria.	[55]
12.	Fucoidan	*Undaria pinnatifida*	Reduces weight gain and fat accumulation and restores the expected level of Firmicutes and Bacteroidetes in mice fed high-fat diets.	[56]
13.	Crude sulfated polysaccharide	*Sargassum fusiforme*	Increases the availability of Faecal bacterium, Phascolarcto bacterium, Ruminococcaeceae, and Lactobacillus	[55]

Hyaluronic Acid

Hyaluronic acid, a glycosaminoglycan found in vertebrate tissues, consists of repeated units of N-acetylglucosamine (NAG) and D-glucuronic acid connected by consecutive β-1,3 and β-1,4 glycosidic linkages, with the chemical formula $(C_{14}H_{21}NO_{11})n$ [75]. Hyaluronic acid is produced *via* microbial fermentation, commonly with *Streptococcus zooepidemicus* [76]. It exhibits notable hydrophilicity, biocompatibility, biodegradability, non-toxicity, and non-immunogenicity, making it ideal for biomedical applications [77]. Modified hyaluronic acid derivatives, synthesized through esterification and the addition of hydrophobic functional groups, have enhanced enzymatic resistance and controlled dissolution [78]. Hydrophobic drugs can be encapsulated by amphiphilic hyaluronic acid derivatives to form supramolecular assemblies that deliver drugs to the colon precisely [79]. Hydrogels and conjugates based on hyaluronic acid, such as those functionalized with norbornene, offer customized mechanical properties and targeted therapeutic potential [80].

Zhang *et al.* developed a pH-sensitive hydrogel drug delivery system consisting of hyaluronic acid and gelatin, integrated with carboxymethyl chitosan microspheres containing curcumin, designed to address the shortcomings of curcumin's low bioavailability and non-specific distribution in the management of IBD. The method utilizes carboxymethyl chitosan microspheres for the precise delivery of the drug to the colon, leveraging the mucosal adhesion properties of carboxymethyl chitosan and the anti-inflammatory and reparative properties of hyaluronic acid. Hyaluronic acid and gelatin hydrogels enabled controlled release, while curcumin-loaded carboxymethyl chitosan microspheres extended drug release (65% over 50 hours) and improved therapeutic efficacy. *In vivo* tests revealed consistent curcumin concentrations in the colon, reduced IL-6 and TNF-α, pro-inflammatory cytokines, and exerted significant anti-inflammatory effects, suggesting the potential for targeted treatment of IBD (Table **2**) [81].

Table 2. Polysaccharides from Fungi and Mushrooms Used in IBD.

Sr. No.	Polysaccharides	Source	Experimental Assay	References
1.	Chitosan	*Saccharomyces boulardii*	A gastric survival rate of approximately **88.75–98.75%**.	[57]
2.	Chitosan oligosaccharide	*Saccharomyces boulardii*	DSS-induced acute colitis in ICR mice. Inhibition of NF- κB signalling pathway and apoptosis in intestinal epithelial cells.	[58]
3.	Polysaccharide GLP	*Hericium erinaceus*	Upregulation: T-SOD and Bacteroidetes; Downregulation: NO, MDA, MPO, IL-6, IL-1β, TNF-α, COX-2, iNOS, p-p65/p65, p-IκBα/IκBα, pAkt/Akt, p-p38/p38, p-ERK/ERK, p-JNK/JNK, Verrucomicrobia, *Actinobacteria, Arthrobacter spp., Methylibiums., Succinivibrio sp., Desulfovibrio sp.*, and *Akkermansia muciniphila*	[59]
4.	Polysaccharide EP-1	*Hericium erinaceus*	Upregulation: MMP, SOD, OCR, ATP, Bcl-2, AA, PA, BA, VA, IBA, IVA, GPR41, GPR43, and IgM; Downregulation: MDA, TNF-α, IL-1, IL-6, ROS, p-p65, p65, caspase-3, and C3	[60]
5.	Polysaccharide CMP33	*Poria cocos*	Upregulation: IL-4, IL-10, and DHT Downregulation: MPO, MDA, TNF-α, IL-6, L-1β, IL-12, IFN-γ, IL-2, IL-17, Hmgcs2, Fabp2, Hp, B4galnt2, B3gnt6, Sap, Ca1, and oleic acid	[61]

(Table 2) cont.....

Sr. No.	Polysaccharides	Source	Experimental Assay	References
6.	Polysaccharide IOP	*Inonotus obliquus*	Upregulation: ZO-1,occludin, IL-4, IL-10, GATA-3, Foxp3. and p-STAT6 Downregulation: p-STAT1, p-STAT3, IFN-γ, IL-17, T-bet, and ROR-γt	[62]
7.	Polysaccharide DIP	*Dictyophora indusiata*	Upregulation: GSH, HO-1, IL-10, Bcl-2, TJP1, and IRF4. Downregulation: MDA,MPO,TNF-α, IL-6, IL-1β, IL-18,NLRP3, p-IκBα,p-STAT3,Bax, IRF5, and CD86	[63]

In another research, Indigo and indirubin were formulated as nanosuspensions co-modified with Pluronic® and hyaluronic acid to surmount the colonic mucus barrier and improve their absorption by inflamed cells, respectively, for the treatment of ulcerative colitis. Inulin functioned as a protective agent during spray-drying and as a modulator of intestinal microbiota, leading to the formation of indurubin/indigo nanocrystals. The nanocrystals demonstrated a 24.3-fold improvement in mucus penetration and a twofold increase in cellular absorption compared to raw indirubin and indigo, thereby providing enhanced efficacy for the treatment of IBD [82].

Vafaei *et al.* investigated the therapeutic effectiveness of budesonide-loaded hyaluronic acid nanoparticles for treating IBD using an acetic acid-induced colitis model in rats. Compared to the free drug (30 μg/kg), budesonide-loaded hyaluronic acid significantly reduced inflammation, TNF-α levels, and MPO activity, while improving histology outcomes. Hyaluronic acid nanoparticles enabled precise drug delivery to the inflamed colon, enhancing therapeutic effectiveness. The findings highlight hyaluronic acid nanoparticles as a feasible polymeric system for IBD therapy by modulating cytokine production, immune responses, and gut microbiota equilibrium [83].

Xanthan Gum

Xanthan gum is chemically an exopolysaccharide produced by oxidative fermentation of primary carbohydrates by Xanthomonas bacteria, predominantly located on Brassica plants [84]. The structure consists of a linear D-glucoseβ-(1,4) linked D-glucose backbone with a tri-saccharide side chain attached by α-(1→3) connections [85]. The presence of carboxylic groups (from pyruvate and glucuronic acid) facilitates chemical modification, hence augmenting its application diversity [86]. Xanthan gum demonstrates remarkable stability throughout an extensive range of pH, temperature, and salt concentrations, and is resistant to enzymatic degradation in the upper GIT [87]. Xanthan gum functions as a release-retardant matrix for colon-targeted drug administration in IBD. The colonic flora partially ferments it, ensuring localized drug delivery, while the stomach and small intestine leave it undigested [88]. This selective decomposition mechanism facilitates the targeted delivery of medicinal medicines to the colon, hence reducing systemic side effects [89]. Moreover, xanthan gum's biocompatibility, biodegradability, and nontoxicity render it an exemplary candidate for hydrogels, tablets, and nanoparticles intended for IBD therapy [90].

Iswandana *et al.* formulated dexamethasone-loaded colon-targeted tablets utilizing probiotics and polysaccharides, including xanthan gum, sodium alginate, and chitosan as primary coatings, with Eudragit L100/S100 as secondary coatings. Xanthan gum was essential for developing its primary coating, providing stability in the upper GIT and facilitating selective drug release in the colon. *In-vitro* dissolution studies indicated the drug release remained unaltered by probiotics and primarily occurred in phosphate buffer at pH 6.8, simulating colon environments. This formulation reduces the systemic adverse effects of dexamethasone, hence improving its effectiveness in treating IBD [91].

Sandu *et al.* developed multi-particulate formulations based on xanthan gum and optimized for colon-targeted delivery of metronidazole for the treatment of IBD. The F6 batch comprised xanthan gum (0.7% w/v) mixed with sodium alginate (2.0% w/v) and cross-linked with glutaraldehyde (0.5 ml) in a 5% w/v calcium chloride solution, resulting in microspheres with a drug entrapment efficiency of 73.63 ± 0.65%. Resistance to enzymatic degradation of xanthan gum guarantees the integrity of the drug in the stomach and small intestine, facilitating its release in the colon *via* microbial enzymatic destruction. The F6 batch adhered to Peppas model kinetics (R^2 = 0.997), indicating regulated drug release with minimal toxicity and biodegradability [92].

Poly-γ-Glutamic Acid (PGA)

PGA is a biodegradable, water-soluble biopolymer formed from D- and L-glutamic acid units interconnected by amide bonds between the α-amino and γ-carboxylic groups [93]. It is primarily synthesized by Bacillus species, including *B. subtilis* and *B. licheniformis*, with strains classified as L-glutamic acid-dependent or independent [94]. PGA demonstrates environmentally favourable, non-toxic, and non-immunogenic properties, rendering it beneficial in pharmaceuticals, medicine, and agriculture [95]. It demonstrates promise in the management of IBD by altering the intestinal environment and diminishing inflammation, owing to its immunomodulatory and protective properties [96, 97].

Sun *et al.* synthesized cysteamine-grafted PGA by conjugating cysteamine with the carboxyl groups of γ-PGA to improve the stability and efficacy of KPV

(Lys–Pro–Val) in the treatment of ulcerative colitis. The PGA hydrogel, formulated *via* self-crosslinking of thiol groups, exhibited excellent mechanical stability and shear-thinning properties, making it suitable for rectal administration. The hydrogel markedly enhanced KPV's stability, prolonged its release, and preserved its anti-inflammatory efficacy. In TNBS-induced colitis rats, the KPV/ poly-γ-glutaric acid hydrogel mitigated colitis symptoms, restored colon shape, diminished inflammatory cytokines, and enhanced treatment results. This formulation emphasizes the role of PGA in stabilizing KPV and augmenting its therapeutic efficacy for IBD [98].

Xu *et al.* formulated a glutamine transaminase-2 crosslinked EMSCs-conditioned medium (EMSCs-CM) hydrogel by incorporating EMSCs-CM into a PGA hydrogel for targeted therapy of ulcerative colitis. The negatively charged γ-PGA hydrogel facilitates retention within the positively charged inflamed colon tissue, allowing for the sustained release of EMSCs-CM during breakdown. *In vitro*, EMSCs-CM exhibited anti-inflammatory properties in IEC-6 cells, but *in vivo*, the EMSCs-CM-Gel markedly diminished inflammatory cytokine expression, maintained intestinal length, and restored the intestinal barrier. This formulation presents an innovative strategy for colon-targeted treatment in ulcerative colitis [99].

β-glucan

β-glucan isolated from Saccharomyces cerevisiae is a glucose polymer characterized by a linear β-(1,3)-glucan backbone and side chain attached *via* β-(1,6) linkage [100]. It emphasizes superior biological activity compared to other glucans and exhibits potential in the treatment of neurological illnesses, obesity, and IBD [101]. Recent studies indicate that low molar mass yeast β-glucans diminish macrophage accumulation, epithelial damage, and colitis in mice triggered by DSS [102]. Despite its therapeutic potential, there are inadequate studies on the preventive and therapeutic effects of yeast β-glucan-derived nanotherapeutics in IBD, notably on their immune-modulatory and gut microbiota-regulating capabilities [103]. Redox-active nanoparticles may improve treatment effectiveness by regulating ROS elevation and reinstating intestinal microbial equilibrium [104].

Researchers developed a prebiotic nanocomposite formulated with yeast-derived β-glucan, functionalized with a bioadhesive polydopamine coating. Oral delivery of the formulation repaired epithelial barriers, inhibited ROS accumulation, and decreased systemic bioavailability, thereby improving therapeutic effectiveness in the murine model of acute colitis. Additionally, 16S rRNA sequencing demonstrated an augmentation in gut microbiota diversity, notably increasing the prevalence of probiotics such as *Lachnospiraceae* NK4A136 and *Bifidobacterium*, which are essential for sustaining gut homeostasis. This formulation illustrates the potential of β-glucan for ROS scavenging and modulation of the intestinal microbiota in the treatment of intestinal disorders (Table **1**) [105].

Algae Polysaccharides

The complex sulphated polymer fucoidan is extracted from brown seaweed cell walls. The disruption of intestinal epithelial cells brought on by oxidative stress and the ensuing rise in paracellular permeability are two examples of such factors in the pathophysiology of IBD. Fucoidan is implicated in preventing stomach ulcers, as evidenced by a growing body of experimental data. By increasing IL-6 and interferon-gamma levels and reducing IL-10 expression, fucoidan protects against aspirin-induced stomach ulcers (Table **1**) [106].

Red Algae Polysaccharides

Unlike the other two types of seaweed, brown and green, which contain polysaccharides, red seaweed is a vital source of numerous advantageous bioactive substances. Sulfated polysaccharides are red algae's primary structural element. Red algae contain common polysaccharides such as xylan, agar, and carrageenan. Red algae contain between 10-50 species, including *Eucheuma, Gigartina, Hypnea*, and *Chondrus*. It is made up of linear polysaccharide chains with sulfate half-esters attached to the sugar units, and it is a part of the intracellular matrix and the exterior cell wall. Carrageenan comes in three general forms: iota, lambda, and kappa. The availability of 3,6-anhydrogalactopyranose and the distribution of sulfate groups on the primary structure serve as the basis for this classification [107].

Ulva Polysaccharide

The ulvan obtained by enzymatic LMW-ulvan synthesis from the green alga U. pertusa is composed of 7.42% glucuronic acid, 57.23% rhamnose, 28.76% xylose, and 1.77% glucose [17]. Its backbone contained (1,3,4)-linked Rha, (1,4)-linked Xyl, and (1,4)-linked GlcA with trace amounts of (1,4)-linked Rha residues. Sulfate substitution took place at C-3 of rhamnose [108]. Additionally, LMW-ulvan reduced the oxidative damage and intestinal inflammation caused by DSS. Meanwhile, LMW-ulvan was able to significantly increase mRNA levels of claudin, occludin, and ZO-1, thereby improving intestinal mucosal permeability. The results of the study thus support the potential application of LMW-ulvan as an IBD functional food ingredient [109].

ANIMAL-DERIVED POLYMERS IN IBD: INDUSTRIAL AND BIOPHARMACEUTICAL APPLICATIONS

Animal-derived polymers, including chitosan, gelatin, collagen, and hyaluronic acid, are essential in the industrial and biopharmaceutical formulation development for IBD [113]. In the pharmaceutical sector, these polymers are extensively employed in colon-targeted drug delivery systems, such as hydrogels, microspheres, and nanoparticles, owing to their mucoadhesive and pH-sensitive properties, which improve localized drug retention at inflamed intestinal regions [114]. Chitosan has been widely utilized to create bioadhesive nanoparticles for the delivery of anti-inflammatory drugs such as mesalamine and corticosteroids [115, 116]. Gelatin and collagen-based scaffolds are investigated for intestinal tissue engineering and wound healing, facilitating mucosal regeneration in ulcerative colitis and Crohn's disease [117]. Hyaluronic acid formulations exhibit anti-inflammatory and barrier-repairing properties, providing therapeutic benefits by reducing oxidative stress and regulating cytokine expression [118]. These biopolymers are valued in industrial applications for their scalability, low toxicity, and ability to produce gels, films, and encapsulating systems, rendering them essential in the development of advanced biopharmaceutical therapies for IBD management [119 - 121].

CONCLUSION

IBD is a complicated illness that is influenced by environmental, microbial, and host variables. Multidisciplinary methods are utilized that link microbial metabolites, microbes, and genetic risk factors to changes in immune responses and epithelial cell activities. The findings from the many studies discussed support the possible development of microbial-generated polymers as future therapies for IBD in humans, demonstrating their intestinal anti-inflammatory properties. In fact, polysaccharide derivatives have demonstrated effectiveness in experimental colitis models, and the mechanisms underlying their positive effects appear to be rather comparable to those documented for medications now utilized in human therapy.

The potential of alginate, hyaluronic acid, xanthan gum, γ-polyglutamic acid, and β-glucan was summarized in this chapter. We anticipate that more research on the interactions between polysaccharides from various algae species, each with a unique structure and molecular weight, as well as intestinal microbes, immune cells, and epithelial cells, will deepen our understanding of their mechanisms and aid in the creation of medications, dietary supplements, and functional foods for the treatment of IBD patients. Recent research has demonstrated the diverse physiological actions of green algal polysaccharides and their substantial influence on human nutrition and health. Drug carriers that target the colon are frequently constructed using polysaccharides like chitosan and pectin to overcome these enzymatic challenges.

DIRECTIONS FOR FUTURE RESEARCH

Future studies on intestinal microbiota, IBD, and microbial-generated polymers must address a number of gaps despite notable advancements. The pathogenic characteristics of IBD and the existing delivery methods that target the inflammatory sites are discussed, followed by a review of the prospects and problems facing this field today. It is envisaged that the disorganized and dispersed study directions can be distilled into a clear structure for further investigation.

REFERENCES

[1] Velikova T, Kaouri IE, Bakopoulou K, *et al.* Mucosal immunity and trained innate immunity of the gut. Gastroenterol Insights 2024; 15(3): 661-75.
[http://dx.doi.org/10.3390/gastroent15030048]

[2] Belkaid Y, Hand TW. Role of the microbiota in immunity and inflammation. Cell 2014; 157(1): 121-41.
[http://dx.doi.org/10.1016/j.cell.2014.03.011] [PMID: 24679531]

[3] Silva FAR, Rodrigues BL, Ayrizono MLS, Leal RF. The immunological basis of inflammatory bowel disease. Gastroenterol Res Pract 2016; 2016: 1-11.
[http://dx.doi.org/10.1155/2016/2097274] [PMID: 28070181]

[4] Guo Q, Jin Y, Chen X, *et al.* NF-κB in biology and targeted therapy: new insights and translational implications. Signal Transduct Target Ther 2024; 9(1): 53.
[http://dx.doi.org/10.1038/s41392-024-01757-9] [PMID: 38433280]

[5] Liu T, Zhang L, Joo D, Sun SC. NF-κB signaling in inflammation. Signal Transduct Target Ther 2017; 2(1): 17023.
[http://dx.doi.org/10.1038/sigtrans.2017.23] [PMID: 29158945]

[6] Jamieson PE, Carbonero F, Stevens JF. Dietary (poly)phenols mitigate inflammatory bowel disease: Therapeutic targets, mechanisms of action, and clinical observations. Curr Res Food Sci 2023; 6: 100521.

[7] M'koma AE. Inflammatory bowel disease: An expanding global health problem. Clin Med Insights Gastroenterol 2013; 14(6): CGast.S12731.
[http://dx.doi.org/10.4137/CGast.S12731]

[8] Hussain Y, Khan H. Immunosuppressive drugs. Encyclopedia of Infection and Immunity. Elsevier 2022; pp. 726-40. Internet
[http://dx.doi.org/10.1016/B978-0-12-818731-9.00068-9]

[9] Zhou Y, Wang D, Yan W. Treatment effects of natural products on inflammatory bowel disease *in vivo* and their mechanisms: Based on animal experiments. Nutrients 2023; 15(4): 1031.
[http://dx.doi.org/10.3390/nu15041031] [PMID: 36839389]

[10] Besednova NN, Zaporozhets TS, Kuznetsova TA, *et al.* Extracts and marine algae polysaccharides in therapy and prevention of inflammatory diseases of the intestine. Mar Drugs 2020; 18(6): 289.
[http://dx.doi.org/10.3390/md18060289] [PMID: 32486405]

[11] Dewangan R, Agrawal N, Lanjhiyana SK, Jaiswal M. Exploring the antineoplastic potential of novel

NSAID derivatives in combatting mammary tumorigenesis: a comprehensive review. Med Chem Res 2025; 34(4): 764-90.
[http://dx.doi.org/10.1007/s00044-025-03377-6]

[12] Li S, Zhang F, Zhang Q. Pathological features-based targeted delivery strategies in IBD therapy: A mini review. Biomed Pharmacother 2022; 151: 113079.
[http://dx.doi.org/10.1016/j.biopha.2022.113079] [PMID: 35605297]

[13] Zheng LX, Chen XQ, Cheong KL. Current trends in marine algae polysaccharides: The digestive tract, microbial catabolism, and prebiotic potential. Int J Biol Macromol 2020; 151: 344-54.
[http://dx.doi.org/10.1016/j.ijbiomac.2020.02.168] [PMID: 32084473]

[14] Imdad A, Pandit NG, Zaman M, Minkoff NZ, Tanner-Smith EE, Gomez-Duarte OG, *et al.* Fecal transplantation for treatment of inflammatory bowel disease. Cochrane Database Syst Rev 2023; 25(4)
[http://dx.doi.org/10.1002/14651858.CD012774.pub3]

[15] Ferrante M, Pouillon L, Mañosa M, *et al.* Results of the eighth scientific workshop of ecco: prevention and treatment of postoperative recurrence in patients with Crohn's Disease undergoing an ileocolonic resection with ileocolonic anastomosis. J Crohn's Colitis 2023; 17(11): 1707-22.
[http://dx.doi.org/10.1093/ecco-jcc/jjad053] [PMID: 37070324]

[16] Njoku GC, Forkan CP, Soltysik FM, Nejsum PL, Pociot F, Yarani R. Unleashing the potential of extracellular vesicles for ulcerative colitis and Crohn's disease therapy. Bioact Mater 2025; 45: 41-57.
[http://dx.doi.org/10.1016/j.bioactmat.2024.11.004] [PMID: 39610953]

[17] Guerreiro CA, Andrade LAD, Fernández-Lainez C, *et al.* Bioactive arabinoxylan oligomers *via* colonic fermentation and enzymatic catalysis: Evidence of interaction with toll-like receptors from *in vitro*, *in silico* and functional analysis. Carbohydr Polym 2025; 352: 123175.
[http://dx.doi.org/10.1016/j.carbpol.2024.123175] [PMID: 39843080]

[18] Li Y, Ye H, Wang T, *et al.* Characterization of low molecular weight sulfate ulva polysaccharide and its protective effect against IBD in mice. Mar Drugs 2020; 18(10): 499.
[http://dx.doi.org/10.3390/md18100499] [PMID: 33003577]

[19] Imbrizi M, Magro F, Coy CSR. Pharmacological therapy in inflammatory bowel diseases: A narrative review of the past 90 years. Pharmaceuticals (Basel) 2023; 16(9): 1272.
[http://dx.doi.org/10.3390/ph16091272] [PMID: 37765080]

[20] Wang CPJ, Byun MJ, Kim SN, *et al.* Biomaterials as therapeutic drug carriers for inflammatory bowel disease treatment. J Control Release 2022; 345: 1-19.
[http://dx.doi.org/10.1016/j.jconrel.2022.02.028] [PMID: 35227764]

[21] Kaur R, Pathak L, Vyas P. Biobased polymers of plant and microbial origin and their applications - a review. Biotechnol Sustain Mater 2024; 1(1): 13.
[http://dx.doi.org/10.1186/s44316-024-00014-x]

[22] Desai N, Rana D, Salave S, *et al.* Chitosan: A potential biopolymer in drug delivery and biomedical applications. Pharmaceutics 2023; 15(4): 1313.
[http://dx.doi.org/10.3390/pharmaceutics15041313] [PMID: 37111795]

[23] Lu P, Ruan D, Huang M, *et al.* Harnessing the potential of hydrogels for advanced therapeutic applications: current achievements and future directions. Signal Transduct Target Ther 2024; 9(1): 166.
[http://dx.doi.org/10.1038/s41392-024-01852-x] [PMID: 38945949]

[24] Tabernero A, Cardea S. Microbial exopolysaccharides as drug carriers. Polymers (Basel) 2020; 12(9): 2142.
[http://dx.doi.org/10.3390/polym12092142] [PMID: 32961830]

[25] Song J, Wang T, Zhang K, *et al.* Natural products-integrated drug delivery systems as innovative therapeutic strategies for inflammatory bowel disease management. Nano Res 2025; 18(10): 94908007.

[http://dx.doi.org/10.26599/NR.2025.94908007]

[26] Fatima SN. Microbial biopolymers: A sustainable alternative to traditional petroleum-based polymers for a greener future. Mater Today Commun 2024; 40: 109846.
[http://dx.doi.org/10.1016/j.mtcomm.2024.109846]

[27] Shendge RS, Zalte TS, Khade SB. Polymeric microspheres redefining the landscape of colon-targeted delivery: A contemporary update. European Journal of Medicinal Chemistry Reports 2024; 11: 100156.
[http://dx.doi.org/10.1016/j.ejmcr.2024.100156]

[28] Yarahmadi A, Dousti B, Karami-Khorramabadi M, Afkhami H. Materials based on biodegradable polymers chitosan/gelatin: a review of potential applications. Front Bioeng Biotechnol 2024; 12: 1397668.
[http://dx.doi.org/10.3389/fbioe.2024.1397668] [PMID: 39157438]

[29] Tan RYH, Lee CS, Pichika MR, Cheng SF, Lam KY. pH responsive polyurethane for the advancement of biomedical and drug delivery. Polymers (Basel) 2022; 14(9): 1672.
[http://dx.doi.org/10.3390/polym14091672] [PMID: 35566843]

[30] Gong T, Liu X, Wang X, Lu Y, Wang X. Applications of polysaccharides in enzyme-triggered oral colon-specific drug delivery systems: A review. Int J Biol Macromol 2024; 275(Pt 1): 133623.
[http://dx.doi.org/10.1016/j.ijbiomac.2024.133623] [PMID: 38969037]

[31] Lai SK, Wang YY, Hanes J. Mucus-penetrating nanoparticles for drug and gene delivery to mucosal tissues. Adv Drug Deliv Rev 2009; 61(2): 158-71.
[http://dx.doi.org/10.1016/j.addr.2008.11.002] [PMID: 19133304]

[32] Patole V, Deshkar S, Baheti R, Giram PS. Gastrointestinal tract environment and its implications on oral drug delivery. Polymers for Oral Drug Delivery Technologies. Elsevier 2025; pp. 3-63. Internet
[http://dx.doi.org/10.1016/B978-0-443-13774-7.00001-3]

[33] Thang NH, Chien TB, Cuong DX. Polymer-based hydrogels applied in drug delivery: An overview. Gels 2023; 9(7): 523.
[http://dx.doi.org/10.3390/gels9070523] [PMID: 37504402]

[34] Jandhyala SM, Talukdar R, Subramanyam C, Vuyyuru H, Sasikala M, Nageshwar Reddy D. Role of the normal gut microbiota. World J Gastroenterol 2015; 21(29): 8787-803.
[http://dx.doi.org/10.3748/wjg.v21.i29.8787] [PMID: 26269668]

[35] Sharma R, Kumar S, Malviya R, *et al.* Recent advances in biopolymer-based mucoadhesive drug delivery systems for oral application. J Drug Deliv Sci Technol 2024; 91: 105227.
[http://dx.doi.org/10.1016/j.jddst.2023.105227]

[36] Deb PK, Kokaz SF, Abed SN, Paradkar A, Tekade RK. Pharmaceutical and biomedical applications of polymers. Basic Fundamentals of Drug Delivery. Elsevier 2019; pp. 203-67. Internet
[http://dx.doi.org/10.1016/B978-0-12-817909-3.00006-6]

[37] Herdiana Y, Wathoni N, Shamsuddin S, Muchtaridi M. Scale-up polymeric-based nanoparticles drug delivery systems: Development and challenges. OpenNano 2022; 7: 100048.
[http://dx.doi.org/10.1016/j.onano.2022.100048]

[38] Farshbaf M, Davaran S, Zarebkohan A, Annabi N, Akbarzadeh A, Salehi R. Significant role of cationic polymers in drug delivery systems. Artif Cells Nanomed Biotechnol 2017; 1-20.
[http://dx.doi.org/10.1080/21691401.2017.1395344] [PMID: 29103306]

[39] Chang RYK, Okamoto Y, Morales S, Kutter E, Chan HK. Hydrogel formulations containing non-ionic polymers for topical delivery of bacteriophages. Int J Pharm 2021; 605: 120850.
[http://dx.doi.org/10.1016/j.ijpharm.2021.120850] [PMID: 34216771]

[40] Moradali MF, Rehm BHA. Bacterial biopolymers: from pathogenesis to advanced materials. Nat Rev Microbiol 2020; 18(4): 195-210.
[http://dx.doi.org/10.1038/s41579-019-0313-3] [PMID: 31992873]

[41] Chen J, Gao Y, Zhang Y, Wang M. Research progress in the treatment of inflammatory bowel disease with natural polysaccharides and related structure–activity relationships. Food Funct 2024; 15(11): 5680-702.
[http://dx.doi.org/10.1039/D3FO04919A] [PMID: 38738935]

[42] Mohammed ASA, Naveed M, Jost N. Polysaccharides; classification, chemical properties, and future perspective applications in fields of pharmacology and biological medicine (a review of current applications and upcoming potentialities). J Polym Environ 2021; 29(8): 2359-71.
[http://dx.doi.org/10.1007/s10924-021-02052-2] [PMID: 33526994]

[43] Blanco FG, Hernández N, Rivero-Buceta V, *et al.* From residues to added-value bacterial biopolymers as nanomaterials for biomedical applications. Nanomaterials (Basel) 2021; 11(6): 1492.
[http://dx.doi.org/10.3390/nano11061492] [PMID: 34200068]

[44] Achbergerová L, Nahálka J. Polyphosphate - an ancient energy source and active metabolic regulator. Microb Cell Fact 2011; 10(1): 63.
[http://dx.doi.org/10.1186/1475-2859-10-63] [PMID: 21816086]

[45] Methacanon P, Madla S, Kirtikara K, Prasitsil M. Structural elucidation of bioactive fungi-derived polymers. Carbohydr Polym 2005; 60(2): 199-203.
[http://dx.doi.org/10.1016/j.carbpol.2004.12.006]

[46] Mahapatra S, Banerjee D. Fungal exopolysaccharide: production, composition and applications. Microbiol Insights 2013; 6: MBI.S10957.
[http://dx.doi.org/10.4137/MBI.S10957] [PMID: 24826070]

[47] Gregory DA, Taylor CS, Fricker ATR, *et al.* Polyhydroxyalkanoates and their advances for biomedical applications. Trends Mol Med 2022; 28(4): 331-42.
[http://dx.doi.org/10.1016/j.molmed.2022.01.007] [PMID: 35232669]

[48] Huang H, Lang Y, Wang S, Zhou M. Microalgae-based drug delivery systems in biomedical applications. Eng Regen 2024; 5(3): 361-74.
[http://dx.doi.org/10.1016/j.engreg.2024.01.002]

[49] Abourehab MAS, Rajendran RR, Singh A, *et al.* Alginate as a promising biopolymer in drug delivery and wound healing: A review of the state-of-the-art. Int J Mol Sci 2022; 23(16): 9035.
[http://dx.doi.org/10.3390/ijms23169035] [PMID: 36012297]

[50] Pacheco-Quito EM, Ruiz-Caro R, Veiga MD. Carrageenan: Drug delivery systems and other biomedical applications. Mar Drugs 2020; 18(11): 583.
[http://dx.doi.org/10.3390/md18110583] [PMID: 33238488]

[51] Mura P, Maestrelli F, Cirri M, Mennini N. Multiple roles of chitosan in mucosal drug delivery: An updated review. Mar Drugs 2022; 20(5): 335.
[http://dx.doi.org/10.3390/md20050335] [PMID: 35621986]

[52] Zhang XW, Liu Q, Thorlacius H. Inhibition of selectin function and leukocyte rolling protects against dextran sodium sulfate-induced murine colitis. Scand J Gastroenterol 2001; 36(3): 270-5.
[http://dx.doi.org/10.1080/003655201750074555] [PMID: 11305514]

[53] Repici A, Hasan A, Capra AP, *et al.* Marine algae and deriving biomolecules for the management of inflammatory bowel diseases: Potential clinical therapeutics to decrease gut inflammatory and oxidative stress markers? Mar Drugs 2024; 22(8): 336.
[http://dx.doi.org/10.3390/md22080336] [PMID: 39195452]

[54] Tabarsa M, You S, Dabaghian EH, Surayot U. Water-soluble polysaccharides from Ulva intestinalis: Molecular properties, structural elucidation and immunomodulatory activities. Yao Wu Shi Pin Fen Xi 2018; 26(2): 599-608.
[http://dx.doi.org/10.1016/j.jfda.2017.07.016] [PMID: 29567229]

[55] Zhu C, Zhang S, Song C, *et al.* Selenium nanoparticles decorated with Ulva lactuca polysaccharide potentially attenuate colitis by inhibiting NF-κB mediated hyper inflammation. J Nanobiotechnology

2017; 15(1): 20.
[http://dx.doi.org/10.1186/s12951-017-0252-y] [PMID: 28270147]

[56] Fritzen-Freire CB, Prudêncio ES, Amboni RDMC, Pinto SS, Negrão-Murakami AN, Murakami FS. Microencapsulation of bifidobacteria by spray drying in the presence of prebiotics. Food Res Int 2012; 45(1): 306-12.
[http://dx.doi.org/10.1016/j.foodres.2011.09.020]

[57] Iraha A, Chinen H, Hokama A, *et al.* Fucoidan enhances intestinal barrier function by upregulating the expression of claudin-1. World J Gastroenterol 2013; 19(33): 5500-7.
[http://dx.doi.org/10.3748/wjg.v19.i33.5500] [PMID: 24023493]

[58] Lu SY, Liu Y, Tang S, *et al. Gracilaria lemaneiformis* polysaccharides alleviate colitis by modulating the gut microbiota and intestinal barrier in mice. Food Chem X 2022; 13: 100197.
[http://dx.doi.org/10.1016/j.fochx.2021.100197] [PMID: 35498989]

[59] Ma ZY, Song XQ, Hu JJ, *et al.* Ketoplatin in triple-negative breast cancer cells MDA-MB-231: High efficacy and low toxicity, and positive impact on inflammatory microenvironment. Biochem Pharmacol 2021; 188: 114523.
[http://dx.doi.org/10.1016/j.bcp.2021.114523] [PMID: 33741331]

[60] Lee SH, Kang MC, Moon SH, Jeon BT, Jeon YJ. Potential use of ultrasound in antioxidant extraction from Ecklonia cava. Algae 2013; 28(4): 371-8.
[http://dx.doi.org/10.4490/algae.2013.28.4.371]

[61] Kong Q, Zhang R, You L, Ma Y, Liao L, Pedisić S. *In vitro* fermentation characteristics of polysaccharide from *Sargassum fusiforme* and its modulation effects on gut microbiota. Food Chem Toxicol 2021; 151: 112145.
[http://dx.doi.org/10.1016/j.fct.2021.112145] [PMID: 33766612]

[62] Zheng W, Duan M, Jia J, Song S, Ai C. Low-molecular alginate improved diet-induced obesity and metabolic syndrome through modulating the gut microbiota in BALB/c mice. Int J Biol Macromol 2021; 187: 811-20.
[http://dx.doi.org/10.1016/j.ijbiomac.2021.08.003] [PMID: 34363822]

[63] Phillips M, Kailasapathy K, Tran L. Viability of commercial probiotic cultures (*L. acidophilus, Bifidobacterium sp., L. casei, L. paracasei and L. rhamnosus*) in cheddar cheese. Int J Food Microbiol 2006; 108(2): 276-80.
[http://dx.doi.org/10.1016/j.ijfoodmicro.2005.12.009] [PMID: 16478637]

[64] Kelesidis T, Pothoulakis C. Efficacy and safety of the probiotic *Saccharomyces boulardii* for the prevention and therapy of gastrointestinal disorders. Therap Adv Gastroenterol 2012; 5(2): 111-25.
[http://dx.doi.org/10.1177/1756283X11428502] [PMID: 22423260]

[65] Ren Y, Sun Q, Gao R, *et al.* Low weight polysaccharide of *Hericium erinaceus* ameliorates colitis *via* inhibiting the NLRP3 inflammasome activation in association with gut microbiota modulation. Nutrients 2023; 15(3): 739.
[http://dx.doi.org/10.3390/nu15030739] [PMID: 36771444]

[66] Shao S, Wang D, Zheng W, *et al.* A unique polysaccharide from *Hericium erinaceus* mycelium ameliorates acetic acid-induced ulcerative colitis rats by modulating the composition of the gut microbiota, short chain fatty acids levels and GPR41/43 respectors. Int Immunopharmacol 2019; 71: 411-22.
[http://dx.doi.org/10.1016/j.intimp.2019.02.038] [PMID: 31059977]

[67] Liu X, Yu X, Xu X, Zhang X, Zhang X. The protective effects of Poria cocos-derived polysaccharide CMP33 against IBD in mice and its molecular mechanism. Food Funct 2018; 9(11): 5936-49.
[http://dx.doi.org/10.1039/C8FO01604F] [PMID: 30378628]

[68] Chen YF, Zheng JJ, Qu C, *et al. Inonotus obliquus* polysaccharide ameliorates dextran sulphate sodium induced colitis involving modulation of Th1/Th2 and Th17/Treg balance. Artif Cells Nanomed Biotechnol 2019; 47(1): 757-66.

[http://dx.doi.org/10.1080/21691401.2019.1577877] [PMID: 30856346]

[69] Kanwal S, Joseph TP, Aliya S, *et al.* Attenuation of DSS induced colitis by Dictyophora indusiata polysaccharide (DIP) *via* modulation of gut microbiota and inflammatory related signaling pathways. J Funct Foods 2020; 64: 103641.
[http://dx.doi.org/10.1016/j.jff.2019.103641]

[70] Lee SH, Bajracharya R, Min JY, Han JW, Park BJ, Han HK. Strategic approaches for colon targeted drug delivery: An overview of recent advancements. Pharmaceutics 2020; 12(1): 68.
[http://dx.doi.org/10.3390/pharmaceutics12010068] [PMID: 31952340]

[71] Begines B, Ortiz T, Pérez-Aranda M, *et al.* Polymeric nanoparticles for drug delivery: Recent developments and future prospects. Nanomaterials (Basel) 2020; 10(7): 1403.
[http://dx.doi.org/10.3390/nano10071403] [PMID: 32707641]

[72] Abka-khajouei R, Tounsi L, Shahabi N, Patel AK, Abdelkafi S, Michaud P. Structures, properties and applications of alginates. Mar Drugs 2022; 20(6): 364.
[http://dx.doi.org/10.3390/md20060364] [PMID: 35736167]

[73] Makarova AO, Derkach SR, Khair T, Kazantseva MA, Zuev YF, Zueva OS. Ion-induced polysaccharide gelation: Peculiarities of alginate egg-box association with different divalent cations. Polymers (Basel) 2023; 15(5): 1243.
[http://dx.doi.org/10.3390/polym15051243] [PMID: 36904484]

[74] Swastha D, Varsha N, Aravind S, *et al.* Alginate-based drug carrier systems to target inflammatory bowel disease: A review. Int J Biol Macromol 2023; 244: 125472.
[http://dx.doi.org/10.1016/j.ijbiomac.2023.125472] [PMID: 37336375]

[75] Qiu L, Shen R, Wei L, *et al.* Designing a microbial fermentation-functionalized alginate microsphere for targeted release of 5-ASA using nano dietary fiber carrier for inflammatory bowel disease treatment. J Nanobiotechnology 2023; 21(1): 344.
[http://dx.doi.org/10.1186/s12951-023-02097-6] [PMID: 37741962]

[76] Ivanovska TP, Mladenovska K, Zhivikj Z, *et al.* Synbiotic loaded chitosan-Ca-alginate microparticles reduces inflammation in the TNBS model of rat colitis. Int J Pharm 2017; 527(1-2): 126-34.
[http://dx.doi.org/10.1016/j.ijpharm.2017.05.049] [PMID: 28552770]

[77] Zhang X, Yuan Z, Wu J, *et al.* An orally-administered nanotherapeutics with carbon monoxide supplying for inflammatory bowel disease therapy by scavenging oxidative stress and restoring gut immune homeostasis. ACS Nano 2023; 17(21): 21116-33.
[http://dx.doi.org/10.1021/acsnano.3c04819] [PMID: 37843108]

[78] Vitulo M, Gnodi E, Meneveri R, Barisani D. Interactions between nanoparticles and intestine. Int J Mol Sci 2022; 23(8): 4339.
[http://dx.doi.org/10.3390/ijms23084339] [PMID: 35457155]

[79] Xu P, Luo S, Song J, Dai Z, Li D, Wu C. Effect of sodium alginate-based hydrogel loaded with lutein on gut microbiota and inflammatory response in DSS-induced colitis mice. Food Sci Hum Wellness 2023; 12(6): 2428-39.
[http://dx.doi.org/10.1016/j.fshw.2023.03.010]

[80] Dicker KT, Gurski LA, Pradhan-Bhatt S, Witt RL, Farach-Carson MC, Jia X. Hyaluronan: A simple polysaccharide with diverse biological functions. Acta Biomater 2014; 10(4): 1558-70.
[http://dx.doi.org/10.1016/j.actbio.2013.12.019] [PMID: 24361428]

[81] Vázquez JA, Montemayor MI, Fraguas J, Murado MA. Hyaluronic acid production by *Streptococcus zooepidemicus* in marine by-products media from mussel processing wastewaters and tuna peptone viscera. Microb Cell Fact 2010; 9(1): 46.
[http://dx.doi.org/10.1186/1475-2859-9-46] [PMID: 20546615]

[82] Iaconisi GN, Lunetti P, Gallo N, *et al.* Hyaluronic acid: A powerful biomolecule with wide-ranging applications—a comprehensive review. Int J Mol Sci 2023; 24(12): 10296.

[http://dx.doi.org/10.3390/ijms241210296] [PMID: 37373443]

[83] Bokatyi AN, Dubashynskaya NV, Skorik YA. Chemical modification of hyaluronic acid as a strategy for the development of advanced drug delivery systems. Carbohydr Polym 2024; 337: 122145. [http://dx.doi.org/10.1016/j.carbpol.2024.122145] [PMID: 38710553]

[84] Payne WM, Svechkarev D, Kyrychenko A, Mohs AM. The role of hydrophobic modification on hyaluronic acid dynamics and self-assembly. Carbohydr Polym 2018; 182: 132-41. [http://dx.doi.org/10.1016/j.carbpol.2017.10.054] [PMID: 29279107]

[85] Wang M, Deng Z, Guo Y, Xu P. Designing functional hyaluronic acid-based hydrogels for cartilage tissue engineering. Mater Today Bio 2022; 17: 100495. [http://dx.doi.org/10.1016/j.mtbio.2022.100495] [PMID: 36420054]

[86] Zhang S, Kang L, Hu S, *et al.* Carboxymethyl chitosan microspheres loaded hyaluronic acid/gelatin hydrogels for controlled drug delivery and the treatment of inflammatory bowel disease. Int J Biol Macromol 2021; 167: 1598-612. [http://dx.doi.org/10.1016/j.ijbiomac.2020.11.117] [PMID: 33220374]

[87] Xie J, Huang Q, Xie H, *et al.* Hyaluronic acid/inulin-based nanocrystals with an optimized ratio of indigo and indirubin for combined ulcerative colitis therapy *via* immune and intestinal flora regulation. Int J Biol Macromol 2023; 252: 126502. [http://dx.doi.org/10.1016/j.ijbiomac.2023.126502] [PMID: 37625742]

[88] Vafaei SY, Abdolghaffari AH, Mahjub R, Eslami SM, Esmaeili M, Abdollahi M, *et al.* Budesonide-Loaded Hyaluronic Acid Nanoparticles for Targeted Delivery to the Inflamed Intestinal Mucosa in a Rodent Model of Colitis. Ahad A, editor Biomed Res Int 2022. [http://dx.doi.org/10.1155/2022/7776092]

[89] Layek B. A comprehensive review of xanthan gum-based oral drug delivery systems. Int J Mol Sci 2024; 25(18): 10143. [http://dx.doi.org/10.3390/ijms251810143] [PMID: 39337626]

[90] Berninger T, Dietz N, González López Ó. Water-soluble polymers in agriculture: xanthan gum as eco-friendly alternative to synthetics. Microb Biotechnol 2021; 14(5): 1881-96. [http://dx.doi.org/10.1111/1751-7915.13867] [PMID: 34196103]

[91] Riaz T, Iqbal MW, Jiang B, Chen J. A review of the enzymatic, physical, and chemical modification techniques of xanthan gum. Int J Biol Macromol 2021; 186: 472-89. [http://dx.doi.org/10.1016/j.ijbiomac.2021.06.196] [PMID: 34217744]

[92] Patel J, Maji B, Moorthy NSHN, Maiti S. Xanthan gum derivatives: review of synthesis, properties and diverse applications. RSC Advances 2020; 10(45): 27103-36. [http://dx.doi.org/10.1039/D0RA04366D] [PMID: 35515783]

[93] Philip A, Philip B. Colon targeted drug delivery systems: a review on primary and novel approaches. Oman Med J 2010; 25(2): 70-8. [http://dx.doi.org/10.5001/omj.2010.24] [PMID: 22125706]

[94] Teruel AH, Gonzalez-Alvarez I, Bermejo M, *et al.* New insights of oral colonic drug delivery systems for inflammatory bowel disease therapy. Int J Mol Sci 2020; 21(18): 6502. [http://dx.doi.org/10.3390/ijms21186502] [PMID: 32899548]

[95] Zhang S, Ermann J, Succi MD, *et al.* An inflammation-targeting hydrogel for local drug delivery in inflammatory bowel disease. Sci Transl Med 2015; 7(300): 300ra128. [http://dx.doi.org/10.1126/scitranslmed.aaa5657] [PMID: 26268315]

[96] Iswandana R, Putri KSS, Anisa HN, Ricardo W, Nurhadi PAS. Formulation of various polysaccharides-based multicoated tablets containing dexamethasone and probiotics for inflammatory bowel disease. J Appl Pharm Sci 2023. [http://dx.doi.org/10.7324/JAPS.2023.129156]

[97] Sandu MKR, Majumdar S, Chatterjee S, Mazumder R. Optimization and characterization of xanthan

gum based multiparticulate formulation for colon targeting. Intell Pharm 2024; 2(3): 339-45. [http://dx.doi.org/10.1016/j.ipha.2024.02.007]

[98] Luo Z, Guo Y, Liu J, *et al.* Microbial synthesis of poly-γ-glutamic acid: current progress, challenges, and future perspectives. Biotechnol Biofuels 2016; 9(1): 134. [http://dx.doi.org/10.1186/s13068-016-0537-7] [PMID: 27366207]

[99] Zhu J, Wang X, Zhao J, *et al.* Genomic characterization and related functional genes of γ- poly glutamic acid producing Bacillus subtilis. BMC Microbiol 2024; 24(1): 125. [http://dx.doi.org/10.1186/s12866-024-03262-z] [PMID: 38622505]

[100] Elbanna K, Alsulami FS, Neyaz LA, Abulreesh HH. Poly (γ) glutamic acid: a unique microbial biopolymer with diverse commercial applicability. Front Microbiol 2024; 15: 1348411. [http://dx.doi.org/10.3389/fmicb.2024.1348411] [PMID: 38414762]

[101] Davaatseren M, Hwang JT, Park JH, Kim MS, Wang S, Sung MJ. Poly-glutamic acid attenuates angiogenesis and inflammation in experimental colitis. Mediators Inflamm 2013; 2013: 1-8. [http://dx.doi.org/10.1155/2013/982383]

[102] Plichta DR, Graham DB, Subramanian S, Xavier RJ. Therapeutic opportunities in inflammatory bowel disease: Mechanistic dissection of host-microbiome relationships. Cell 2019; 178(5): 1041-56. [http://dx.doi.org/10.1016/j.cell.2019.07.045] [PMID: 31442399]

[103] Sun J, Xue P, Liu J, *et al.* Self-cross-linked hydrogel of cysteamine-grafted γ-polyglutamic acid stabilized tripeptide KPV for alleviating TNBS-induced ulcerative colitis in rats. ACS Biomater Sci Eng 2021; 7(10): 4859-69. [http://dx.doi.org/10.1021/acsbiomaterials.1c00792] [PMID: 34547895]

[104] Yang W, Zhang X, Qi L, *et al.* Colon-targeted EMSCs conditional medium hydrogel for treatment of ulcerative colitis in mice. Biomed Mater 2023; 18(6): 065010. [http://dx.doi.org/10.1088/1748-605X/acfadb] [PMID: 37722391]

[105] Aimanianda V, Clavaud C, Simenel C, Fontaine T, Delepierre M, Latgé JP. Cell wall β-(1,6)-glucan of Saccharomyces cerevisiae: structural characterization and *in situ* synthesis. J Biol Chem 2009; 284(20): 13401-12. [http://dx.doi.org/10.1074/jbc.M807667200] [PMID: 19279004]

[106] Muro P, Zhang L, Li S, *et al.* The emerging role of oxidative stress in inflammatory bowel disease. Front Endocrinol (Lausanne) 2024; 15: 1390351. [http://dx.doi.org/10.3389/fendo.2024.1390351] [PMID: 39076514]

[107] Xie Y, Shao F, Duan X, *et al.* Whole β-glucan particle attenuates AOM/DSS-induced colorectal tumorigenesis in mice *via* inhibition of intestinal inflammation. Front Pharmacol 2023; 14: 1017475. [http://dx.doi.org/10.3389/fphar.2023.1017475] [PMID: 36713833]

[108] Murphy EJ, Rezoagli E, Major I, Rowan NJ, Laffey JG. β-glucan metabolic and immunomodulatory properties and potential for clinical application. J Fungi (Basel) 2020; 6(4): 356. [http://dx.doi.org/10.3390/jof6040356] [PMID: 33322069]

[109] Ren Q, Sun S, Zhang XD. Redox-active nanoparticles for inflammatory bowel disease. Nano Res 2021; 14(8): 2535-57. [http://dx.doi.org/10.1007/s12274-021-3303-5]

[110] Yang F, Su Y, Yan C, Chen T, Cheung PCK. Attenuation of inflammatory bowel disease by oral administration of mucoadhesive polydopamine-coated yeast β-glucan *via* ROS scavenging and gut microbiota regulation. J Nanobiotechnology 2024; 22(1): 166. [http://dx.doi.org/10.1186/s12951-024-02434-3] [PMID: 38610032]

[111] Wang Y, Xing M, Cao Q, Ji A, Liang H, Song S. Biological activities of fucoidan and the factors mediating its therapeutic effects: A review of recent studies. Mar Drugs 2019; 17(3): 183. [http://dx.doi.org/10.3390/md17030183] [PMID: 30897733]

[112] Liyanage NM, Nagahawatta DP, Jayawardena TU, Jeon YJ. The role of seaweed polysaccharides in

gastrointestinal health: Protective effect against inflammatory bowel disease. Life (Basel) 2023; 13(4): 1026.
[http://dx.doi.org/10.3390/life13041026] [PMID: 37109555]

[113] Kidgell JT, Glasson CRK, Magnusson M, *et al.* Ulvans are not equal - Linkage and substitution patterns in ulvan polysaccharides differ with Ulva morphology. Carbohydr Polym 2024; 333: 121962.
[http://dx.doi.org/10.1016/j.carbpol.2024.121962] [PMID: 38494219]

[114] Kruidenier L, Kuiper I, Lamers CBHW, Verspaget HW. Intestinal oxidative damage in inflammatory bowel disease: semi-quantification, localization, and association with mucosal antioxidants. J Pathol 2003; 201(1): 28-36.
[http://dx.doi.org/10.1002/path.1409] [PMID: 12950014]

[115] Ouyang Y, Zhao J, Wang S. Multifunctional hydrogels based on chitosan, hyaluronic acid and other biological macromolecules for the treatment of inflammatory bowel disease: A review. Int J Biol Macromol 2023; 227: 505-23.
[http://dx.doi.org/10.1016/j ijbiomac.2022.12.032] [PMID: 36495992]

[116] Zhao S, Zhang J, Qiu M, *et al.* Mucoadhesive and thermosensitive Bletilla striata polysaccharide/chitosan hydrogel loaded nanoparticles for rectal drug delivery in ulcerative colitis. Int J Biol Macromol 2024; 254(Pt 1): 127761.
[http://dx.doi.org/10.1016/j.ijbiomac.2023.127761] [PMID: 38287598]

[117] Varshosaz J, Jaffarian Dehkordi A, Golafshan S. Colon-specific delivery of mesalazine chitosan microspheres. J Microencapsul 2006; 23(3): 329-39.
[http://dx.doi.org/10.1080/02652040600612405] [PMID: 16801244]

[118] Ahmed T, Aljaeid B. Preparation, characterization, and potential application of chitosan, chitosan derivatives, and chitosan metal nanoparticles in pharmaceutical drug delivery. Drug Des Devel Ther 2016; 10(Jan): 483-507.
[http://dx.doi.org/10.2147/DDDT.S99651] [PMID: 26869768]

[119] La Monica F, Campora S, Ghersi G. Collagen-based scaffolds for chronic skin wound treatment. Gels 2024; 10(2): 137.
[http://dx.doi.org/10.3390/gels10020137] [PMID: 38391467]

[120] Dovedytis M, Liu ZJ, Bartlett S. Hyaluronic acid and its biomedical applications: A review. Eng Regen 2020; 1: 102-3.
[http://dx.doi.org/10.1016/j.engreg.2020.10.001]

[121] Varma K, Gopi S. Biopolymers and their role in medicinal and pharmaceutical applications. Biopolymers and their Industrial Applications. Elsevier 2021; pp. 175-91. Internet
[http://dx.doi.org/10.1016/B978-0-12-819240-5.00007-9]

CHAPTER 7

Advancements in Nano Drug Delivery Systems Using Natural Polymers

Nidhi Agrawal[1], **Rashmi Dewangan**[1], **Mohammad Akbar Siddiqui**[1], **Sakshi Gupta**[1], **S.K. Lanjhiyana**[1] and **Meenakshi Jaiswal**[1,*]

[1] *Department of Pharmacy, Guru Ghasidas Vishwavidyalaya, Bilaspur 495009, Chhattisgarh, India*

Abstract: With improvements in therapeutic efficacy, accuracy, and safety, nano Drug Delivery (DD) technologies have brought about a revolution in the pharmaceutical and healthcare sectors. Natural polymers have garnered a substantial amount of attention among the different materials that have been investigated for the purpose of nano DD. The utilization of these systems has become significant in nanomedicine for targeted drug administration, enhancing biocompatibility, safety, permeability, retention time, and reducing toxicity. An appropriate biodegradable polymer can be used as the drug carrier for targeted and sustained DD. This chapter summarizes current research and new developments in the field, highlighting the promise of natural polymer-based nano-DD methods and emerging polymers with unique characteristics suitable for DD applications.

Keywords: Biodegradable polymer, Controlled release, Nano drug delivery, Natural polymers, Targeted therapy.

INTRODUCTION

Biodegradable Polymers (BDP) found in nature are extensively utilized in drug delivery due to their natural abundance, biodegradability, biocompatibility, and reduced toxicity [1 - 4]. These encompass protein-based polymers such as albumin, gelatine, soy, and collagen, as well as polysaccharides like chitosan, agarose, dextran, hyaluronic acid, alginate, carrageenan, and cyclodextrin. Nevertheless, the use of natural polymers as drug carriers poses challenges due to their extensive molecular weight ranges and heterogeneity across batches (Fig. **1**) [5 - 9]. These polymers have a wide range of proven medicinal actions, including antioxidant, wound healing, antimicrobial, and anti-inflammatory, fields has

* **Corresponding author Meenakshi Jaiswal**: Department of Pharmacy, Guru Ghasidas Vishwavidyalaya, Bilaspur 495009, Chhattisgarh, India; E-mail: jaiswalmeenakshiggu@gmail.com

fostered growing confidence over its potential to significantly enhance clinical detection and treatment of diseases. Such a system encompasses *in vitro* and *in vivo* features, fabrication of advanced biocompatible materials, nutraceuticals, and medication delivery systems [10 - 16]. The primary motivation for interest in Nanoparticles (NPs) for medical applications is their distinctive characteristics, including a high surface-to-mass ratio, quantum properties, and their capacity to adsorb or serve as carriers for other materials [17, 18].

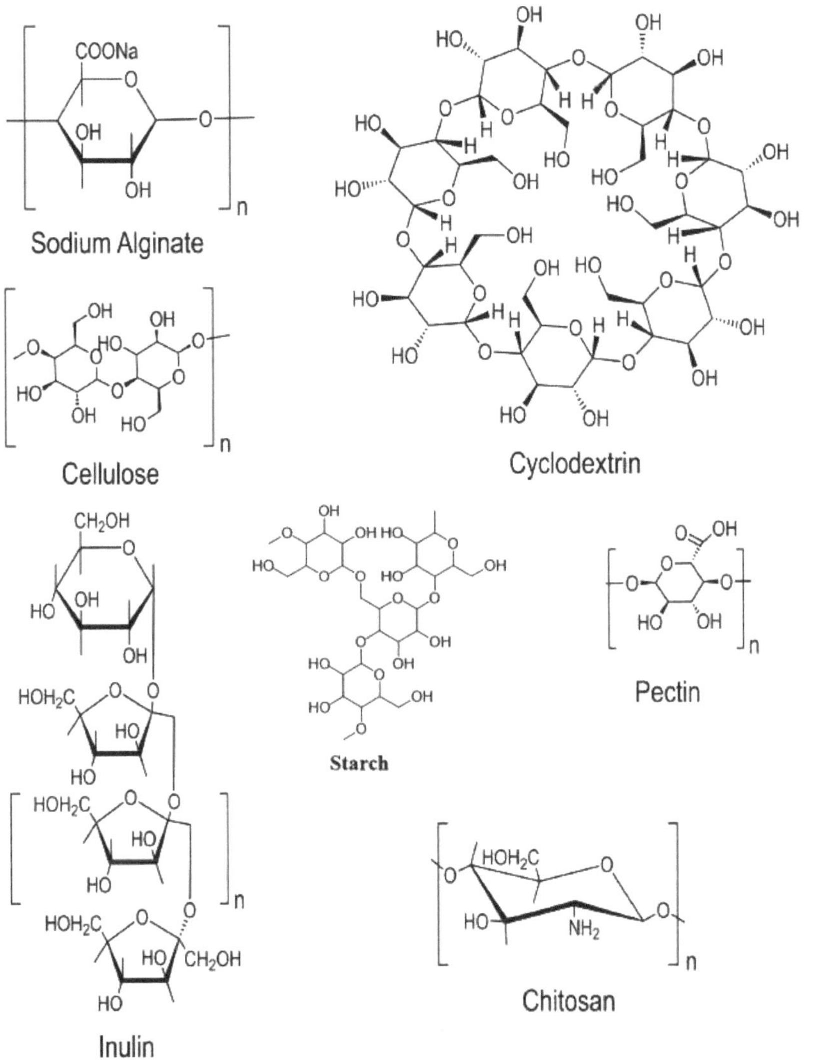

Fig. (1). Chemical structures of some natural polymers used in DD.

NATURAL POLYMERS USED IN NANO DD SYSTEMS

Cyclodextrins

β-Cyclodextrins (βCD), a type of cyclic oligosaccharide, are widely used, particularly for the delivery of hydrophobic drugs. These oligosaccharides are composed of 7 glucose units and have a hydrophilic outer layer and a hydrophobic interior. In one of the cyclodextrin-based nanoformulations, ginsenoside Rg3 and quercetin are successfully co-delivered, increasing the efficiency of chemo-immunotherapy for colorectal cancer. This method improves DD and malignant targeting and extends survival in animal models when used in combination with anti-PD-L1 therapy [19].

A novel βCD–Mel–AgNPs nanosystem was developed by the researchers, which improves the therapeutic potential of Melphalan. The formation of a robust complex with βCD markedly enhanced the drug's stability and solubility, minimizing its hydrolysis and degradation. The integration of Silver Nanoparticles (AgNPs) into the βCD–Mel complex not only enhanced the stability of the NPs but also offered a viable platform for targeted DD [20]. Also, the βCD@DB complex, combined with plasmonic gold NPs and polyethylene glycol, represents a notable progression in improving the delivery and effectiveness of Dacarbazine in cancer treatment. This advanced nanosystem overcomes the shortcomings of Dacarbazine, including poor solubility and instability, while enhancing its biocompatibility and controlled release properties [21].

Cellulose

Cellulose, the primary skeletal element in plants, is a nearly limitless polymeric raw material characterized by its intriguing structure and properties. They are hydrophilic, chiral, biodegradable, chemically modifying, and capable of creating diverse semicrystalline fibre morphologies [22]. An investigation demonstrates the feasibility of using Vetiver zizanioides root agro-waste for the enzymatic synthesis of Cellulose Nanoparticles (CNPs). The results demonstrate that pectinase and viscozyme are proficient in generating crystalline cellulose nanocrystals, whereas cellulase produces cellulose nanofibers. The synthesized CNPs demonstrate favourable characteristics, including non-toxicity, biodegradability, and biocompatibility, rendering them appropriate for use in textile and drug-delivery systems. This research highlights the beneficial utilization of agro-waste while adhering to green chemistry principles, thereby fostering sustainable practices in material production [23]. One of the research reports effectively synthesized and characterized a novel micellar DD system utilizing ethyl cellulose grafted with polyethylene glycol. The resultant nanomicelles exhibited advantageous characteristics, such as optimal size, minimal cytotoxicity of the blank micelles, and efficient drug release kinetics, especially at acidic pH levels [24]. The researchers have also effectively enhanced a DD system using N-Trimethyl Chitosan (TMC) and carboxylate-containing cellulose derivatives, illustrating the crucial role of both organic and inorganic cross-linkers in regulating the release of Ciprofloxacin (CPX). The results demonstrated that the organic crosslinking of TMC with Carboxymethyl Cellulose (CMC) produced a more stable and efficient delivery system than conventional formulations [25].

Starch

In the field of DD systems, starch has been widely used as a binder, disintegrant, and filler. It is the second most abundant natural polymer ever discovered. However, due to the poor functional qualities of natural starch, its utilization is restricted to certain contexts [26]. A novel delivery method integrating porous starch with self-assembled nanocarriers was developed to enhance the oral absorption of lipophilic drugs. The lipophilic probucol-loaded porous starch-based self-assembled nano-delivery (PSN) technology enhanced the water solubility of probucol by more than 50,000 times and achieved cumulative release exceeding 80% in Gastrointestinal (GI) fluids [27].

The controlled release of functional substances in food and digestive systems can be accomplished using starch, a non-allergenic, Generally Recognized as Safe (GRAS), and inexpensive natural carbohydrate polymer. Starch can be modified to acquire specific properties, and various wall materials can be incorporated with starch for encapsulation. Methods such as electrospinning, spray drying, and nano-emulsification can improve the controlled release of food components [28]. Few researchers have developed a new nano-DD system utilizing ligand-functionalized NPs, called p-Coumaric acid-loaded aptamer-conjugated starch nanoparticles (Apt-p-CA-AStNPs), for targeted therapy of triple-negative breast cancer. These NPs exhibited notable cytotoxicity against MDA-MB-231 cells, underscoring their ability to trigger apoptosis *via* several cellular pathways [29].

Inulin

Inulin is a type of storage polysaccharide that is water-soluble and is classified as a fructan, which is a collection of types of carbohydrates that are not digested. Inulin has been granted GRAS status in the United States of America and is widely available in approximately 36,000 plant species [30, 31]. The fabrication of core-shell Lipidic Nanoparticles (LNPs) utilizing lecithin sodium acetate and quaternized inulin has yielded encouraging outcomes for DD applications. The quaternized inulin coating enhanced the uptake of NPs in breast cancer cells and produced a superior toxicity profile relative to uncoated LNPs [32]. The Inulin-Stearic Acid (INU-SA) compound was also synthesized and tested for site-specific Genistein (GEN) administration for colon cancer therapy. To release the GEN site-specifically, modified INU-SA self-assembles into drug-releasing NPs. GNP has a lower IC50 than pure GEN against HCT 116 human colorectal cancer cells [33].

Pectin

Pectin acts as a gelling and stabilizing polymer in a wide variety of foods and specialized items, and it also has favourable effects on human health and many biomedical applications [34 - 36]. The research demonstrates the remarkable potential of pectin-based NPs for delivering drugs in oncological treatment. The excellent self-assembly of doxorubicin-conjugated hydrophilic pectin with dihydroartemisinin demonstrates a proficient approach for targeted drug release under acidic conditions, hence improving therapeutic efficacy against cancers [37]. Also, the fabrication of Selenium Nanoparticles (SeNPs) and a Selenium Nanocomposite (SeNC) was investigated to enhance DD. The SeNC, including pectin, keratin, and ferulic acid, exhibited significant encapsulation efficiency and prolonged drug release [38]. The advancement of a new nanoparticle-based DD system, particularly pectin-coated polymeric NPs containing the peptide Ac2-26, offers a potential strategy to improve anastomotic healing in surgical patients with inflammatory bowel disease. The study's results demonstrate that these NPs significantly diminish postoperative colitis activity, accelerate wound closure, and improve healing outcomes [39].

Guar Gum

Guar gum, a naturally occurring polymer, possesses a substantial number of hydroxyl groups, which augment its hydrogen bonding capacity when dissolved in water, hence enhancing the viscosity and gelling qualities of the guar gum solution. Guar gum is utilized across several sectors, including textile, culinary, petrochemical, mining, and paper, for diverse applications due to its characteristics [40 - 43]. A guar gum-pectin-based Solid Self-nanoemulsifying DD System (S-SNEDDS) containing curcumin and faecal microbiota extract was developed to treat Polycystic Ovarian Syndrome (PCOS). Pharmacokinetic and pharmacodynamic tests in letrozole-treated female Wistar rats showed increased bioavailability and therapeutic effectiveness with the improved formulation. The findings suggest that this novel delivery strategy may be a successful adjuvant therapy for PCOS, opening the door to research on gut microbiota regulation and metabolic disease treatment [44]. Another study also indicates that guar gum NPs encapsulated with vanadium oxide sulfate (GVNs) exhibit enhanced antioxidant activities relative to other investigated compounds, including non-encapsulated guar gum NPs and vanadium oxide sulfate alone [45].

Chitosan

Chitosan, an amino polysaccharide derived from natural chitin biomass, has garnered a lot of attention as one of the developing pharmaceutical excipients and DD vehicles. It has been reported that chitosan may be utilized in DD systems to produce pharmaceuticals that have improved mucoadhesiveness, penetration, absorption, and bioavailability (Table 1) [46 - 48]. The research reveals that chitosan-based nanoparticles adorned with PEGylated zinc oxide nanoparticles (CS-AMP-P-ZnO NPs) significantly improve the antibacterial efficacy of ampicillin against drug-resistant pathogens such as *E. coli.* The formulation has advantageous characteristics, including reduced aggregation, improved stability, and enhanced biocompatibility, positioning it as a viable option for addressing bacterial infections with minimal harm to human cells or other biological systems [49].

Table 1. List of some nano DD systems that utilize natural polymers for DD.

Types of Delivery system	Drug used	Polymer used	Outcome of the research	References
Chitosan-based nanoparticles adorned with PEGylated zinc oxide nanoparticles (CS-AMP-P-ZnO NPs)	Ampicillin	Chitosan and PEGylated zinc oxide	Improvement of antibacterial efficacy	[49]
Chitosan-based Nanoparticles (ChNPs)	Paclitaxel	Chitosan	Optimized cellular uptake, drug accumulation, cytotoxicity, and selectivity	[54]
Quaternary ammonium—chitosan nanoparticles and their S-protected thiolated derivative	Fluorescein isothiocyanate dextran (FD4)	Chitosan (Ch), hyaluronic acid (HA)	NP QA-Ch-S-pro was found to be superior to NP QA-Ch in terms of mucoadhesiveness	[55]
Combinational Mucoadhesive Nanoparticle for Intranasal Delivery	Rivastigmine and insulin,	Chitosan	A promising approach for enhancing nasal transport efficiency	[56]
Mucoadhesive nanoparticles	Gemcitabine	PLGA, chitosan	CH-GEM-NPs are suitable delivery systems for GEM, both as a single therapy and as a chemosensitizer to the GBM gold standard therapy	[57]

(Table 1) cont.....

Types of Delivery system	Drug used	Polymer used	Outcome of the research	References
Nanofibers	Resveratrol	Chitosan, gelrite	Scanning electron microscopy (SEM) showed that the diameters of the formulated fibres were 166 ± 37 nm for 95:5% w/v (Chitosan: gelrite) and 291 ± 41 nm for 95:10% w/v (Chitosan:gelrite). Encapsulation efficiency was found to be 86 ± 6%, out of which 43–51% was delivered to the intestine only	[58]

Breast cancer represents a significant global health issue, and the identification of cost-effective and targeted treatment strategies poses considerable challenges. Chitosan-based Nanoparticles (ChNPs) exhibit potential for targeted DD systems, facilitating the transfer of antitumor drugs to specific sites. Researchers have enhanced ChNPs to optimize cellular uptake, drug accumulation, cytotoxicity, and selectivity. The modifications exploit the Enhanced Permeability and Retention (EPR) effect, along with biological ligands [50 - 53].

Gelatine

Gelatine has been extensively utilized in the food, pharmaceutical, and cosmetic sectors owing to its superior biocompatibility, facile biodegradability, and low antigenicity [59, 60]. Researchers succeeded in producing an innovative nano-in nanofiber DD system employing temozolomide-loaded gelatine NPs encapsulated within polyvinyl alcohol nanofibers. This novel method exhibited efficient prolonged drug release over seven days and markedly improved cellular uptake in U87MG glioma cells [61]. Gelatine Nanocomposites (GNCs) with different amounts of Carbon Dots (CDs) were developed utilizing solvent-casting techniques. CDs functioned as a cross-linker and chromophore, reducing the need for hazardous cross-linkers. The GNC hydrogel was utilized to investigate the release of the antibacterial agent cefadroxil under stomach and intestinal pH environments [62].

Alginate

Alginates are a type of biopolymer that are often derived from brown seaweed, brown algae (*Ochrophyta* and *Phaeophyceae*), and bacteria (*Azotobacter vinelandii* and *Pseudomonas* species) that are members of the polycationic copolymer family. The molecular mass of commercial grades of these biopolymers ranges from 32,000 to 40,000 g/mol, and they are bio-degradable, biocompatible, non-antigenic, and non-hazardous [63, 64]. Alginate serves a function in the formulation of resveratrol-loaded PLGA nanoparticles (RES-PCAC-NPs) for the management of Ulcerative Colitis (UC). Employing layer-by layer self-assembly technology, alginate facilitates the development of a polyelectrolyte film that improves the stability and transport of NPs through the gastric environment to the specified sites of inflammation [65]. An advanced oral DD system for anti-TNF-α antibodies, particularly Infliximab (IFX), is designed for the treatment of Inflammatory Bowel Disease (IBD). Integrating alginate into the nano-in-microparticle formulation with chitosan and carboxymethyl chitosan successfully protects IFX from the adverse circumstances of the GI tract. This protection is vital for ensuring that the therapeutic drug reaches the inflamed intestinal tissues, where it can exert its anti-inflammatory effects [66].

MECHANISM OF DRUG RELEASE FROM NANO FORMULATIONS

The fundamental objective of controlled DD systems is to maintain therapeutic drug levels in the bloodstream while reducing dose frequency through sustained and predictable release, ideally adhering to a zero-order kinetic profile. The release of drugs from nanocarriers is affected by the type and ratio of the drug, polymer, and excipients, their physicochemical interactions, and the production technique. Polymeric nanoparticle systems have attracted considerable interest owing to their adjustable physicochemical properties, biocompatibility, and ability to encapsulate both hydrophilic and hydrophobic medicines, thereby facilitating precise regulation of release kinetics and targeted administration (Fig. **2**).

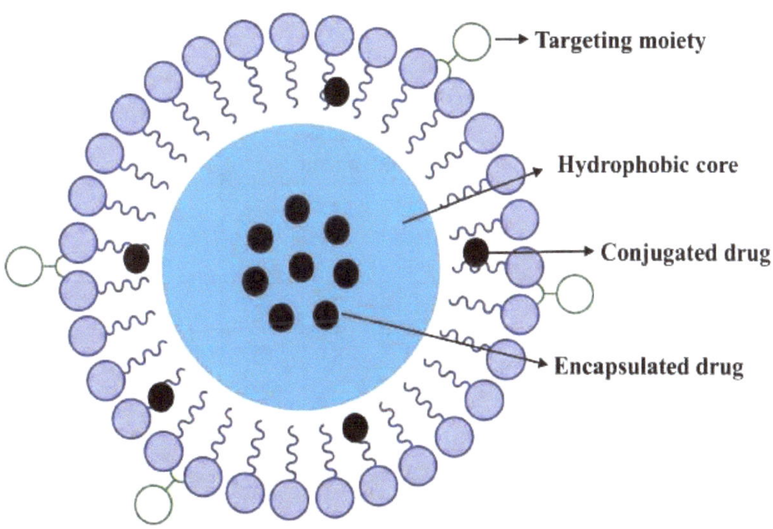

Fig. (2). Schematic illustration of the polymeric nanoparticle system used in DD.

Drug release can be classified into diffusion-controlled, solvent-controlled, degradation-controlled, and stimuli-responsive (pH-controlled) systems based on the underlying mechanism [67]. In diffusion-controlled systems, drugs permeate a membrane or polymer matrix driven by concentration gradients, whereas solvent-controlled systems, such as osmotic and swelling-controlled carriers, manage release *via* solvent penetration and polymer network expansion, frequently characterized by the Peppas model. By utilizing biodegradable polymers, degradation-controlled systems allow for the release of drugs through the process of hydrolytic or enzymatic polymer erosion. Stimuli-responsive systems release drugs in response to external or internal stimuli like pH, temperature, magnetic fields, or ultrasound, facilitating site-specific delivery, especially beneficial for targeting tumour microenvironments [68]. In combination, these strategies may have meticulous regulation of drug kinetics, augmenting therapeutic effectiveness and patient adherence.

RECENT PATENTS AND MARKETED NANOFORMULATIONS USING NATURAL POLYMERS

Natural polymers, including chitosan, alginate, gelatine, and hyaluronic acid, have emerged as promising biomaterials for nano-DD owing to their biodegradability, biocompatibility, and rapid chemical modification. Recent trends have indicated a transition from exclusively synthetic carriers to hybrid and green nanotechnologies that utilize natural biopolymers to enhance therapeutic efficacy and mitigate toxicity (Table **2**).

Table 2. Examples of some marketed nanoformulations using natural polymers.

Formulation	Natural Polymer	Formulation Mechanism	Regulatory Status	Clinical Trial Outcome
Abraxane	Albumin	Nanoparticle-bound paclitaxel using albumin for solubility	FDA-approved	Improved survival in breast and pancreatic cancer
Onivyde	Natural lipids	PEGylated liposomal irinotecan for sustained release	FDA-approved	Enhanced retention and reduced toxicity
α-Mangostin hydrogel film	Chitosan + Alginate	Hydrogel film	Phase 2 (clinical)	For oral/oral-mucosal recurrent aphthous stomatitis
OSSIXA(r) VOLUMAX	Collagen	Membrane/scaffold	FDA-approved	Guided bone & tissue regeneration

(Table 2) cont.....

Formulation	Natural Polymer	Formulation Mechanism	Regulatory Status	Clinical Trial Outcome
JuvA(c)derm VolbellaA(r) XC	Hyaluronic Acid	Gel injection	FDA-approved	Lip augmentation and facial wrinkles
RestylaneA(r)	Hyaluronic acid	Injectable gel	FDA-approved	Perioral lines and lip enhancement
Plenity$_{TM}$	Modified Cellulose	Hydrogel capsule	FDA-approved	Weight loss (obesity management)
LacrimeraA(r)	Chitosan-N-acetylcysteine	Eye drops	Approved for use in the European market	Dry eye disease treatment

Chitosan-based nanoparticles containing paclitaxel were shown to exhibit enhanced anticancer efficacy and reduced haemolytic toxicity compared to traditional formulations, whereas heparin-berberine conjugates show potential against *Helicobacter pylori* infections with reduced cytotoxicity [69, 70]. Likewise, ellagic acid-stabilized solid lipid nanoparticles containing vancomycin reduced nephrotoxicity, while polymeric micelles of quercetin facilitated sustained drug release for up to 10 days [71, 72]. Numerous FDA-approved nanomedicines, such as DoxilA(r) (liposomal doxorubicin) and AbraxaneA(r) (albumin-bound paclitaxel), have facilitated the development of natural polymer-based systems, stimulating additional advancements in bio-derived nanocarriers [73]. Liu *et al.* have invented a temperature and redox-responsive nano hydrogel termed "disulfide cross-linked polyisopropylacrylamide grafted dextran. The final product was prepared by synthesizing 2-dodecyltrithiocarbonyl-2-methylpropionic acid, grafting it onto dextran, and then polymerizing it. This method utilizes reversible addition-fragmentation chain transfer radical polymerization, which enables the controlled polymerization with non-toxic reagents and precision molecular structures [74].

In another patent, inventors have presented a cellulose aerogel that consists of cellulose nanoparticles, ideally comprising at least 50% to 80% cellulose nanocrystals by weight, with densities ranging from 0.001 to 1.59 g/cm^3 and an average pore diameter of less than 100 nm. This innovation has shown high porosity, low density, and a significant surface area, enabling diverse applications in medicinal, cosmetic, and environmental fields by incorporating functional additives like carbon nanotubes and metal nanoparticles, thus promoting sustainable practices in materials science [75]. Likewise, in 2019, inventors presented an innovative approach to addressing atrophic Age-related Macular Degeneration (AMD) *via* a sustained-release DD system. This invention provides a formulation for a drug delivery system, capable of releasing therapeutic doses of the anti-neovascular agent over a prolonged duration, hence decreasing the necessity for frequent injections and mitigating the risk of complications associated with repeated treatments. This patent represents a substantial advancement in the management of dry AMD, offering a promising strategy for a condition that currently lacks appropriate therapeutic options [76].

Despite significant advancements, numerous challenges remain regarding regulatory approval, scalability, and the long-term stability of these systems. The diversity in natural polymer sources, inconsistencies across batches, and the risk of microbial contamination can affect the reproducibility of formulations. Therefore, ongoing research is aimed at standardizing polymer purification, managing crosslinking, and understanding the mechanisms of degradation pathway [77]. Continuous advancements in polymer engineering, manufacturing techniques, and clinical validation are progressively transforming natural polymer-based nanocarriers from the laboratory into clinically applicable and economically viable nanomedicine platforms.

CONCLUSION

In conclusion, the exploration of biodegradable natural polymers in DD systems has revealed significant potential to advance therapeutic efficacy while minimizing toxicity. Various natural polymers, including cyclodextrins, cellulose, starch, inulin, pectin, guar gum, chitosan, gelatine, and alginate, have been effectively utilized to develop innovative nanoparticle-based DD systems. These systems exploit the exclusive properties of each polymer to improve drug solubility, stability, and targeted delivery, particularly in the treatment of complex diseases, *viz*., tumour and IBD conditions. Advancements in nanotechnology, coupled with the sustainable use of natural resources, highlight the potential for these BDPs to revolutionize DD methods, ultimately leading to more effective and safer therapeutic options. Continued research and development in this field are essential to overcome existing challenges and fully understand the benefits of these natural polymers in clinical applications.

REFERENCES

[1] Bhovi VK, Melinmath SP, Gowda R. Biodegradable polymers and their applications: A review. Mini Rev Med Chem 2022; 22(16): 2081-101.
[http://dx.doi.org/10.2174/1389557522666220128152847] [PMID: 35088668]

[2] Fiandra EF, Shaw L, Starck M, McGurk CJ, Mahon CS. Designing biodegradable alternatives to commodity polymers. Chem Soc Rev 2023; 52(23): 8085-105.
[http://dx.doi.org/10.1039/D3CS00556A] [PMID: 37885416]

[3] Oleksy M, Dynarowicz K, Aebisher D. Advances in biodegradable polymers and biomaterials for medical applications-a review. Molecules 2023; 28(17): 6213.
[http://dx.doi.org/10.3390/molecules28176213] [PMID: 37687042]

[4] Nath PC, Sharma R, Debnath S, *et al.* Recent trends in polysaccharide-based biodegradable polymers for smart food packaging industry. Int J Biol Macromol 2023; 253(Pt 8): 127524.
[http://dx.doi.org/10.1016/j.ijbiomac.2023.127524] [PMID: 37865365]

[5] Hu L, Sun Y, Wu Y. Advances in chitosan-based drug delivery vehicles. Nanoscale 2013; 5(8): 3103-11.
[http://dx.doi.org/10.1039/c3nr00338h] [PMID: 23515527]

[6] Park JH, Saravanakumar G, Kim K, Kwon IC. Targeted delivery of low molecular drugs using chitosan and its derivatives. Adv Drug Deliv Rev 2010; 62(1): 28-41.
[http://dx.doi.org/10.1016/j.addr.2009.10.003] [PMID: 19874862]

[7] Jiang Z, Song Z, Cao C, *et al.* Multiple natural polymers in drug and gene delivery systems. Curr Med Chem 2024; 31(13): 1691-715.
[http://dx.doi.org/10.2174/0929867330666230316094540] [PMID: 36927424]

[8] Kruk K, Winnicka K. Alginates combined with natural polymers as valuable drug delivery platforms. Mar Drugs 2022; 21(1): 11.
[http://dx.doi.org/10.3390/md21010011] [PMID: 36662184]

[9] George A, Shah PA, Shrivastav PS. Natural biodegradable polymers based nano-formulations for drug delivery: A review. Int J Pharm 2019; 561: 244-64.
[http://dx.doi.org/10.1016/j.ijpharm.2019.03.011] [PMID: 30851391]

[10] Houacine C, Yousaf SS, Khan I, Khurana RK, Singh KK. Potential of natural biomaterials in nano-scale drug delivery. Curr Pharm Des 2019; 24(43): 5188-206.
[http://dx.doi.org/10.2174/1381612825666190118153057] [PMID: 30657035]

[11] Haque SE, Iqubal A, Iqubal MK, Fazal SA, Pottoo FH. Nutraceuticals and their derived nano-formulations for the prevention and treatment of alzheimer's disease. Curr Mol Pharmacol 2021; 15(1): 23-50.
[http://dx.doi.org/10.2174/1874467214666210309115605] [PMID: 33687906]

[12] Ozogul Y, Karsli GT, Durmus M, *et al.* Recent developments in industrial applications of nanoemulsions. Adv Colloid Interface Sci 2022; 304: 102685.
[http://dx.doi.org/10.1016/j.cis.2022.102685] [PMID: 35504214]

[13] Zhang Y, Wu Y, Du H, *et al.* Nano-drug delivery systems in oral cancer therapy: Recent developments and prospective. Pharmaceutics 2023; 16(1): 7.
[http://dx.doi.org/10.3390/pharmaceutics16010007] [PMID: 38276483]

[14] Yasmin F, Najeeb H, Shaikh S, *et al.* Novel drug delivery systems for inflammatory bowel disease. World J Gastroenterol 2022; 28(18): 1922-33.
[http://dx.doi.org/10.3748/wjg.v28.i18.1922] [PMID: 35664964]

[15] Kamath PR, Sunil D. Nano-chitosan particles in anticancer drug delivery: An up-to-date review. Mini Rev Med Chem 2017; 17(15): 1457-87.
[http://dx.doi.org/10.2174/1389557516666170228105731] [PMID: 28245780]

[16] Agrawal N, Siddiqui MA, Gupta S, Jaiswal M, Lanjhiyana SK. Exploring recent advances in colon-targeted drug delivery systems: From traditional methods to advanced technologies. Curr Gastroenterol Rep 2025; 27(1): 67.
[http://dx.doi.org/10.1007/s11894-025-01019-w] [PMID: 41082057]

[17] De Jong . Drug delivery and nanoparticles: Applications and hazards. Int J Nanomedicine 2008; 133: 133.
[http://dx.doi.org/10.2147/IJN.S596]

[18] Ferrari M. Cancer nanotechnology: opportunities and challenges. Nat Rev Cancer 2005; 5(3): 161-71.
[http://dx.doi.org/10.1038/nrc1566] [PMID: 15738981]

[19] Sun D, Zou Y, Song L, *et al.* A cyclodextrin-based nanoformulation achieves co-delivery of

ginsenoside Rg3 and quercetin for chemo-immunotherapy in colorectal cancer. Acta Pharm Sin B 2022; 12(1): 378-93.
[http://dx.doi.org/10.1016/j.apsb.2021.06.005] [PMID: 35127393]

[20] Sierpe R, Donoso-González O, Lang E, *et al.* Solid-state formation of a potential melphalan delivery nanosystem based on β-cyclodextrin and silver nanoparticles. Int J Mol Sci 2023; 24(4): 3990.
[http://dx.doi.org/10.3390/ijms24043990] [PMID: 36835401]

[21] Quintana-Contardo S, Donoso-González O, Lang E, *et al.* Optimizing dacarbazine therapy: Design of a laser-triggered delivery system based on β-cyclodextrin and plasmonic gold nanoparticles. Pharmaceutics 2023; 15(2): 458.
[http://dx.doi.org/10.3390/pharmaceutics15020458] [PMID: 36839779]

[22] Klemm D, Heublein B, Fink HP, Bohn A. Cellulose: fascinating biopolymer and sustainable raw material. Angew Chem Int Ed 2005; 44(22): 3358-93.
[http://dx.doi.org/10.1002/anie.200460587] [PMID: 15861454]

[23] Seth R, Meena A, Meena R. Enzyme-based green synthesis, characterisation, and toxicity studies of cellulose nanocrystals/fibres produced from the Vetiveria zizanioides roots agro-waste. Environ Sci Pollut Res Int 2022; 30(55): 116984-99.
[http://dx.doi.org/10.1007/s11356-022-24455-x] [PMID: 36484940]

[24] Singam A, Killi N, Patel PR, Gundloori RVN. PEGylated ethyl cellulose micelles as a nanocarrier for drug delivery. RSC Advances 2021; 11(49): 30532-43.
[http://dx.doi.org/10.1039/D1RA04242D] [PMID: 35479870]

[25] Lotfy VF, Basta AH. Optimizing the chitosan-cellulose based drug delivery system for controlling the ciprofloxacin release versus organic/inorganic crosslinker, characterization and kinetic study. Int J Biol Macromol 2020; 165(Pt A): 1496-506.
[http://dx.doi.org/10.1016/j.ijbiomac.2020.10.047] [PMID: 33058976]

[26] Odeniyi MA, Omoteso OA, Adepoju AO, Jaiyeoba KT. Starch nanoparticles in drug delivery: A review. Polim Med 2018; 48(1): 41-5.
[http://dx.doi.org/10.17219/pim/99993] [PMID: 30657657]

[27] Zhang Z, Huang J, Jiang S, *et al.* Porous starch based self-assembled nano-delivery system improves the oral absorption of lipophilic drug. Int J Pharm 2013; 444(1-2): 162-8.
[http://dx.doi.org/10.1016/j.ijpharm.2013.01.021] [PMID: 23340325]

[28] Zhu F. Encapsulation and delivery of food ingredients using starch based systems. Food Chem 2017; 229: 542-52.
[http://dx.doi.org/10.1016/j.foodchem.2017.02.101] [PMID: 28372213]

[29] Mariadoss AVA, Saravanakumar K, Sathiyaseelan A, Karthikkumar V, Wang MH. Smart drug delivery of p-Coumaric acid loaded aptamer conjugated starch nanoparticles for effective triple-negative breast cancer therapy. Int J Biol Macromol 2022; 195: 22-9.
[http://dx.doi.org/10.1016/j.ijbiomac.2021.11.170] [PMID: 34861273]

[30] Shoaib M, Shehzad A, Omar M, *et al.* Inulin: Properties, health benefits and food applications. Carbohydr Polym 2016; 147: 444-54.
[http://dx.doi.org/10.1016/j.carbpol.2016.04.020] [PMID: 27178951]

[31] Le Bastard Q, Chapelet G, Javaudin F, Lepelletier D, Batard E, Montassier E. The effects of inulin on gut microbial composition: a systematic review of evidence from human studies. Eur J Clin Microbiol Infect Dis 2020; 39(3): 403-13.
[http://dx.doi.org/10.1007/s10096-019-03721-w] [PMID: 31707507]

[32] Vatansever O, Bahadori F, Bulut S, Eroglu MS. Coating with cationic inulin enhances the drug release profile and *in vitro* anticancer activity of lecithin-based nano drug delivery systems. Int J Biol Macromol 2023; 237: 123955.
[http://dx.doi.org/10.1016/j.ijbiomac.2023.123955] [PMID: 36906213]

[33] Jangid AK, Solanki R, Patel S, Pooja D, Kulhari H. Genistein encapsulated inulin-stearic acid bioconjugate nanoparticles: Formulation development, characterization and anticancer activity. Int J Biol Macromol 2022; 206: 213-21.
[http://dx.doi.org/10.1016/j.ijbiomac.2022.02.031] [PMID: 35181329]

[34] Mohnen D. Pectin structure and biosynthesis. Curr Opin Plant Biol 2008; 11(3): 266-77.
[http://dx.doi.org/10.1016/j.pbi.2008.03.006] [PMID: 18486536]

[35] Thakur BR, Singh RK, Handa AK, Rao MA. Chemistry and uses of pectin - A review. Crit Rev Food Sci Nutr 1997; 37(1): 47-73.
[http://dx.doi.org/10.1080/10408399709527767] [PMID: 9067088]

[36] Emran TB, Islam F, Mitra S, *et al.* Pectin: A bioactive food polysaccharide with cancer preventive potential. Molecules 2022; 27(21): 7405.
[http://dx.doi.org/10.3390/molecules27217405] [PMID: 36364232]

[37] Tao Y, Zheng D, Zhao J, *et al.* Self-assembling ph-responsive nanoparticle platform based on pectin–doxorubicin conjugates for codelivery of anticancer drugs. ACS Omega 2021; 6(15): 9998-10004.
[http://dx.doi.org/10.1021/acsomega.0c06131] [PMID: 34056155]

[38] Baburao C, Selvasudha N, Kishore K, *et al.* Design, fabrication, and evaluation of keratin and pectin incorporated supramolecular structured zero-oxidation state selenium nanogel blended 3D printed transdermal patch. Int J Biol Macromol 2024; 268(Pt 1): 131769.
[http://dx.doi.org/10.1016/j.ijbiomac.2024.131769] [PMID: 38692999]

[39] Lee JH, Reischl S, Walter RL, *et al.* Orally delivered biodegradable targeted inflammation resolving pectin-coated nanoparticles induce anastomotic healing post intestinal surgery. Sci Rep 2024; 14(1): 29253.
[http://dx.doi.org/10.1038/s41598-024-80886-1] [PMID: 39587209]

[40] Sharma G, Sharma S, Kumar A, *et al.* Guar gum and its composites as potential materials for diverse applications: A review. Carbohydr Polym 2018; 199: 534-45.
[http://dx.doi.org/10.1016/j.carbpol.2018.07.053] [PMID: 30143160]

[41] Thombare N, Jha U, Mishra S, Siddiqui MZ. Guar gum as a promising starting material for diverse applications: A review. Int J Biol Macromol 2016; 88: 361-72.
[http://dx.doi.org/10.1016/j.ijbiomac.2016.04.001] [PMID: 27044346]

[42] Mandal S, Hwang S, Shi SQ. Guar gum, a low-cost sustainable biopolymer, for wastewater treatment: A review. Int J Biol Macromol 2023; 226: 368-82.
[http://dx.doi.org/10.1016/j.ijbiomac.2022.12.039] [PMID: 36513177]

[43] Garg SS, Gupta J. Guar gum-based nanoformulations: Implications for improving drug delivery. Int J Biol Macromol 2023; 229: 476-85.
[http://dx.doi.org/10.1016/j.ijbiomac.2022.12.271] [PMID: 36603711]

[44] Choi H, Lim J, Hong J, *et al.* Curcumin interrupts the interaction between the androgen receptor and Wnt/β-catenin signaling pathway in LNCaP prostate cancer cells. Prostate Cancer Prostatic Dis 2010; 13: 343-9.
[http://dx.doi.org/10.1007/s00210-024-03029-3] [PMID: 38507103]

[45] Soumya RS, Reshmi R, Jomon S, Antu KA, Riya MP, Raghu KG. Synthesis, characterization and evaluation of the antioxidant potential of vanadium encapsulated guar gum nanoparticles. Food Funct 2014; 5(3): 535-44.
[http://dx.doi.org/10.1039/c3fo60339c] [PMID: 24463743]

[46] Khan MIH, An X, Dai L, Li H, Khan A, Ni Y. Chitosan-based polymer matrix for pharmaceutical excipients and drug delivery. Curr Med Chem 2019; 26(14): 2502-13.
[http://dx.doi.org/10.2174/0929867325666180927100817] [PMID: 30259805]

[47] Muxika A, Etxabide A, Uranga J, Guerrero P, de la Caba K. Chitosan as a bioactive polymer:

Processing, properties and applications. Int J Biol Macromol 2017; 105(Pt 2): 1358-68.
[http://dx.doi.org/10.1016/j.ijbiomac.2017.07.087] [PMID: 28735006]

[48] Matalqah SM, Aiedeh K, Mhaidat NM, Alzoubi KH, Bustanji Y, Hamad I. Chitosan nanoparticles as a novel drug delivery system: A review article. Curr Drug Targets 2020; 21(15): 1613-24.
[http://dx.doi.org/10.2174/1389450121666200711172536] [PMID: 32651965]

[49] Sathiyaseelan A, Saravanakumar K, Zhang X, Naveen KV, Wang MH. Ampicillin-resistant bacterial pathogens targeted chitosan nano-drug delivery system (CS-AMP-P-ZnO) for combinational antibacterial treatment. Int J Biol Macromol 2023; 237: 124129.
[http://dx.doi.org/10.1016/j.ijbiomac.2023.124129] [PMID: 36958450]

[50] Herdiana Y, Wathoni N, Shamsuddin S, Joni IM, Muchtaridi M. Chitosan-based nanoparticles of targeted drug delivery system in breast cancer treatment. Polymers (Basel) 2021; 13(11): 1717.
[http://dx.doi.org/10.3390/polym13111717] [PMID: 34074020]

[51] Shanmuganathan R, Edison TNJI, LewisOscar F, Kumar P, Shanmugam S, Pugazhendhi A. Chitosan nanopolymers: An overview of drug delivery against cancer. Int J Biol Macromol 2019; 130: 727-36.
[http://dx.doi.org/10.1016/j.ijbiomac.2019.02.060] [PMID: 30771392]

[52] Liyanage PY, Hettiarachchi SD, Zhou Y, *et al.* Nanoparticle-mediated targeted drug delivery for breast cancer treatment. Biochim Biophys Acta Rev Cancer 2019; 1871(2): 419-33.
[http://dx.doi.org/10.1016/j.bbcan.2019.04.006] [PMID: 31034927]

[53] F ud Din, W Aman, I Ullah, OS Qureshi, O Mustapha, S Shafique. Effective use of nanocarriers as drug delivery systems for the treatment of selected tumors. Int J Nanomedicine 2017; 12: 7291-309.
[http://dx.doi.org/10.2147/IJN.S146315]

[54] Zhang X, Niu S, Williams GR, *et al.* Dual-responsive nanoparticles based on chitosan for enhanced breast cancer therapy. Carbohydr Polym 2019; 221: 84-93.
[http://dx.doi.org/10.1016/j.carbpol.2019.05.081] [PMID: 31227170]

[55] Fabiano A, Piras AM, Uccello-Barretta G, *et al.* Impact of mucoadhesive polymeric nanoparticulate systems on oral bioavailability of a macromolecular model drug. Eur J Pharm Biopharm 2018; 130: 281-9.
[http://dx.doi.org/10.1016/j.ejpb.2018.07.010] [PMID: 30006244]

[56] Jamshidnejad-Tosaramandani T, Kashanian S, Karimi I, SchiAth HB. Synthesis of a rivastigmine and insulin combinational mucoadhesive nanoparticle for intranasal delivery. Polymers (Basel) 2024; 16(4): 510.
[http://dx.doi.org/10.3390/polym16040510] [PMID: 38399888]

[57] Ramalho MJ, Serra A%, Lima J, Loureiro JA, Pereira MC. Chitosan-PLGA mucoadhesive nanoparticles for gemcitabine repurposing for glioblastoma therapy. Eur J Pharm Biopharm 2024; 200: 114326.
[http://dx.doi.org/10.1016/j.ejpb.2024.114326] [PMID: 38759897]

[58] Rostami M, Ghorbani M, Aman mohammadi M, Delavar M, Tabibiazar M, Ramezani S. Development of resveratrol loaded chitosan-gellan nanofiber as a novel gastrointestinal delivery system. Int J Biol Macromol 2019; 135: 698-705.
[http://dx.doi.org/10.1016/j.ijbiomac.2019.05.187] [PMID: 31145955]

[59] Liu D, Nikoo M, Boran G, Zhou P, Regenstein JM. Collagen and gelatin. Annu Rev Food Sci Technol 2015; 6(1): 527-57.
[http://dx.doi.org/10.1146/annurev-food-031414-111800] [PMID: 25884286]

[60] Salahuddin B, Wang S, Sangian D, Aziz S, Gu Q. Hybrid gelatin hydrogels in nanomedicine applications. ACS Appl Bio Mater 2021; 4(4): 2886-906.
[http://dx.doi.org/10.1021/acsabm.0c01630] [PMID: 35014383]

[61] Shetty K, Yadav KS. Temozolomide nano-in-nanofiber delivery system with sustained release and enhanced cellular uptake by U87MG cells. Drug Dev Ind Pharm 2024; 50(5): 420-31.

[http://dx.doi.org/10.1080/03639045.2024.2332906] [PMID: 38502031]

[62] Bhattacharyya SK, Dule M, Paul R, *et al.* Carbon dot cross-linked gelatin nanocomposite hydrogel for pH-sensing and pH-responsive drug delivery. ACS Biomater Sci Eng 2020; 6(10): 5662-74. [http://dx.doi.org/10.1021/acsbiomaterials.0c00982] [PMID: 33320568]

[63] Kothale D, Verma U, Dewangan N, Jana P, Jain A, Jain D. Alginate as promising natural polymer for pharmaceutical, food, and biomedical applications. Curr Drug Deliv 2020; 17(9): 755-75. [http://dx.doi.org/10.2174/1567201817666200810110226] [PMID: 32778024]

[64] Severino P, da Silva CF, Andrade LN, de Lima Oliveira D, Campos J, Souto EB. Alginate nanoparticles for drug delivery and targeting. Curr Pharm Des 2019; 25(11): 1312-34. [http://dx.doi.org/10.2174/1381612825666190425163424] [PMID: 31465282]

[65] Jin M, Li S, Wu Y, Li D, Han Y. Construction of chitosan/alginate nano-drug delivery system for improving dextran sodium sulfate-induced colitis in mice. Nanomaterials (Basel) 2021; 11(8): 1884. [http://dx.doi.org/10.3390/nano11081884] [PMID: 34443715]

[66] Li X, Yu M, Zhu Z, *et al.* Oral delivery of infliximab using nano-in-microparticles for the treatment of inflammatory bowel disease. Carbohydr Polym 2021; 273: 118556. [http://dx.doi.org/10.1016/j.carbpol.2021.118556] [PMID: 34560967]

[67] Langer R, Peppas N. Chemical and physical structure of polymers as carriers for controlled release of bioactive agents: A review. J Macromol Sci Part C Polym Rev 1983; 23(1): 61-126. [http://dx.doi.org/10.1080/07366578308079439]

[68] Son GH, Lee BJ, Cho CW. Mechanisms of drug release from advanced drug formulations such as polymeric-based drug-delivery systems and lipid nanoparticles. J Pharm Investig 2017; 47(4): 287-96. [http://dx.doi.org/10.1007/s40005-017-0320-1]

[69] Hong SP, Kang SH, Kim DK, Kang BS. Paramagnetic nanoparticle-based targeting theranostic agent for c6 rat glioma cell. J Nanomater 2016; 2016: 1-10. [http://dx.doi.org/10.1155/2016/7617894]

[70] Chang CH, Huang WY, Lai CH, *et al.* Development of novel nanoparticles shelled with heparin for berberine delivery to treat Helicobacter pylori. Acta Biomater 2011; 7(2): 593-603. [http://dx.doi.org/10.1016/j.actbio.2010.08.028] [PMID: 20813208]

[71] Aldawsari HM, Hosny KM. Solid lipid nanoparticles of Vancomycin loaded with Ellagic acid as a tool for overcoming nephrotoxic side effects: Preparation, characterization, and nephrotoxicity evaluation. J Drug Deliv Sci Technol 2018; 45: 76-80. [http://dx.doi.org/10.1016/j.jddst.2018.02.016]

[72] Dian L, Yu E, Chen X, *et al.* Enhancing oral bioavailability of quercetin using novel soluplus polymeric micelles. Nanoscale Res Lett 2014; 9(1): 684. [http://dx.doi.org/10.1186/1556-276X-9-684] [PMID: 26088982]

[73] Maeng JH, Lee DH, Jung KH, *et al.* Multifunctional doxorubicin loaded superparamagnetic iron oxide nanoparticles for chemotherapy and magnetic resonance imaging in liver cancer. Biomaterials 2010; 31(18): 4995-5006. [http://dx.doi.org/10.1016/j.biomaterials.2010.02.068] [PMID: 20347138]

[74] Shuoqi Liu, Fengbao Zhang, Weipeng Lü, Yang Wang, Guoliang Zhang. Temperature and redox stimuli responsive nano-hydrogel and preparation method thereof. CN102391427A 2019.

[75] Rebecca Davies. Thielemans Wim Albert Wilfried Irene. Cellulose nanoparticle aerogels, hydrogels and organogels US20130018112A1 2019.

[76] Scott M. Whitcup, Michael R. Robinson, Wendy M. Blanda, Patrick M. Hughes, James A. Burke. Method for treating atrophic age related macular degeneration. US Patent 2022; US 20190336441A1.

[77] Harun-Or-Rashid M, Aktar MN, Hossain MS, *et al.* Recent advances in micro- and nano-drug delivery systems based on natural and synthetic biomaterials. Polymers (Basel) 2023; 15(23): 4563. [http://dx.doi.org/10.3390/polym15234563] [PMID: 38231996]

CHAPTER 8

Natural Polymers in Combination Therapies for Inflammatory Bowel Disease Management

Mohammad Akbar Siddiqui[1], **Nidhi Agrawal**[1], **Sakshi Gupta**[1], **Meenakshi Jaiswal**[1] and **S. K. Lanjhiyana**[1,*]

[1] *Department of Pharmacy, Guru Ghasidas Vishwavidyalaya, Bilaspur 495009, Chhattisgarh, India*

Abstract: Inflammatory Bowel Disease (IBD) is a chronic Gastrointestinal (GI) condition characterized by relapsing inflammation, which significantly impacts patients' quality of life. Despite advancements in treatment, current therapeutic strategies face limitations in achieving targeted drug delivery to the inflamed intestinal regions. Combination therapies integrating natural polymers have emerged as a promising approach to enhance drug efficacy, stability, and bioavailability while minimizing systemic side effects. This chapter explores the pathophysiology of IBD, the challenges associated with conventional treatments, and the role of combination therapies utilizing natural polymers. Specifically, the discussion highlights the potential of polymer-based drug delivery systems incorporating small molecules, probiotics, and biologics. Natural polymers such as alginate, chitosan, and pectin offer biocompatibility and colon-specific degradation, making them ideal carriers for drug targeting. The synergistic effects of polymer-based combination therapies offer a novel therapeutic avenue for improving IBD management. Future studies should prioritize refining formulation methods and undertaking comprehensive clinical trials to ensure these approaches are both effective and safe.

Keywords: Biologics, Combination therapy, Inflammatory bowel disease, Natural polymers, Probiotics, Small molecule.

INTRODUCTION

Overview of Inflammatory Bowel Disease (IBD)

IBD is a long-term, recurring disorder that impacts the GI tract. This condition is marked by non-infectious, chronic inflammation that primarily impacts the lining of the GI tract, leading to ongoing structural and functional damage of the

* **Corresponding author S. K. Lanjhiyana:** Department of Pharmacy, Guru Ghasidas Vishwavidyalaya, Bilaspur 495009, Chhattisgarh, India; E-mail: sklanjh1975@gmail.com

Meenakshi Jaiswal & S.K. Lanjhiyana (Eds.)

epithelium with few common symptoms such as abdominal pain with cramping, bloody diarrhoea, and weight loss, which necessitates long-term therapy [1]. IBD is categorized into two primary subtypes based on pathological characteristics and disease manifestation. Ulcerative Colitis (UC) predominantly targets the mucosal layer of the colon, causing inflammation in a continuous pattern along the inner lining. In contrast, Crohn's Disease (CD) may affect various locations within the GI tract in a discontinuous manner, with the terminal ileum being the most commonly impacted region. These subtypes represent distinct clinical entities, necessitating tailored treatment strategies [2]. Though the specific causes of IBD are unclear, it is believed that genetic, immune system, and environmental factors are involved. The IBD is more prevalent in developed countries, with incidence rates ranging from around 5.3 to 63.6 per 100,000 individuals [3].

Pathophysiology of UC and CD

Patients with UC exhibited reduced diversity of Firmicutes and increased levels of γ-proteobacteria, Enterobacteriaceae, and sulfite-reducing deltaproteobacteria. The role of these changes in intestinal inflammation is still uncertain. Interleukin (IL-13), produced by T helper (Th2) and natural killer T cells, works with Tumour Necrosis Factor-α (TNF-α) to regulate tight junction gene expression and affects membrane integrity, thereby increasing gut permeability. Activated antigen-presenting cells (APCs), recognizing commensal microbiota through Toll-like Receptors (TLR2 and TLR4), initiate the differentiation of CD4+ T cells into effector subsets such as Th2, Th9, and Treg [4]. Th2-associated cytokines like IL-5 and IL-13 dominate in UC, although the overall role of Th2 cells is inconclusive. Th9 cells, producing IL-9, also contribute to UC by hindering mucosal healing and disrupting the mucus layer's protective functions. The CD is driven by Th1 cells, leading to small bowel inflammation and increased proinflammatory cytokines (IFN-γ and IL-17A) [5]. The Th17 pathway, influenced by cytokines like IL-6 and IL-23, interacts with the Th1 response. Increased levels of transcription factors (*e.g.*, STAT4, T-bet) and cytokine receptors (IL-12Rβ2) promote Th1 differentiation. Consequently, both Th1 and Th17 pathways contribute to CD development, with mortality mainly due to pulmonary disease and certain cancers [6].

Diagnosis

Precise identification of IBD is essential for effective management. Nevertheless, no serum or faecal biomarkers are sufficient for assessing suspicious and confirmed IBD cases. Innovative methods for identifying biomarkers, such as genetic expression technology using the Applied Biosystems GeneChip system in peripheral blood [7], tissue biopsies from mucous membranes [8], assessment of mRNA expression levels in bloodstream leukocyte cell RNA [9], and c-microRNAs [10], have demonstrated encouraging results. Following diagnosis, many IBD medications fail to achieve clinical remission and frequently result in side effects, including diarrhea, renal dysfunction, and opportunistic infections like TB. Additionally, evaluating inflammation through endoscopy is both costly and invasive. The initial method of combining phenotype and serology information is inadequate for differentiating CD from UC; thus, it is complicated to predict accurate clinical outcomes [11].

The study of metabolism is becoming an effective technique for analyzing metabolites in biological samples. It can significantly impact the early identification of IBD, the establishment of therapeutic targets, and the implementation of targeted therapies [12]. For instance, T1259 serum biochemical levels can distinguish IBD from normal individuals [13]. Likewise, serological and fecal biochemical screening has shown promise for distinguishing juvenile IBD from healthy individuals by measuring Fecal Calprotectin (FC) and metabolites like choline [14]. Fecal FC assessment is not limited to pediatric cases; in patients with UC. FC exceeds C-Reactive Protein (CRP) in predicting clinical outcomes and therapeutic response, including inflammation and mucosal healing. The comprehensive functions of FC in IBD patients, such as therapy forecasting, prediction of disease recurrence, and relapse after surgical intervention, are reviewed by Mumolo *et al.* [15]. Metabolic assessment serves as a valuable tool for identifying specific biomarkers that distinguish among IBD subclasses. By employing diverse statistical methods, researchers can analyze metabolites to uncover both the similarities and variations in their profiles, thereby characterizing disease phenotypes. For instance, biopsies from individuals with active UC exhibit elevated levels of glutamine and glutathione when evaluated against control tissues or those from individuals with inactive UC [16]. Nevertheless, the high cost of biochemical methods and spectroscopic instruments poses significant challenges to their accessibility, particularly in developing countries.

Challenges in Current IBD Treatments

A primary challenge in the management of IBD is the limited ability of therapeutically active agents to reach the colonic region effectively. Minimizing drug releases in the upper GI tract is critical due to the significantly different pH values of the GI tract, *i.e.*, low/acidic to high/alkaline pH, as well as varying transit times [17, 18]. In IBD, particularly Ulcerative Colitis (UC), the colonic pH can decrease, which poses a significant challenge for effective treatment. Optimizing drug release in the colonic region with high enzymatic degradation and a pH environment, results in poor absorption of drugs in the inflamed colon segment. These factors can complicate the design of colon-targeted delivery systems based on a single approach [19]. Hence, utilizing combinations of one or more approaches for drug targeting to the colon might be a solution to overcome these complications. Single-unit dosage forms have several disadvantages, such as unpredictable disintegration, dose dumping, and irritation. To overcome these challenges, multiparticulate systems are designed. Due to their smaller size, multiparticulate dose forms allow for fast distribution throughout the GI tract, resulting in more uniform and safe drug absorption [20].

ROLE OF COMBINATION THERAPY IN IBD

The management of IBD disease has a wide area of research for healthcare researchers, emphasizing the development of a delivery system for its management. Over the past 6 years, the European Medicines Agency (EMA) has approved multiple therapeutic agents for IBD, with some currently in clinical trials and expected to be available in the coming years [21]. Due to the intricate pathophysiology of IBD, which involves various inflammatory pathways that are simultaneously activated in the GI mucosa, inhibiting a single target is insufficient for optimal inflammation management in each patient. Drug candidates used as monotherapy that are effective in treating luminal disease may not be as successful in managing co-existing extraintestinal manifestations or other autoimmune diseases. The researchers have begun to investigate whether combining two advanced therapies may enhance efficacy [22]. Combined targeted therapy with different mechanisms of action is an essential therapeutic approach proposed for the management of IBD. It involves using a combination of therapeutic agents, predominantly immunosuppressive agents combined with biologics and biologics with small-molecule drugs [23]. These therapeutic approaches have been employed for the management of IBD patients who exhibit resistance to treatment or those with inactive disease presenting complex extraintestinal manifestations. In the first scenario, the therapeutic benefit is due to an additive or synergistic impact. Conversely, in the second scenario, combination therapies enhance patients' odds of responding to particular drugs [24, 25].

COMBINATION THERAPIES USING NATURAL POLYMERS

Natural polymers attracted attention due to concerns about the toxicity of synthetic polymers. They are biodegradable, non-toxic, highly stable, easy to handle, more economical, and are degraded specifically in the colon, which makes them more qualified for transporting drugs aimed at treating IBD [26]. Natural polymer-based combination therapies entail the concurrent delivery of multiple therapeutic agents within a single system developed from naturally derived polymers [27, 28]. The main natural polymers used in the release of drugs are alginate, amylose, albumin, carrageenan, cellulose, cyclodextrin, collagen, chitosan, chondroitin, dextran, gelatin, hyaluronic acid, inulin, pectin, starch, guar gum, xanthan gum, cashew gum, and zein [29, 30].

Combination Therapy with Small Molecules

Combination therapy employing natural polymer-based carriers with small molecules has shown significant clinical outcomes in IBD models. Small-Molecule Pharmaceuticals (SMPs) are naturally occurring chemical molecules with molecular weights in the range of 100 to 900 Da. Due to their small size, SMPs can easily cross the cell membrane. These pharmaceutical compounds exhibit anti-inflammatory and immunosuppressive properties by modulating leukocyte migration and cellular signalling. Small molecular pharmaceuticals have distinct chemical properties and exhibit significant pharmacokinetic differences compared to other biological drugs [31]. As they are administered orally, they offer undeniable benefits in terms of therapeutic compliance and improving overall well-being. However, their short half-life necessitates daily oral administration, unlike biologics, which require less frequent dosing. Their compact size allows for efficient passage through cell membranes, resulting in a quicker onset of action, more consistent effects, and reduced immunogenicity [32]. As a result, they offer the potential for a more prolonged therapeutic effect while minimizing the likelihood of anti-drug antibody development. At present, SMPs are categorised into two groups based on their targeted pathways into two groups: those that inhibit cellular signaling (*e.g.*, JAK inhibitors like tofacitinib, SMAD blockers, and Phosphodiesterase 4 inhibitors) and those that interfere with leukocyte trafficking (*e.g.*, Sphingosine-1-Phosphate modulators) [33, 34]. Natural polymers protect labile small molecules from premature degradation and enable their sustained release at the inflammation site, thereby enhancing drug stability, therapeutic efficacy, and local bioavailability. However, certain challenges persist, including batch-to-batch variability in polymer composition, limited scalability during formulation development, and difficulties in achieving consistent and reproducible drug loading, which may affect product uniformity and clinical translation [29].

Combination Therapy with Probiotic

Natural polymers (such as chitosan, alginate, xanthan gum, guar gum, and pectin) protect probiotics against gastric acidity and bile salts, allowing their controlled release in the colon. Probiotics are live microorganisms that, when consumed in sufficient quantities, confer a therapeutic effect to the host. Probiotic therapy involves the deliberate incorporation of beneficial bacteria into the gut microbiota, facilitating competition for nutrients among beneficial bacteria and suppressing pathogenic bacteria [35]. Probiotics participate in a variety of physiological activities that promote health, particularly by supporting gut health. The most commonly used probiotic strains recognized for their positive health impacts include *Enterococcus faecium, Bifidobacterium, Bacillus, Lactobacillus*, *Pediococcus,* and the non-pathogenic yeast *Saccharomyces boulardii (S. boulardii)* [36]. The biological mechanisms underlying the beneficial efficacy of these probiotics include the biosynthesis of butyrate and Short-chain Fatty Acids (SCFAs); activation of stimulatory signaling proteins; release of extracellular proteins capable of reducing pro-inflammatory cytokine levels; upregulation of mucin-2 expression; enhancement of autophagy; and increased production of host-defense peptides [37]. Although their potential has been well-demonstrated in both preclinical and clinical studies, probiotics are not without theoretical risks. These have been highlighted in various case reports, clinical trial findings, and experimental models. Identified risks include systemic infections, undesirable metabolic activities, immune system overstimulation in vulnerable individuals, gene transfer, and gastrointestinal complications [38]. The potential of probiotics in treating Ulcerative Colitis (UC) has garnered growing interest. Nevertheless, further research is necessary to provide researchers with guidance on the appropriate selection and application of probiotics. We suggest that combining multiple probiotics with varying functions can effectively reduce intestinal inflammation [39]. Numerous reports exist on natural polymer-based carrier systems, such as chitosan-alginate microspheres/ hydrogels, pectin-chitosan hydrogels, and xanthan gum-based carrier systems, for the delivery of probiotics in IBD management, highlighting their efficacy. Many of these studies show positive results and predominantly feature *Lactobacillus, Bifidobacterium*, and *Saccharomyces* strains [40]. The combination of natural polymers exhibits a synergistic effect by integrating the distinct physicochemical properties of each polymer to enhance encapsulation efficiency, improve the stability and controlled release of probiotics, and increase their therapeutic efficacy in formulations such as capsules, gels, and coated tablets. However, certain limitations exist, including potential gastrointestinal discomfort such as bloating or constipation and the risk of allergic reactions in individuals sensitive to shellfish, which may restrict the broader clinical application of chitosan-based delivery systems.

Combination Therapy with Biologics

Currently, infliximab, vedolizumab, and adalimumab are approved by the US FDA for the management of IBD. The parenteral administration of most biologics and biosimilars presents various disadvantages, including an increased risk of infections, hypersensitivity reactions, autoimmunity, malignancy development, liver damage, and exacerbation of heart failure. Embedding biologics in combined natural polymer matrix systems significantly enhances their local bioavailability, as these systems can protect biologics from proteolytic enzymes and provide controlled release at diseased sites [41]. Dual biologic therapy refers to the concurrent use of two biologics or a biologic(s) along with a small-molecule therapeutic agent in individuals with IBD. In contrast, combined treatment technology involves the use of biological agents alongside other medications, predominantly immunosuppressants [42]. These targeting strategies have been implemented in treatment-resistant IBD patients or those with remission phase, accompanied by challenging symptoms beyond the GI tract. Recent evidence suggests that dual biologic therapy offers a safe and effective alternative for individuals who fail to respond to individual biological treatments and for cases with difficult-to-manage complications beyond the GI tract [43]. The commonly used combined therapy to date has been the simultaneous use of anti-TNF molecules with vedolizumab or ustekinumab. These combinations were chosen based on their satisfactory safety profiles and the level of effectiveness they exhibit when used individually [44]. Table **1** summarizes examples of different combination therapies in the management of IBD.

Table 1. Different combination therapy for the management of IBD.

Combination type	IBD type	Types of study	Efficacy	Refs.
Vedolizumab and adalimumab	CD	Case report	Clinical remission and endoscopic improvement	[52]
Infliximab and natalizumab	CD	Randomized controlled trial	Clinical remission	[53]
Infliximab and azathioprine	CD	randomized, double-blind trial	Clinical remission	[54]
Vedolizumab and tofacitinib	UC	Retrospective cohort	Clinical remission	[55]
Anti-TNF and ustekinumab	CD and UC	retrospective study	Clinical remission	[56, 57]
Ocrelizumab and vedolizumab	UC	Retrospective cohort	Clinical, biomarker remission, and endoscopic improvement	[58]
Sulfasalazine and extracts of *E. humifusa*	UC	Research study	Effects of probiotics	[59]

Combination Therapy with Antibiotics

Antibiotics such as ciprofloxacin and metronidazole are widely used to treat severe IBD symptoms, but systemic exposure causes dysbiosis and adverse effects. Polymer-based formulations contribute to localized antibiotic release. Chitosan-heparin nanoparticles loaded with ciprofloxacin improved their stability under gastric pH conditions and exhibited excellent antibacterial activity [45]. Similarly, guar gum microsphere encapsulated with metronidazole showed low drug release at gastric pH and higher drug release at colonic pH [46].

Antibiotics are only prescribed when there is a "serious suspicion of septic complications." However, this guideline has limited experimental value. In cases of severe relapse, stool and blood cultures take a minimum of three days to provide results, leaving the patient to endure symptoms such as bloody diarrhea, fever, anorexia, vomiting, and abdominal pain during this period [47]. Moreover, microbial sepsis may not always be detected in the cultures. Therefore, most clinical gastroenterologists worldwide prefer the "blind" empirical administration of a combined antibiotic therapy (primarily metronidazole and ciprofloxacin) for at least 5 days in severe UC cases alongside the intensive treatment regimen [48].

Currently, three clinical reports have explored the use of combined antibiotic therapy in individuals with acute UC. The earliest study examined the oral delivery of three antibiotics (amoxicillin, tetracycline, and metronidazole) in 30 individuals with acute UC who were either corticosteroid-resistant or corticosteroid-dependent [49]. The subsequent investigation assessed the combination treatment of two therapeutic molecules (ceftriaxone and metronidazole or placebo) as a supplemental treatment in 50 patients suffering from a serious UC recurrence [50]. Meanwhile, Rhodes *et al.* explored the efficacy and safety of an antibiotic regimen comprising ciprofloxacin, doxycycline, and hydroxychloroquine, followed by a maintenance phase with doxycycline and hydroxychloroquine, in 39 patients with CD [51].

CONCLUSION AND FUTURE PERSPECTIVES

The management of IBD remains a challenge due to its complex etiology and the limitations of conventional treatments. Combination therapies involving natural polymers provide a targeted, effective, and safer alternative by facilitating site-specific drug release while reducing systemic toxicity. This chapter has examined the potential of natural polymer-based targeting systems to enhance the therapeutic outcomes of small molecules, probiotics, and biologics. The ability of natural polymers to protect active pharmaceutical agents and control their release in the colon underscores their value in IBD treatment. However, further research is needed to refine these systems, optimize their pharmacokinetics, and establish their long-term clinical benefits. Future advancements in polymer science and nanotechnology will likely drive the next generation of IBD therapeutics, offering improved patient outcomes and expanded treatment options.

REFERENCES

[1] Lanjhiyana SK, Bajpayee P, Kesavan K, Lanjhiyana S, Muthu MS. Chitosan–sodium alginate blended polyelectrolyte complexes as potential multiparticulate carrier system: colon-targeted delivery and gamma scintigraphic imaging. Expert Opin Drug Deliv 2013; 10(1): 5-15. [http://dx.doi.org/10.1517/17425247.2013.734805] [PMID: 23106236]

[2] Karlinger K, Györke T, Makö E, Mester Á, Tarján Z. The epidemiology and the pathogenesis of inflammatory bowel disease. Eur J Radiol 2000; 35(3): 154-67. [http://dx.doi.org/10.1016/S0720-048X(00)00238-2] [PMID: 11000558]

[3] Jarmakiewicz-Czaja S, Zielińska M, Sokal A, Filip R. Genetic and epigenetic etiology of inflammatory bowel disease: An update. Genes (Basel) 2022; 13(12): 2388. [http://dx.doi.org/10.3390/genes13122388] [PMID: 36553655]

[4] Yeshi K, Ruscher R, Hunter L, Daly NL, Loukas A, Wangchuk P. Revisiting inflammatory bowel disease: Pathology, treatments, challenges and emerging therapeutics including drug leads from natural products. Journal of Clinical Medicine MDPI; 2020 2020; 9

[5] Vebr M, Pomahačová R, Sýkora J, Schwarz J. A narrative review of cytokine networks: pathophysiological and therapeutic implications for inflammatory bowel disease pathogenesis. Biomedicines 2023; 11(12): 3229. [http://dx.doi.org/10.3390/biomedicines11123229] [PMID: 38137450]

[6] Harbour SN, Maynard CL, Zindl CL, Schoeb TR, Weaver CT. Th17 cells give rise to Th1 cells that are required for the pathogenesis of colitis. Proc Natl Acad Sci USA 2015; 112(22): 7061-6. [http://dx.doi.org/10.1073/pnas.1415675112] [PMID: 26038559]

[7] Burakoff R, Pabby V, Onyewadume L, *et al.* Blood-based biomarkers used to predict disease activity in Crohn's disease and ulcerative colitis. Inflamm Bowel Dis 2015; 21(5): 1132-40. [http://dx.doi.org/10.1097/MIB.0000000000000340] [PMID: 25895006]

[8] Dieckgraefe BK, Stenson WF, Korzenik JR, Swanson PE, Harrington CA. Analysis of mucosal gene expression in inflammatory bowel disease by parallel oligonucleotide arrays. Physiol Genomics 2000; 4(1): 1-11. [http://dx.doi.org/10.1152/physiolgenomics.2000.4.1.1] [PMID: 11074008]

[9] Wu F, Guo NJ, Tian H, *et al.* Peripheral blood MicroRNAs distinguish active ulcerative colitis and Crohn's disease. Inflamm Bowel Dis 2011; 17(1): 241-50. [http://dx.doi.org/10.1002/ibd.21450] [PMID: 20812331]

[10] Burczynski ME, Peterson RL, Twine NC, *et al.* Molecular classification of Crohn's disease and ulcerative colitis patients using transcriptional profiles in peripheral blood mononuclear cells. J Mol Diagn 2006; 8(1): 51-61. [http://dx.doi.org/10.2353/jmoldx.2006.050079] [PMID: 16436634]

[11] Hong SM, Baek DH. Diagnostic procedures for inflammatory bowel disease: laboratory, endoscopy, pathology, imaging, and beyond. Diagnostics (Basel) 2024; 14(13): 1384. [http://dx.doi.org/10.3390/diagnostics14131384] [PMID: 39001273]

[12] Ning L, Zhou YL, Sun H, *et al.* Microbiome and metabolome features in inflammatory bowel disease *via* multi-omics integration analyses across cohorts. Nat Commun 2023; 14(1): 7135. [http://dx.doi.org/10.1038/s41467-023-42788-0] [PMID: 37932270]

[13] Johnston C, Dunn W, Broadhurst D, *et al.* T1259 serum metabolite profiles differentiate Crohn's Disease from ulcerative colitis and from healthy controls. Gastroenterology 2010; 138(5): S-523. [http://dx.doi.org/10.1016/S0016-5085(10)62414-6]

[14] Al-Beltagi M, Saeed NK, Bediwy AS, Elbeltagi R. Fecal calprotectin in pediatric gastrointestinal diseases: Pros and cons. World J Clin Pediatr 2024; 13(2): 93341. [http://dx.doi.org/10.5409/wjcp.v13.i2.93341] [PMID: 38948001]

[15] Mumolo MG, Bertani L, Ceccarelli L, *et al.* From bench to bedside: Fecal calprotectin in inflammatory bowel diseases clinical setting. World J Gastroenterol 2018; 24(33): 3681-94. [http://dx.doi.org/10.3748/wjg.v24.i33.3681] [PMID: 30197475]

[16] Ruan EA, Rao S, Burdick JS, *et al.* Glutathione levels in chronic inflammatory disorders of the human colon. Nutr Res 1997; 17(3): 463-73. [http://dx.doi.org/10.1016/S0271-5317(97)00007-9]

[17] Agrawal N, Jaiswal M. Synthesis and pharmacological characterization of new curcumin ester pro-drugs with enhanced anti-inflammatory, anti-ulcerogenic and improved tissue distribution. Journal of Medical Pharmaceutical and Allied Sciences 2023; 12(5): 6066-74. [http://dx.doi.org/10.55522/jmpas.V12I5.5264]

[18] Agrawal N, Jaiswal M. Synthesis and pharmacological characterization of new curcumin ester pro-drugs with enhanced anti-inflammatory, anti-ulcerogenic and improved tissue distribution. Journal of Medical pharmaceutical and allied sciences 2023; 12(5): 6066-74. [http://dx.doi.org/10.55522/jmpas.V12I5.5264]

[19] Balderramo D. Role of the combination of biologics and/or small molecules in the treatment of patients with inflammatory bowel disease. World Journal of Gastroenterology Baishideng Publishing Group Inc. 2022; Vol. 28: pp. 6743-51.

[20] Katz S, Liu Y. Challenges in the Management of Inflammatory Bowel Disease. Geriatric Gastroenterology. Cham: Springer International Publishing 2021; pp. 1675-90. [http://dx.doi.org/10.1007/978-3-030-30192-7_66]

[21] Cai Z, Wang S, Li J. Treatment of inflammatory bowel disease: A comprehensive review. Front Med (Lausanne) 2021; 8: 765474. [http://dx.doi.org/10.3389/fmed.2021.765474] [PMID: 34988090]

[22] Saez A, Herrero-Fernandez B, Gomez-Bris R, Sánchez-Martinez H, Gonzalez-Granado JM. Pathophysiology of inflammatory bowel disease: Innate immune system. Int J Mol Sci 2023; 24(2): 1526. [http://dx.doi.org/10.3390/ijms24021526] [PMID: 36675038]

[23] Dai C, Huang YH, Jiang M. Combination therapy in inflammatory bowel disease: Current evidence and perspectives. Int Immunopharmacol 2023; 114: 109545. [http://dx.doi.org/10.1016/j.intimp.2022.109545] [PMID: 36508920]

[24] Sun W, Sanderson PE, Zheng W. Drug combination therapy increases successful drug repositioning. Drug Discov Today 2016; 21(7): 1189-95. [http://dx.doi.org/10.1016/j.drudis.2016.05.015] [PMID: 27240777]

[25] De Bernardi A, Bezzio C, Puricelli M, Gilardi D, Saibeni S. Combining advanced targeted therapy in inflammatory bowel disease: Current practice and future directions. J Clin Med 2025; 14(2): 590. [http://dx.doi.org/10.3390/jcm14020590] [PMID: 39860594]

[26] Lima L, Barreiro E. Bioisosterism: A useful strategy for molecular modification and drug design. Curr Med Chem 2005; 12(1): 23-49. [http://dx.doi.org/10.2174/0929867053363540] [PMID: 15638729]

[27] Kruk K, Winnicka K. Alginates combined with natural polymers as valuable drug delivery platforms. Mar Drugs 2022; 21(1): 11. [http://dx.doi.org/10.3390/md21010011] [PMID: 36662184]

[28] Lima IBC, Moreno LCGAI, Silva-Filho EC, Irache JM, Veiga FJB, Rolim HML, *et al.* Development of nanostructured systems using natural polymers to optimize the treatment of inflammatory bowel diseases: A prospective study. Journal of Drug Delivery Science and Technology Editions de Sante 2021. [http://dx.doi.org/10.1016/j.jddst.2021.102590]

[29] Shah BM, Palakurthi SS, Khare T, Khare S, Palakurthi S. Natural proteins and polysaccharides in the

development of micro/nano delivery systems for the treatment of inflammatory bowel disease. International Journal of Biological Macromolecules Elsevier BV. 2020; Vol. 165: pp. 722-37.

[30] Satchanska G, Davidova S, Petrov PD. Natural and synthetic polymers for biomedical and environmental applications. Polymers Multidisciplinary Digital Publishing Institute (MDPI). 2024. [http://dx.doi.org/10.3390/polym16081159]

[31] Manrai M, Jha AA, Dawra S, Pachisia AV. Biologics, small molecules and more in inflammatory bowel disease: The present and the future. Future Pharmacology 2024; 4(1): 279-316. [http://dx.doi.org/10.3390/futurepharmacol4010017]

[32] Li P, Zheng Y, Chen X. Drugs for autoimmune inflammatory diseases: from small molecule compounds to anti-TNF biologics. Front Pharmacol 2017; 8: 460. [http://dx.doi.org/10.3389/fphar.2017.00460] [PMID: 28785220]

[33] Higashiyama M, Hokari R. New and emerging treatments for inflammatory bowel disease. Digestion 2023; 104(1): 74-81. [http://dx.doi.org/10.1159/000527422] [PMID: 36366823]

[34] Penagini F, Lonoce L, Abbattista L, *et al.* Dual biological therapy and small molecules in pediatric inflammatory bowel disease. Pharmacol Res 2023; 196: 106935. [http://dx.doi.org/10.1016/j.phrs.2023.106935] [PMID: 37748559]

[35] Isaacs K, Herfarth H. Role of probiotic therapy in IBD. Inflamm Bowel Dis 2008; 14(11): 1597-605. [http://dx.doi.org/10.1002/ibd.20465] [PMID: 18421762]

[36] Latif A, Shehzad A, Niazi S, *et al.* Probiotics: mechanism of action, health benefits and their application in food industries. Front Microbiol 2023; 14: 1216674. [http://dx.doi.org/10.3389/fmicb.2023.1216674] [PMID: 37664108]

[37] Roy S, Dhaneshwar S. Role of prebiotics, probiotics, and synbiotics in management of inflammatory bowel disease: Current perspectives. World Journal of Gastroenterology Baishideng Publishing Group Inc. 2023; Vol. 29: pp. 2078-100.

[38] Jakubczyk D, Leszczyńska K, Górska S. The effectiveness of probiotics in the treatment of Inflammatory Bowel Disease (IBD)—a critical review. Nutrients 2020; 12(7): 1973. [http://dx.doi.org/10.3390/nu12071973] [PMID: 32630805]

[39] Wang Y, Xie Q, Zhang Y, *et al.* Combination of probiotics with different functions alleviate DSS-induced colitis by regulating intestinal microbiota, IL-10, and barrier function. Appl Microbiol Biotechnol 2020; 104(1): 335-49. [http://dx.doi.org/10.1007/s00253-019-10259-6] [PMID: 31758237]

[40] Fan H, Du J, Liu X, *et al.* Effects of pentasa-combined probiotics on the microflora structure and prognosis of patients with inflammatory bowel disease. Turk J Gastroenterol 2019; 30(8): 680-5. [http://dx.doi.org/10.5152/tjg.2019.18426] [PMID: 31418411]

[41] Aljabri A, Soliman GM, Ramadan YN, Medhat MA, Hetta HF. Biosimilars versus biological therapy in inflammatory bowel disease: challenges and targeting strategies using drug delivery systems. Clin Exp Med 2025; 25(1): 107. [http://dx.doi.org/10.1007/s10238-025-01558-6] [PMID: 40186719]

[42] Xu YH, Zhu WM, Guo Z. Current status of novel biologics and small molecule drugs in the individualized treatment of inflammatory bowel disease. World Journal of Gastroenterology Baishideng Publishing Group Inc. 2022; Vol. 28: pp. 6888-99.

[43] Ben-Horin S, Kopylov U, Chowers Y. Optimizing anti-TNF treatments in inflammatory bowel disease. Autoimmun Rev 2014; 13(1): 24-30. [http://dx.doi.org/10.1016/j.autrev.2013.06.002] [PMID: 23792214]

[44] Hirten RP, Iacucci M, Shah S, Ghosh S, Colombel JF. Combining biologics in inflammatory bowel disease and other immune mediated inflammatory disorders. Clin Gastroenterol Hepatol 2018; 16(9): 1374-84.

[http://dx.doi.org/10.1016/j.cgh.2018.02.024] [PMID: 29481970]

[45] Dewint P, Hansen BE, Verhey E, *et al.* Adalimumab combined with ciprofloxacin is superior to adalimumab monotherapy in perianal fistula closure in Crohn's disease: a randomised, double-blind, placebo controlled trial (ADAFI). Gut 2014; 63(2): 292-9.
[http://dx.doi.org/10.1136/gutjnl-2013-304488] [PMID: 23525574]

[46] Kumar GV, Su CH, Velusamy P. Ciprofloxacin loaded genipin cross-linked chitosan/heparin nanoparticles for drug delivery application. Mater Lett 2016; 180: 119-22.
[http://dx.doi.org/10.1016/j.matlet.2016.05.108]

[47] Shukla RK, Tiwari A. Design and development of microparticulate delivery system of metronidazole: Experimental design methodology. J Appl Polym Sci 2012; 126(1): 304-14.
[http://dx.doi.org/10.1002/app.36900]

[48] Alayo QA, Fenster M, Altayar O, *et al.* Systematic review with meta-analysis: Safety and effectiveness of combining biologics and small molecules in inflammatory bowel disease. Crohn's & Colitis 360 2022; 4(1): otac002.
[http://dx.doi.org/10.1093/crocol/otac002] [PMID: 35310082]

[49] Kato K, Ohkusa T, Terao S, *et al.* Adjunct antibiotic combination therapy for steroid-refractory or -dependent ulcerative colitis: an open-label multicentre study. Aliment Pharmacol Ther 2014; 39(9): 949-56.
[http://dx.doi.org/10.1111/apt.12688] [PMID: 24628398]

[50] Mishra S, Mandavdhare HS, Singh H, *et al.* Adjuvant use of combination of antibiotics in acute severe ulcerative colitis: A placebo controlled randomized trial. Expert Rev Anti Infect Ther 2021; 19(7): 949-55.
[http://dx.doi.org/10.1080/14787210.2021.1856656] [PMID: 33245002]

[51] Rhodes JM, Subramanian S, Flanagan PK, *et al.* Randomized trial of ciprofloxacin doxycycline and hydroxychloroquine versus budesonide in Active Crohn's Disease. Dig Dis Sci 2021; 66(8): 2700-11.
[http://dx.doi.org/10.1007/s10620-020-06477-y] [PMID: 32681228]

[52] Solitano V, Ma C, Hanžel J, Panaccione R, Feagan BG, Jairath V. Advanced combination treatment with biologic agents and novel small molecule drugs for inflammatory bowel disease. Gastroenterol Hepatol (N Y) 2023; 19(5): 251-63.
[PMID: 37799456]

[53] Sands BE, Kozarek R, Spainhour J, *et al.* Safety and tolerability of concurrent natalizumab treatment for patients with Crohn's disease not in remission while receiving infliximab. Inflamm Bowel Dis 2007; 13(1): 2-11.
[http://dx.doi.org/10.1002/ibd.20014] [PMID: 17206633]

[54] Colombel JF, Sandborn WJ, Reinisch W, *et al.* Infliximab, azathioprine, or combination therapy for Crohn's disease. N Engl J Med 2010; 362(15): 1383-95.
[http://dx.doi.org/10.1056/NEJMoa0904492] [PMID: 20393175]

[55] Dolinger MT, Spencer EA, Lai J, Dunkin D, Dubinsky MC. Dual biologic and small molecule therapy for the treatment of refractory pediatric inflammatory bowel disease. Inflamm Bowel Dis 2021; 27(8): 1210-4.
[http://dx.doi.org/10.1093/ibd/izaa277] [PMID: 33125058]

[56] Yerushalmy-Feler A, Olbjorn C, Kolho KL, *et al.* Dual biologic or small molecule therapy in refractory pediatric inflammatory bowel disease (DOUBLE-PIBD): A multicenter study from the pediatric IBD porto group of ESPGHAN. Inflamm Bowel Dis 2024; 30(2): 159-66.
[http://dx.doi.org/10.1093/ibd/izad064] [PMID: 37042978]

[57] Guo C, Zhou J, Wang G, Wu J. Dual biologic or small molecule therapy in pediatric inflammatory bowel disease: A single center experience. Children (Basel) 2025; 12(1): 75.
[http://dx.doi.org/10.3390/children12010075] [PMID: 39857906]

[58] Fumery M, Yzet C, Brazier F. Letter: combination of biologics in inflammatory bowel diseases. Aliment Pharmacol Ther 2020; 52(3): 566-7.
[http://dx.doi.org/10.1111/apt.15891] [PMID: 32656825]

[59] Wang Y, Xie Q, Zhang Y, *et al.* Combination of probiotics with different functions alleviate DSS-induced colitis by regulating intestinal microbiota, IL-10, and barrier function. Appl Microbiol Biotechnol 2020; 104(1): 335-49.
[http://dx.doi.org/10.1007/s00253-019-10259-6] [PMID: 31758237]

CHAPTER 9

Advancement in Bioengineered Natural Polymers for Combating IBD: Current Progress and Future Prospects

Shibangi Mukhopadhyay[1], **Yogesh Vaishnav**[1], **Achal Mishra**[1], **Sanjay Kumar Bharti**[1], **Rajkumar**[1] and **Meenakshi Jaiswal**[1,*]

[1] *Department of Pharmacy, Guru Ghasidas Vishwavidyalaya, Bilaspur 495009, Chhattisgarh, India*

Abstract: Inflammatory Bowel Disease (IBD) is a persistent, relapsing, and untreatable disorder that impacts the intestines. The ineffectiveness of prolonged therapy, substantial side effects due to systemic exposure, and increased risks of infection and malignancy from immunosuppression are obstacles to contemporary clinical treatments. To reduce the systemic toxicity of these medicinal agents and enhance intestinal adhesion and retention while targeting the mucosa, polymeric systems have been developed as delivery approaches. To address IBD, we elucidated pharmaceutical delivery techniques derived from polymers. Smart bionanomaterials, which are biocompatible nanoscale substances that respond to environmental stimuli, can facilitate treatment and diagnostics. These materials can deliver live probiotics and drugs, mostly amino salicylates and corticosteroids, to the inflamed regions of the gastrointestinal tract, particularly the colon, in the context of IBD. Smart bionanomaterials offer several advantages, such as regulated release, stimulus responsiveness, targeted dispersion, and encapsulation. These attributes make them an indispensable adjunct in the diagnosis and treatment of IBD. The improvement of therapeutic intervention techniques and sophisticated delivery technology offers insights into the design and development of polymeric systems for medication administration from bench to bedside in the treatment of IBD.

Keywords: Amino salicylates, biocompatibility, colon-targeted therapy, drug delivery techniques, encapsulation, environmental stimuli.

INTRODUCTION

Colon-targeted diseases encompass a group of autoimmune disorders, with Inflammatory Bowel Diseases (IBD) being the most significant. IBD is

* **Corresponding author Meenakshi Jaiswal**: Department of Pharmacy, Guru Ghasidas Vishwavidyalaya, Bilaspur 495009, Chhattisgarh, India; E-mail: jaiswalmeenakshiggu@gmail.com

Meenakshi Jaiswal & S.K. Lanjhiyana (Eds.)

characterised by chronic and acute inflammatory conditions, mucosal ulceration, oedema, and haemorrhage within the Gastrointestinal (GI) tract. IBD is becoming more and more common among young people and is becoming a dangerous condition that makes them much more likely to get colon cancer [1]. The causes of IBD are still being studied. Some of the most important ones are genetic predispositions, environmental factors, and the integrity of the intestinal mucosal barrier. Compared to healthy colon mucosa, a sick colon disrupts the equilibrium among the gut bacteria, the immune system, and the internal environment of the intestine. This makes the inflammation in the intestine worse. Sometimes, an imbalance of Reactive Oxygen Species (ROS) and the breakdown of tight junctions make intestinal tissues more permeable. This raises the levels of oxygen and antigens, which can make the immune system work too hard. This enhancement of the immune system facilitates colon-targeted cancer therapy. IBD is largely divided into two variants: Ulcerative Colitis (UC) and Crohn's disease (CD). UC is less detrimental as it is localised to a specific region of the mucosal layer in the colon; CD is a chronic and aggressive form of inflammation that penetrates deeper into the intestinal wall and impacts the GI tract [2]. The principal aims of IBD treatment are to maintain remission from inflammatory episodes and prevent recurrent inflammation. Conventional therapeutic regimens for IBD include 5-aminosalicylic acid-based anti-inflammatory agents, corticosteroids, immunosuppressive drugs (tacrolimus, cyclosporine-A, methotrexate, azathioprine, and 6-mercaptopurine), and antibiotics (ciprofloxacin and metronidazole). The advancement of biological therapeutics utilising monoclonal antibodies has enhanced the clinical efficiency of IBD treatment [3].

It is problematic to regulate IBD, specifically in sensitive and elderly individuals, because long-term use of standard drugs has been linked to the most common side effects, such as pancreatitis, allergic responses, nausea, and elevated liver enzymes. Although the drugs indicated above provide clinical remission, they are ineffective and have severe side effects over time. Drug Delivery Systems (DDSs) are being developed to rigorously distribute payloads to the inflammatory intestinal mucosa. These systems can usually be delivered orally, intraperitoneally, intrarectally, or intravenously. Intrarectal administration is unsuccessful elsewhere but effective for treating distal lesions. More importantly, in developing countries, inappropriate needle overuse increases the risk of AIDS. Inserting needles is painful, invasive, and not very popular [2]. After reading most publications, it is evident that the more recent technologies employed in various delivery systems to treat IBD rely entirely on the usage of various polymers that increase the effectiveness of various medication combinations. Due to their self-assembled hierarchical structure, ease of manufacturing, and ability to alter chemical properties, polymeric DDSs have shown clinical efficacy and widespread use in a range of illnesses, with exceptional biodegradability and biocompatibility [4].

When it comes to tackling IBD, both natural and synthetic polymers have a role to play. Polysaccharides and other naturally occurring polymers are highly valued not only because they are cost-effective and biodegradable, but also due to their adhesive properties, which allow them to remain at target sites where they are needed most. Research into synthetic polymers has been robust due to their adaptability in terms of chemical composition, molecular weight, structure, and post-modification ease. IBD is a group of conditions that includes UC and CD, and recently developed synthetic polymers are helping to improve therapy for these conditions. One of the main obstacles to IBD is the lack of appropriate materials for targeted drug delivery, controlled release, and the mitigation of systemic adverse effects. Such synthetic polymers include polyphenols, cationic polymers, Polyethylene Glycol (PEG), polyesters (PLGA, PCL, *etc.*), and polyacrylates, among others [5]. Drug delivery techniques for IBD frequently use synthetic polymers, which have limited systemic bioavailability and poor oral absorption. Consequently, a considerable amount of the drug might not reach the intended sites in the intestines, thereby reducing its therapeutic efficacy. An increase in intestinal inflammation and disruption of gut microbiota are two ways in which some of these polymers, such as polyethylene microplastics, exacerbate inflammatory bowel disease symptoms. They could interact badly with the gut flora or create toxic by-products. One example is the potential for inflammation and other gastrointestinal problems caused by some emulsifiers used in synthetic formulations, which might undermine the integrity of the gut barrier. Due to their less damaging nature, natural polymers have been used far more than synthetic polymers. For hydrogels that exhibit low toxicity potential, biodegradability, and sensitivity to particular environmental stimuli, natural polymers are usually the way to go because they are more environmentally friendly. Proteins such as gelatin, chondroitin sulphate, and hyaluronic acid, and carbohydrates such as pectin, chitosan, and alginate are examples of natural polymers. There are a number of advantages to using these natural polymers for drug delivery rather than manufactured polymers. It is difficult to modify them to meet the needs of drug deliverydue to their inadequate mechanical properties and tensile strength. And because they are already there, they might provoke immune responses that would make them useless as biomaterials for oral drug delivery [6].

The creation of innovative bionanomaterials, which are safe nanoscale materials that respond to environmental cues, has made it much easier to find and treat illnesses. In recent decades, smart materials have gained prominence and are particularly intriguing for medical applications. Conductive hydrogel cardiac patches composed of smart materials have demonstrated encouraging outcomes in the treatment of myocardial infarction. Hyaluronic acid-based hydrogels have excellent biocompatibility and possess significant potential for the bioprinting of flexible connective tissues. Certain materials are termed bionanomaterials due to their biocompatibility, as specified by governing bodies such as the European Medicines Agency and the US Food and Drug Administration (USFDA), together with their nanoscale dimensions. The development of medication delivery methods, especially for oral administration, can be aided by bionanomaterials. These materials enhance the effectiveness of delivery methods by encapsulating various active compounds with healing properties [7].

This chapter discusses traditional therapies and the incorporation of polymers to improve medication administration through effective delivery methods. Upon evaluating the merits and drawbacks of synthetic and natural polymers, our analysis concludes that natural polymers exhibit superior effectiveness with less toxicity. This chapter highlights recent breakthroughs in the use of polymer-based biomaterials for the treatment of IBD [8].

TYPES OF SYNTHETIC POLYMERS USED TO UPHOLD CONVENTIONAL METHODS TO TREAT IBD

Synthetic polymers are essential for enhancing IBD treatment by offering customised medication delivery techniques that improve effectiveness and reduce systemic side effects. The primary objective of IBD treatment is to precisely target the inflamed areas of the colon with anti-inflammatory drugs. Synthetic polymers offer several benefits for this purpose, and the applications of different polymeric formulations are described in Table **1**. The principal types of synthetic polymers are as follows:

Table 1. Applications of different types of synthetic polymers used in formulations.

Sl. No.	Synthetic Polymer Used	Formulation Prepared	Applications	References
1	PLGA	PLGA-Tofacitinib citrate (TFA) nanoparticles; hyaluronic acid-conjugated PLGA nanoparticles	JAK inhibitors alter intracellular signal transductions that are essential for the development of inflammatory and immunological responses; for UC treatment, target activated macrophages after HA-CD44 interacts with resident colonic epithelial cells to target inflammatory colitis tissue.	[9, 15]

(Table 1) cont.....

Sl. No.	Synthetic Polymer Used	Formulation Prepared	Applications	References
2	PEG	PEG-functionalized microparticles	These microparticles have the potential to increase therapeutic effectiveness and decrease side effects by acting as a targeted therapy approach to inflammatory mucosal regions in IBD.	[16]
3	Polyphenols	Uniform and multifunctional polyphenol-based colloidal particles	Polyphenol spheres effectively deplete ROS and demonstrate outstanding thermal and chemical durability, as well as high activity. This is useful for *in vivo* ROS control for inflammatory therapeutics.	[17]
4	Polyacrylates	Eudragit-coated chitosan microspheres for the delivery of Curcumin (CUR)	Eudragit S-100-coated microspheres were used to successfully transport CUR to the colon in a pH-triggered manner. CUR's distribution to the large intestine was improved by encapsulating it in microspheres. When compared to free CUR, the pharmacological action of CUR delivered colonically *via* microspheres was much stronger.	[12]
5	PLA	PLA-based injectable microspheres	They can be employed as embolic agents in transcatheter arterial embolization, a tumor management technique that works well.	[14]

Poly Lactic-co-glycolic Acid (PLGA)

PLGA is formed from the repetitive monomer units of lactic acid and glycolic acid, resulting in a biocompatible and biodegradable polymer. Because it can tolerate diverse ratios of Lactic Acid (LA) to Glycolic Acid (GA), which affect its hydrolytic breakdown kinetics, PLGA is a versatile material for drug delivery. The ester bonds in PLGA undergo hydrolysis *in vivo*, yielding naturally occurring lactic and glycolic acids, which are subsequently eliminated from the body as carbon dioxide *via* the Krebs cycle metabolism and water. Due to its unique properties, PLGA is an advantageous option for controlled drug release applications and has received FDA approval for pharmaceutical use. The synthesis of nanoparticles and the oral delivery of diverse compounds have both significantly utilised PLGA. Besides its recognised role as a drug delivery system, PLGA has recently been noted for its effects on colonic health and gut microbial diversity. A low Molecular Weight (MW) grade (2000–2500 g/mol) of PLGA is metabolized into lactate, a precursor for the human colonic microbiota to produce Short-chain Fatty Acids (SCFAs). It lowers the expression of inflammatory markers (IL-8 and IL-10), according to recent findings in an *in vitro* model of colonic inflammation. Despite the hydrolysable nature of PLGA, studies have revealed that PEGylated or hyaluronic acid-functionalized PLGA nanoparticles may sustain stability for colonic targeting in the upper gastrointestinal tract [9].

Polyethylene Glycol (PEG)

PEGylation, the method of attaching PEG chains to nanoparticles, is commonly employed to enhance the stability and circulation time of drug carriers while simultaneously reducing immunogenicity and early clearance, despite PEG not typically being used in isolation for pharmaceutical encapsulation. It is characterized by recurring units of ethylene oxide and, notably, polyethylene molecules such as PEG obtained by chemical synthesis. They provide a hydrophilic surface, creating favourable conditions for formulation. They can convey carrier system characteristics such as particle translocation and facilitate the intracellular transport of genetic material. PEG is primarily employed to enhance the compactness of nucleic acid-based therapeutics and can be included in many formulations due to its cost-effectiveness [10]. PEG is commonly employed as a drug carrier due to its aqueous solubility, biocompatibility, and ability to protect pharmaceuticals from enzymatic degradation. To enhance the stability of biologic drugs, such as monoclonal antibodies, and prolong their half-life in the body, Polyethylene Glycol (PEG) can be conjugated to them. PEG-functionalized nanoparticles facilitate the targeted delivery of anti-inflammatory drugs to inflamed intestinal tissues, enhancing their efficacy and reducing systemic side effects.

Polyphenols

The anti-inflammatory and antioxidant properties of polyphenols have made them a viable choice for the treatment or inhibition of chronic inflammatory diseases. The majority of research has focused on animal models of colitis, such as intestinal cell lines treated with lipid oxidation products or pro-inflammatory cytokines, animals lacking anti-inflammatory mediators, or pharmacological inducers. By modulating cell signaling pathways, which are mostly triggered in response to oxidative and inflammatory stimuli, and with NF-kB as the main downstream effector, these studies show that polyphenols can effectively reduce intestinal inflammation. This is despite the fact that there is currently minimal information on the use of polyphenols in the management of human IBD. Polyphenols may thus be able to stop or slow the progression of IBD, particularly as their concentration in the gut is higher than in other tissues [11]. Several studies have shown that polyphenols' beneficial effects on human health are due to mechanisms other than their simple antioxidant role. Much emphasis has been placed on a novel theory of how these substances work biologically: they interact with certain signaling proteins that regulate gene expression in response to inflammation and oxidative stress. Among the signals these substances seem to control are MEK, ERK, p38 MAPK, PI-3K/Akt, and STAT-1. Although polyphenol-mediated cellular regulation involves many signaling pathways, NF-kB appears to be the main downstream transcription factor.

Polyacrylates

Eudragit and its derivatives that comprise polymerised acrylic acid, methacrylic acid, or their esters are the most common types of polyacrylates. These are the substances made by various forms of chemical synthesis and derived from polymethacrylate. They are mostly sensitive to pH, and environmental conditions can also affect them. To serve at the right pH and mask the flavour, they are enterically coated. Enterically bounded polymers of this kind exhibit colon-targeted effects [10]. Since UC mostly affects the distal colon, medication may be released in the distal ileum *via* Eudragit S-100, a pH-sensitive polymer with a threshold pH greater than 7 [12].

Polylactic Acid (PLA)

The repeating units of lactic acid are known as PLA. This type of polymer is mostly produced by fermenting carbohydrates, which may be found in readily available and practical sources such as tapioca roots and maize starch. PLA may particularly absorb the microparticles within dendritic cells and macrophages and is primarily biodegradable. Among the many advantages of PLA are its biocompatibility, biodegradability, and ease of hydrolysis at elevated temperatures. It comes from renewable agricultural resources. Additionally, the agriculture economy benefits from this latter circumstance. Compared to conventional petroleum-based commodity plastics, it reduces carbon dioxide emissions because it captures a lot of it. The most important aspect of PLA is its ability to adjust its composition to modify its physical properties [13]. PLA can also be altered by mixing it with other substances and copolymerizing the lactide with hydrophilic macromonomers such as PEG, lactone-type monomers, or monomers containing functional groups, such as amino and carboxylic groups. A single polymer may be used in a variety of applications with just slight modifications to its physical-chemical structure due to the vast range of PLA's applications. Mixing or copolymerising the polymer with other polymeric or non-polymeric components is a common way to get the desired behaviour. The surface properties of materials are essential for defining their applications, particularly for biomaterials in terms of biocompatibility. PLA biomaterials have been surface-modified using a range of methods, including chemical, physical, plasma, and radiation-induced procedures, to achieve the necessary surface properties [14].

FROM FACING CHALLENGES TO INNOVATION: THE RISE OF REVOLUTIONIZING NATURAL POLYMERS WITH ENGINEERED SOLUTIONS TO COMBAT IBD

Synthetic polymers are studied extensively due to their versatile molecular weight, architecture, chemical composition, and ease of post-modification. Synthetic polymers, while commonly employed in the conventional treatment of IBD, present several limitations. Their potential for cytotoxicity and adverse immunological reactions, which may lead to inflammation and unintended side effects, is a primary concern. Synthetic polymers often exhibit a lack of biodegradability, resulting in accumulation within the body and potential long-term toxicity. Poor biocompatibility may hinder drug absorption and efficacy, thereby reducing treatment effectiveness. Moreover, their high manufacturing costs and complex synthesis processes limit their availability for widespread clinical application. The identified disadvantages indicate the necessity for alternative, more biocompatible drug delivery methods in the treatment of IBD [2]. Additionally, synthetic polymers exhibit several disadvantages, including inadequate drug loading, abnormal burst release, high costs, aggregation within formulations, diminished mechanical strength, ineffective drug release in the colonic environment, challenges in *in vivo* release, electrolyte imbalance, cytotoxic potential, enzyme-mediated degradation in the upper gastrointestinal tract, and toxicity concerns [10]. Compared to natural polymers, synthetic polymers like polyesters, polypeptides, and polyphosphazenes typically exhibit superior mechanical strength and controlled degradation rates. Natural and synthetic polymers often lack ideal properties when used independently; therefore, their combination is employed to effectively create hydrogels with enhanced characteristics for ulcerative colitis and colon targeting [6]. Researchers have looked into gut microbiota modulators, naturally bioactive small compounds, and reactive oxygen species scavengers as possible substitutes for systemic polymers, which pose difficulties in the traditional therapy of IBD. Advanced polymeric drug delivery systems have been designed to specifically target the intestinal mucosa, improving adhesion and retention within the gastrointestinal tract. This strategy aims to enhance drug bioavailability and therapeutic efficacy while minimizing systemic toxicity. This article examines polymer-based drug delivery approaches for IBD management, highlighting key design principles for developing hierarchical, mucosa-targeting, and bioresponsive systems. Additionally, it explores innovative drug delivery technologies and therapeutic strategies [18]. The different types of engineered polymer-based systems for IBD treatment are discussed below and illustrated in Figs. (**1** and **2**).

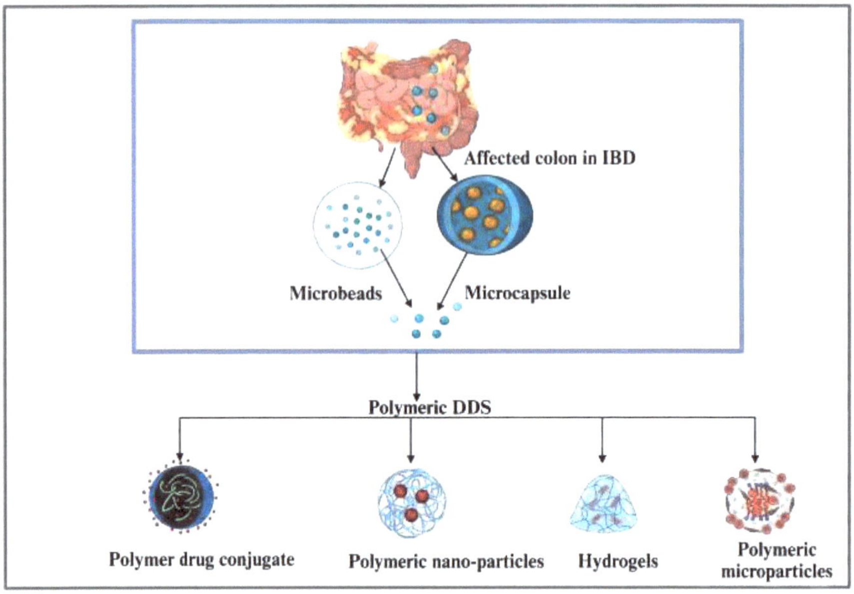

Fig. (1). Innovative polymeric systems for different types of drug delivery.

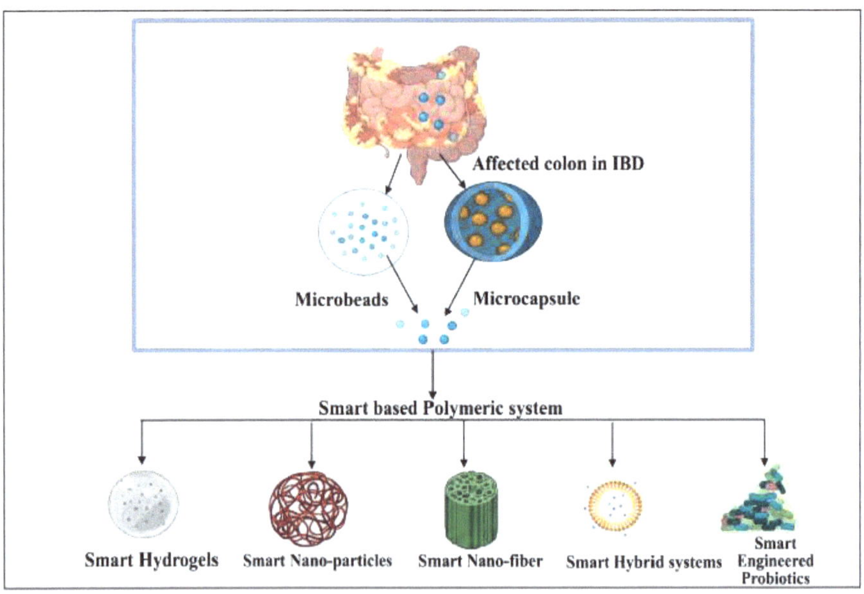

Fig. (2). Evolving role of polymers as smart-responsive drug delivery systems.

Challenges in Scale-up and Manufacturing

The introduction of novel polymer topologies derived from biopolymers and synthetic polymers, the capacity of macromolecules to form supramolecular assemblies with distinct properties, and the application of supercritical fluids, high-pressure processes, and catalytic processes utilizing specially designed carriers have significantly advanced the bio-inspired synthesis of innovative synthetic biopolymers with complex properties.

Polymers with homogeneous structures are defined by a limited Molecular Weight Distribution (MWD). Uniformity is characterized by chemical structure concerning (1) monomer orientation, sequence, and stereoregularity, (2) polymer shape and morphology, and (3) chemical functionality. Although achieving the same high degree of consistency in synthetic polymers as in proteins remains impractical, nature efficiently employs other polymers with lower uniformity, such as polysaccharides, poly (amino acids), and polyhydroxyalkanoates. In recent years, it has been feasible to produce enough amounts of polymers exhibiting several characteristics of homogeneity using realistic experimental techniques [19, 20].

Some of the challenges in scale-up and manufacturing of bioengineered polymers are as follows:

1. Strain Development and Stability

Genetic instability: The various microbial strains or cells used for the biosynthesis of polymers may lose productivity due to plasmid loss, mutations, or metabolic burden.

Reproducibility: The main problem with scalability is maintaining a consistent polymer composition and molecular weight, even with small metabolic shifts that change monomer ratios.

Regulatory gene control: It is difficult and cost-intensive to scale up tightly regulated promoters or induction systems (such as IPTG, temperature-sensitive).

2. Process Optimization and Scale-Up Challenges

Oxygen and nutrient transfer limitations: On larger scales, gradients of oxygen and substrates are established, and heterogeneity in polymer yield and structure occurs.

Viscosity and rheology problems: The accumulation of high-molecular-weight polymers increases broth viscosity, which negatively affects mixing and mass transfer.

Limitations of bioreactor design: Conditions optimized at the laboratory scale such as shear rate, temperature, and pH may translate differently at the pilot or industrial scale, resulting in altered polymer properties.

3. Feedstock and Raw Material Variability

Feedstock variability: Bio-based feedstocks may differ in composition or impurities, such as glycerol, sugars, or hydrolysates. These feedstocks affect yield and reproducibility.

Affordable substrate supply: Raw materials used must be sustainable and of low cost to make the process economically feasible.

The primary role of a biodegradable polymer-based scaffold must be to remain at the implantation site while preserving its physical properties and integrity, and to facilitate the attachment, proliferation, and differentiation of cells until the regeneration of tissues at the damaged location. The degradation rate of the scaffold should ideally align with the rate of neo-tissue synthesis to ensure a seamless transition of load transfer from the scaffold to the tissue. A recent study indicates that the breakdown rate of certain biodegradable polymers varies depending on polymer composition, loading conditions, and environmental factors. Enzymatic degradation begins at the polymer's surface; hence, the surface area and condition (porosity) of the polymer are critical parameters influencing the degradation rate. Currently, several methods exist for the fabrication of porous scaffolds, including porogen leaching, emulsion freeze-drying, expansion in high-temperature gas, 3D printing, phase separation techniques, and thermal phase separation [21].

Polymeric Drug Delivery Systems

The different types of polymeric drug delivery systems are depicted in Fig. (**1**) and explained as follows.

Polymer-drug Conjugate

A polymeric drug conjugate is a drug delivery approach that improves drug solubility, stability, and controlled release through the chemical attachment of a medicinal molecule to a polymer. These conjugates enhance pharmacokinetics in cancer treatment and chronic illnesses by prolonging circulation duration, reducing toxicity, and enabling targeted distribution. Polymers such as Chitosan, Polyethylene Glycol (PEG), and Polyglutamic Acid (PGA) are commonly utilised as carriers due to their biocompatibility and capability to improve drug efficacy. Polymeric drug conjugates can be created with particular ligands for active targeting or can take advantage of passive targeting processes, such as the Enhanced Permeability and Retention (EPR) effect in malignancies. While these conjugates offer significant benefits, challenges related to polymer accumulation, biodegradability, and complex synthesis remain areas of active investigation. Advances in nanotechnology and personalized medicine are driving the development of next-generation polymeric drug conjugates to improve both safety and therapeutic efficacy. Typically, drugs are linked to polymers *via* cleavable linkers that respond to physiological stimuli, including pH fluctuations or enzymatic activity, thereby facilitating controlled drug release [22]. The covalent attachment of therapeutic agents to polymer carriers minimizes premature drug leakage.

Amphiphilic polymer-drug couples linked covalently can self-assemble into Nanoparticles (NPs), thereby enhancing their stability and delivery efficiency. The conjugation of 5-Aminosalicylic acid (5-ASA) and its azo prodrugs to polymers through ester linkers is relatively straightforward. Colonic bacteria produce azoreductase, an enzyme capable of cleaving the azo bond, thereby facilitating the release of 5-ASA. In one study, dextran with molecular weights of 10, 70, and 500 kDa was successfully conjugated to Budesonide (BUD), with the 70 kDa dextran-conjugate exhibiting superior stability, solubility, and drug release efficiency. Notably, only 10% of the conjugated BUD was released in the upper gastrointestinal tract, whereas colonic delivery showed a twofold increase in drug concentration [23].

Physical Encapsulation of the Drug in Polymeric Nanoparticles

Beyond covalent conjugation, hydrophobic and electrostatic interactions also allow for the physical encapsulation of drugs within polymeric nanoparticles. Due to their negative charge, these nanoparticles can interact with cationic polymers to form nanoscale assemblies or incorporate hydrophobic drugs through non-covalent interactions. Furthermore, cationic small molecules can form lipophilic macromolecules by interacting with polymeric nanoparticles [24]. In the treatment of IBD, studies have shown that polyphenol-based polymers work well as protein and nucleic acid nanocarriers. Even in aqueous conditions, polyphenols and pharmaceuticals form strong hydrogen bonds and hydrophobic interactions, thereby improving drug loading efficiency. Polymeric nanoparticles are produced using a variety of techniques, such as double emulsion-solvent evaporation, film creation and rehydration [25], and nanoprecipitation [26]. Lipid-polymer hybrid nanoparticles have emerged as versatile carriers, offering improved drug loading capacity, stability, and cellular uptake. Furthermore, macromolecular therapeutics such as nucleic acids and antioxidant enzymes can effectively bind to cationic lipids, thereby enhancing their therapeutic potential [27].

Polymer Microparticles and Hydrogels

One of the well-controlled drug release methods is polymeric microparticles, which are readily prepared by solvent evaporation and spray drying. Common applications for CS/Alg composite microparticles include colon-targeted drug delivery, and because of the two polymers' ionotropic gelation/polyelectrolyte complexation, they are produced *via* spray drying [28]. Drug leaking in the stomach results from the CS/Alg composite microparticle's inability to withstand severe acidic conditions. As a result, enteric coatings, such as Eudragit® polymers, are frequently used to stop medication degradation and premature release [29]. Both drug delivery and tissue engineering extensively use PLGA, a biodegradable aliphatic polyester [30]. Pathak and associates created polylactic acid microspheres and wrapped them in mesenchymal stem cells that had immunomodulatory and anti-inflammatory qualities. To treat colitis caused by Dextran Sodium Sulfate (DSS), the coated microspheres were used to administer an intraperitoneal injection of IDN6556, a broad-spectrum caspase inhibitor [31]. Because of their micron-size, microparticles are appealing for delivering macromolecules and nanoparticles, such as monoclonal antibodies and antioxidant enzymes. A Catalase (CAT)-loaded microsphere with dual shells composed of polydopamine and dextran sulfate effectively maintained enzyme activity in stomach fluid before reaching the colon for broad-spectrum ROS scavenging [32, 33].

Smart Polymer-based Systems

The different types of smart polymer-based systems are depicted in Fig. (**2**) and explained as follows.

Smart Hydrogels

Three-dimensional networks of hydrophilic polymers called hydrogels have the ability to expand in water and hold a significant amount of water while retaining their structural integrity through chemical or physical cross-linking of separate polymer chains [34]. Because of their great capacity to absorb water, porosity, pliability, soft structure, controlled release, and resemblance to biological tissues, hydrogels can be used for a variety of biomedical applications, including wound treatment, tissue engineering, and drug administration. The kind of polymer, its concentration, and the reaction conditions can all be changed to modify these characteristics [35, 36]. Smart hydrogels contain active chemicals, including dexamethasone, HA, and 5-Aminosalicylic Acid (5-ASA), which are anti-inflammatory. Furthermore, the smart hydrogel contains microorganisms, including Lactobacillus acidophilus and Lactobacillus reuteri, to mimic IBD. IBD is diagnosed and treated using smart hydrogels that react to environmental stimuli, including pH, temperature, enzymes, and ROS [37, 38].

Smart Nanoparticles

A large family of materials with sizes less than 100 nm is called nanoparticles. They fall under the following categories: semiconductor, metal, ceramic, lipid, carbon, and polymeric nanoparticles [39]. Most smart nanoparticles for IBD are polymeric; they can target specific cells, reduce side effects, and protect the drug by encapsulating it. They also respond to a variety of physical, chemical, and biological stimuli, such as ROS, pH, ligands, magnetic fields, and gut microbiota, and thus provide controlled release [40]. Their usage is restricted by chemical instability and particle aggregation, despite their good mucoadhesive and biocompatible properties and ease of preparation [41]. Lipid nanoparticles are more cost-effective, readily scalable, biodegradable, and have superior biocompatibility as compared to polymeric nanoparticles. However, they are restricted by their reduced loading capacity as a result of the medications' decreased solubility [42]. Because of their favourable optical and magnetic characteristics, inorganic nanoparticles can be used to treat IBD. Smart nanoparticles control microbiota balance or transport anti-inflammatory drugs to the colon. *In vitro* and *in vivo*, the majority of smart nanoparticles work by blocking proinflammatory cytokines and efficiently localizing in the intestines' inflammatory region [43].

Smart Nanofibers

Smart nanofibers are produced by electrospinning nanometer-diameter polymeric fibers with high surface-to-volume ratios, low weight, and tunable, high porosity [44]. Smart nanofibers may carry small molecular drugs in addition to larger biological medicines, including proteins, nucleic acids, bacteria, and even stem cells [45, 46]. Like other smart bionanomaterials, smart nanofibers can respond to environmental stimuli and allow for controlled and targeted drug delivery. Prolonged manufacturing times and low production efficiency are two drawbacks of electrospinning; however, they may be avoided by employing nozzle-less electrospinning and multiple jets [47]. Smart nanofibers were developed for the treatment of IBD in order to deliver probiotic bacteria like *Lactobacillus plantarum* and *Lactobacillus rhamnosus*, as well as anti-inflammatory medications, including prednisolone, diclofenac sodium, and budesonide [48].

Smart Hybrid Bionanomaterials

To improve the effectiveness and reduce the negative effects of medications supplied, smart hybrid bionanomaterials integrate two or more bionanomaterials

[49]. A combination of two or more bionanomaterials can enhance their ability to deliver active chemicals to the inflammatory bowel, which will help with IBD diagnosis and/or therapy. The majority of intelligent hybrid bionanomaterials blend hydrogels and nanoparticles [50]. They react to environmental stimuli like magnetic fields, pH, ROS, and biomolecules. In order to help diagnose IBD, smart hybrid devices can sample the microbiota or inject active substances into the colon [51, 52].

Smart Probiotics

Smart probiotics, or genetically modified safe bacteria, are living organisms rather than inanimate smart bionanomaterials. Similar to intelligent bionanomaterials, probiotics can respond to external stimuli and release active compounds capable of diagnosing and treating IBD [53]. This is frequently achieved through the controlled production of anti-inflammatory recombinant proteins. By modulating the gut microbiota and interacting with the immune system, probiotics exhibit immunoregulatory properties that contribute to alleviating IBD symptoms and maintaining microbial balance. The delivery of therapeutic and diagnostic recombinant proteins further strengthens these beneficial effects [54, 55].

PATENT-BASED NEWER TECHNOLOGY TO TREAT IBD

The chronic nature and difficulty of managing IBD, which includes disorders like UC and CD, provide substantial obstacles. While immunosuppressive drugs are a common component of conventional treatment plans, they are not always appropriate for individuals and can have serious adverse effects. New patent-based technologies have emerged in response to these difficulties, with the goal of revolutionising current approaches to treating IBD. Innovative, patent-protected technology is a prime example of the multi-pronged strategy now in place to better treat inflammatory bowel disease, which is discussed in detail in Table **2**. These developments have the ability to enhance patient outcomes and quality of life for individuals impacted by this disabling ailment by combining pharmacological discoveries with bioengineering and nanotechnology.

MARKETED FORMULATIONS USING ENGINEERED NATURAL POLYMERS

IBD was once thought to be limited to the Western/developed world, but during the past ten or so years, the number of cases reported in Asian countries has significantly increased. This is partly due to the availability of sophisticated detection methods, like colonoscopy and endoscopy, which were not widely available in the past, particularly in the 1980s. Additionally, linked to the increase in illness incidence is industrialization, which began in the West and is currently rapidly expanding in Asian nations [66]. Polymers are highly versatile materials with desirable physical and chemical properties, making them valuable for usage in therapeutic applications, drug delivery systems, and medical devices. As a result, the potential of functional polymers for medicinal applications has attracted significant interest recently. Biomaterials based on polymers have found effective applications in tissue engineering, dentistry, medical device components, and artificial organs. Research on the use of biomedical polymers for therapeutic purposes is also expanding. Polymers have been used in these applications as carriers to transfer proteins, antibodies, plasmid DNA, siRNA, and active medicinal compounds [67, 68]. Significant progress in polymer-based drug delivery systems and polymeric prodrugs has improved the therapeutic effectiveness of various pharmaceuticals and biotherapies, resulting in the development of several commercially successful products. Notable examples of these marketed formulations include Gliadel®, CYPHER®, Neulasta®, PegIntron®, PEGASYS®, Cimzia®, ABRAXANE®, and others [69]. Thus, repurposing the currently available and proven safe anti-inflammatory drugs might be a practical strategy to enhance the therapeutic care of the illness by utilizing innovative delivery techniques to overcome their translational obstacles [70]. The various types of marketed products designed to enhance the drug delivery systems and can induce tissue healing properties are depicted in Fig. (**3**) and explained as follows:

Table 2. Patent-driven innovations in natural polymers for IBD management.

Sl. No.	Application No.	Title of Patent	Theory of Invention	Application(s)	References
1	US 9,642,914 B2	Photo-crosslinked biodegradable hydrogel	A variety of natural polymer macromers, crosslinked with a variety of degradable crosslinks, can be mixed into the photo-crosslinked biodegradable hydrogel.	Exhibit cytocompatibility and significantly produce non-toxic products after decomposition.	[56]

(Table 2) cont.....

Sl. No.	Application No.	Title of Patent	Theory of Invention	Application(s)	References
2	US 10, 434, 139 B2	Oral pharmaceutical composition	Specifically, azo-crosslinked polymers are microbially degradable polymers that have been studied for use in medication delivery to the colon.	Orally administered drugs coated with pH-sensitive polymers enhance stability and increase hydrophilicity.	[57]
3	EP 3 551 194 B1	Glycan polymers and related methods thereof	In order to treat IBD, the invention offers a glycosyl polymer preparation that may be used in a protocol to treat a patient with a disease or ailment linked to an undesired amount of a metabolite.	They help treat the disease by modulating the production or levels of metabolites.	[58]
4	US20250017883A1	Use of short-chain fatty acids for the treatment and prevention of diseases and disorders	The invention involves Short-chain Fatty Acids (SCFAs) as the primary byproduct of anaerobic bacterial fermentation in the gut, which have been demonstrated to regulate a variety of Gastrointestinal (GI) tract activities, including homeostasis and metabolic processes.	SCFAs and related therapeutic compounds and other compounds are used for the treatment or prevention of diseases or disorders.	[59]

(Table 2) cont.....

Sl. No.	Application No.	Title of Patent	Theory of Invention	Application(s)	References
5	US 11,759,442 B2	Use of short-chain fatty acids for the treatment and prevention of diseases and disorders	In this invention, the SCFA precursor moiety comprises a combination of an acetyl-CoA carboxylase inhibitor and vitamin D, and in other embodiments, one additional moiety of SCFA comprises PEG.	This kind of additional treatment shows therapeutic efficacy in the treatment of autoimmune diseases.	[60]
6	US 10, 130, 695 B2	Compositions containing combinations of bioactive molecules derived from microbiota for the treatment of disease	The purpose of this disclosure is to offer products that are effective, can be produced to the same quality standards as pharmaceuticals, and mitigate the negative consequences of changes in the microbiota on human health.	The formulations are helpful for the prevention and treatment of illnesses, including inflammatory, autoimmune, and infectious disorders, when taken orally *via* colonic delivery.	[61]
7	CA2785658C	Compositions and methods for treatment and prophylaxis of inflammatory bowel disease	In order to cure IBD symptoms and lower the chance of recurrence, the invention proposes using probiotic formulations in conjunction with antibiotics.	By combining probiotics with antibiotics to prepare a unitary dosage form to improve patient compliance with treatment protocols.	[62]

(Table 2) cont.....

Sl. No.	Application No.	Title of Patent	Theory of Invention	Application(s)	References
8	EP2555760B1	Chitosan derivatives for the treatment of mucositis or ulceration	The innovation concerns soluble chitosans, their derivatives, and their applications.	Many techniques have been proposed to enhance wound healing, such as covering the wound with reticulated foam, especially with antimicrobial compounds, as a dressing, and utilizing devices that provide positive and/or negative pressure at the wound site.	[63]
9	CN102196807B	Water-insoluble polymer: starch-based film coatings for colon targeting	A controlled-release dosage form for an active ingredient is provided by the current invention. It consists of an active ingredient coated with a polymeric mixture that contains a water-insoluble polymer and a starch group containing amylose.	Many pharmacotherapies, including those for inflammatory bowel conditions like Crohn's disease (CD) and Ulcerative Colitis (UC), can benefit greatly by targeting the segmented intestine.	[64]

(Table 2) cont.....

Sl. No.	Application No.	Title of Patent	Theory of Invention	Application(s)	References
10	US 20190374650 A1	Compositions and methods for delivery of polymer/biomacromolecule conjugates	Compositions including polymer moieties (such as poly (L-glutamic acid moieties)) linked to biomacromolecule agents, techniques for creating such polymer conjugates, and systems and procedures using such conjugates are the focus of the current invention.	Polymers linked to biomacromolecule agents (*e.g.*, peptides, neo-antigens, adjuvant molecules, nucleic acids, *etc.*) that are complexed, conjugated, encapsulated, absorbed, adsorbed, or admixed and designed to cure, prevent, or improve a variety of illnesses	[65]

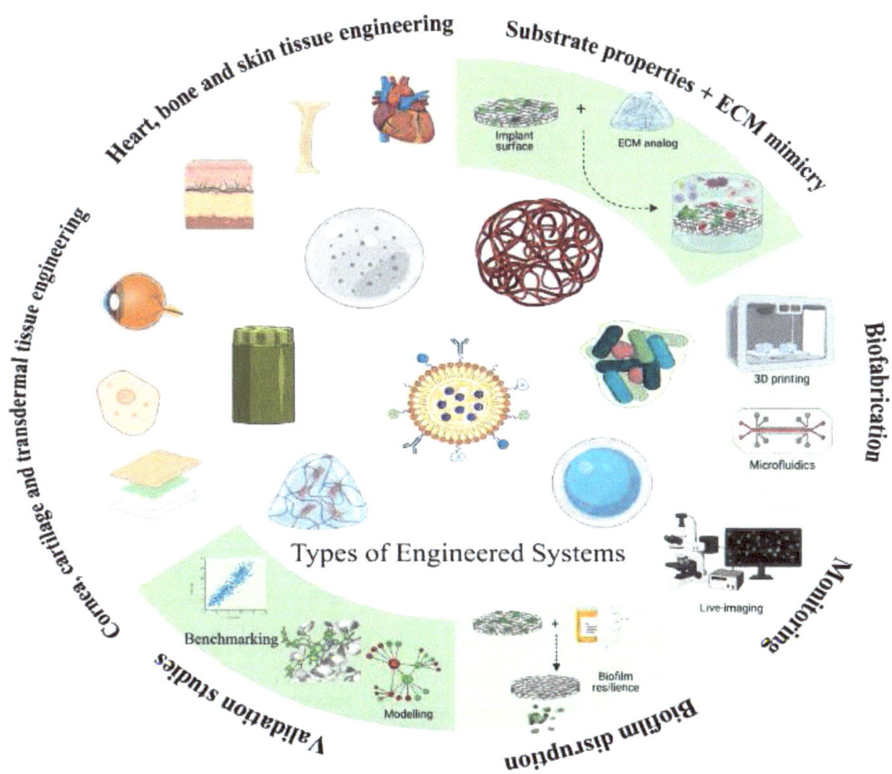

Fig. (3). Types of different engineered systems and their applications.

Iron-sequestering Polymers for the Treatment of Iron Overload Disorders

The development of systemically non-absorbed iron chelators that are taken orally and that selectively bind and extract excess dietary iron from the gastrointestinal tract is a potential strategy for treating iron insufficiency. Desferrioxamine is now regarded as the gold standard for iron chelation treatment. Non-absorbed polymeric ligands have the potential to be used as therapeutic agents to treat certain iron overload illnesses because they efficiently sequester and remove dietary iron. These polymeric ligands must have high capacity, selectivity, and affinity for iron in both oxidation states, while causing the least disruption to vital metal ions required for human physiology, to be therapeutically useful [71].

Azopolymers used as Colon-specific Drug Delivery

Numerous physiological triggers have been suggested for the colon's targeted medication release. One strategy has been to use the abundance of microbes that inhabit the lower gastrointestinal system. The reduction of water-soluble azo dyes like Prontosil is one of the several metabolic processes that these organisms may mediate. It has also been demonstrated that the prodrug sulphasalazine undergoes reductive cleavage due to microbial azo reduction [72].

Eudragit-coated Formulations

Ora-Curcumin-S(OCS), a highly water-soluble curcumin polymer-drug combination with a hydrophilic pH-dependent Eudragit® S100 polymer, was developed to address some of the limitations. OCS effectively transports curcumin, an anti-inflammatory, to the colon's luminal side while having no effect on blood flow. This approach involves the formulation of a polymer-curcumin based Toll-like receptor-4 (TLR4) antagonist, supported by strong preclinical evidence. These findings highlight curcumin's long-sought therapeutic potential to improve IBD pathology and reduce the risk of colon cancer [1].

Certolizumab Pegol (Cimzia)

PEGylated proteins have significantly improved the management of Rheumatoid Arthritis (RA) and other chronic conditions, including UC associated with RA. Certolizumab pegol is the only PEGylated drug targeting Tumour Necrosis Factor (TNF)-α. This medication is a humanized, antigen-binding monoclonal antibody fragment that has undergone PEGylation to enhance its therapeutic properties [73].

Programmable Polymers for Tissue Healing

Nowadays, a large number of biocompatible, nondegradable Shape Memory Polymers (SMPs) are used in clinical settings to enhance surgical handling during minimally invasive operations and to address previously unresolvable issues and unhealthy geometries. Despite being authorized for a number of uses, these nonbiodegradable polymers remain in the patient's body and are either incorporated or encapsulated as long-lasting relics, which support the creation of a 3D-fabricated biomaterial scaffold (bioscaffold) that modulates inflammation intrinsically for soft tissue healing [74].

Nanostructures manufactured from natural polymers might be a wonderful choice for drug delivery and for optimizing IBD therapy because of their properties, which are intended to completely and progressively overcome the numerous barriers to efficiently release the medication in the inflamed colon [75].

CONCLUSION

Finally, the complicated aetiology of IBD, including genetic, environmental, and microbial components, poses substantial difficulties in the therapeutic management of the disease, especially UC and CD. IBD cases, particularly in younger age groups, highlighting the critical need for efficient treatment approaches to reduce the likelihood of colon cancer and other severe consequences. Although 5-aminosalicylic acid derivatives, corticosteroids, and immunosuppressants are effective in inducing remission, the side effects associated with their long-term usage typically make them unfeasible; thus, we need to find alternatives. An encouraging new direction for improving the effectiveness of inflammatory bowel disease treatments is the development of drug delivery systems that use both synthetic and natural polymers. These advancements aim to improve drug targeting, bioavailability, and the mitigation of systemic adverse effects, encompassing the creation of smart hydrogels and hybrid bionanomaterials. In addition, there is hope for a paradigm shift in IBD management and therapy thanks to the incorporation of bioengineering and nanotechnology into the creation of therapeutic drugs. Improving the quality of life for persons affected by this chronic and debilitating ailment requires ongoing study to improve these tactics and optimise patient outcomes.

REFERENCES

[1] Kesharwani SS, Ahmad R, Bakkari MA, *et al.* Site-directed non-covalent polymer-drug complexes for Inflammatory Bowel Disease (IBD): Formulation development, characterization and pharmacological evaluation. J Control Release 2018; 290: 165-79. [http://dx.doi.org/10.1016/j.jconrel.2018.08.004] [PMID: 30142410]

[2] Pu Y, Fan X, Zhang Z, *et al.* Harnessing polymer-derived drug delivery systems for combating

inflammatory bowel disease. J Control Release 2023; 354: 1-18.
[http://dx.doi.org/10.1016/j.jconrel.2022.12.044] [PMID: 36566845]

[3] Khare T, Palakurthi SS, Shah BM, Palakurthi S, Khare S. Natural product-based nanomedicine in treatment of inflammatory bowel disease. Int J Mol Sci 2020; 21(11): 3956.
[http://dx.doi.org/10.3390/ijms21113956] [PMID: 32486445]

[4] Li H, Sun J, Zhu H, *et al.* Recent advances in development of dendritic polymer-based nanomedicines for cancer diagnosis. Wiley Interdiscip Rev Nanomed Nanobiotechnol 2021; 13(2): e1670.
[http://dx.doi.org/10.1002/wnan.1670] [PMID: 32949116]

[5] Khan S, McCabe J, Hill K, Beales PA. Biodegradable hybrid block copolymer – lipid vesicles as potential drug delivery systems. J Colloid Interface Sci 2020; 562: 418-28.
[http://dx.doi.org/10.1016/j.jcis.2019.11.101] [PMID: 31806358]

[6] Sohail M, Mudassir , Minhas MU, *et al.* Natural and synthetic polymer-based smart biomaterials for management of ulcerative colitis: a review of recent developments and future prospects. Drug Deliv Transl Res 2019; 9(2): 595-614.
[http://dx.doi.org/10.1007/s13346-018-0512-x] [PMID: 29611113]

[7] Stojanov S, Berlec A. Smart bionanomaterials for treatment and diagnosis of inflammatory bowel disease. Nanotechnol Rev 2024; 13(1): 20240057.
[http://dx.doi.org/10.1515/ntrev-2024-0057]

[8] Wang CPJ, Byun MJ, Kim SN, *et al.* Biomaterials as therapeutic drug carriers for inflammatory bowel disease treatment. J Control Release 2022; 345: 1-19.
[http://dx.doi.org/10.1016/j.jconrel.2022.02.028] [PMID: 35227764]

[9] Seegobin N, McCoubrey LE, Vignal C, *et al.* Dual action tofacitinib-loaded PLGA nanoparticles alleviate colitis in an IBD mouse model. Drug Deliv Transl Res 2024; 1-8.
[PMID: 39527394]

[10] Dar MJ, Ali H, Khan A, Khan GM. Polymer-based drug delivery: the quest for local targeting of inflamed intestinal mucosa. J Drug Target 2017; 25(7): 582-96.
[http://dx.doi.org/10.1080/1061186X.2017.1298601] [PMID: 28277824]

[11] Biasi F, Astegiano M, Maina M, Leonarduzzi G, Poli G. Polyphenol supplementation as a complementary medicinal approach to treating inflammatory bowel disease. Curr Med Chem 2011; 18(31): 4851-65.
[http://dx.doi.org/10.2174/092986711797535263] [PMID: 21919842]

[12] Sareen R, Jain N, Rajkumari A, Dhar KL. pH triggered delivery of curcumin from Eudragit-coated chitosan microspheres for inflammatory bowel disease: characterization and pharmacodynamic evaluation. Drug Deliv 2016; 23(1): 55-62.
[http://dx.doi.org/10.3109/10717544.2014.903534] [PMID: 24758141]

[13] Gupta B, Revagade N, Hilborn J. Poly(lactic acid) fiber: An overview. Prog Polym Sci 2007; 32(4): 455-82.
[http://dx.doi.org/10.1016/j.progpolymsci.2007.01.005]

[14] Lasprilla AJR, Martinez GAR, Lunelli BH, Jardini AL, Filho RM. Poly-lactic acid synthesis for application in biomedical devices — A review. Biotechnol Adv 2012; 30(1): 321-8.
[http://dx.doi.org/10.1016/j.biotechadv.2011.06.019] [PMID: 21756992]

[15] Hlaing SP, Cao J, Lee J, *et al.* Hyaluronic acid-conjugated PLGA nanoparticles alleviate ulcerative colitis *via* CD44-mediated dual targeting to inflamed colitis tissue and macrophages. Pharmaceutics 2022; 14(10): 2118.
[http://dx.doi.org/10.3390/pharmaceutics14102118] [PMID: 36297553]

[16] Lautenschläger C, Schmidt C, Lehr CM, Fischer D, Stallmach A. PEG-functionalized microparticles selectively target inflamed mucosa in inflammatory bowel disease. Eur J Pharm Biopharm 2013; 85(3): 578-86.

[http://dx.doi.org/10.1016/j.ejpb.2013.09.016] [PMID: 24084650]

[17] Liu Z, Yu W, Sheng W, *et al.* Controllable synthesis of polyphenol spheres *via* amine-catalyzed polymerization-induced self-assembly. Biomacromolecules 2022; 23(1): 140-9.
[http://dx.doi.org/10.1021/acs.biomac.1c01158] [PMID: 34910461]

[18] Alatab S, Sepanlou SG, Ikuta K, *et al.* The global, regional, and national burden of inflammatory bowel disease in 195 countries and territories, 1990–2017: a systematic analysis for the Global Burden of Disease Study 2017. Lancet Gastroenterol Hepatol 2020; 5(1): 17-30.
[http://dx.doi.org/10.1016/S2468-1253(19)30333-4] [PMID: 31648971]

[19] Ali M, Brocchini S. Synthetic approaches to uniform polymers. Adv Drug Deliv Rev 2006; 58(15): 1671-87.
[http://dx.doi.org/10.1016/j.addr.2006.10.002] [PMID: 17125883]

[20] Nilsen A, Braslau R. Nitroxide decomposition: Implications toward nitroxide design for applications in living free-radical polymerization. J Polym Sci A Polym Chem 2006; 44(2): 697-717.
[http://dx.doi.org/10.1002/pola.21207]

[21] Mizuno K, Kido H, Narita T, Dohmoto M, Ogawa T, Osawa S. Control of degradation rate of porous biodegradable Polymers InProceedings of the 8th polymer for advanced technologies international symposium 2005; 13-6.

[22] Canevari M, Castagliuolo I, Brun P, *et al.* Poly(ethylene glycol)-mesalazine conjugate for colon specific delivery. Int J Pharm 2009; 368(1-2): 171-7.
[http://dx.doi.org/10.1016/j.ijpharm.2008.09.058] [PMID: 18996458]

[23] Priyam A, Shivhare K, Yadav S, Sharma AK, Kumar P. Enhanced solubility and self-assembly of amphiphilic sulfasalazine-PEG-OMe (S-PEG) conjugate into core-shell nanostructures useful for colonic drug delivery. Colloids Surf A Physicochem Eng Asp 2018; 547: 157-67.
[http://dx.doi.org/10.1016/j.colsurfa.2018.03.048]

[24] Zeng Z, He X, Li C, *et al.* Oral delivery of antioxidant enzymes for effective treatment of inflammatory disease. Biomaterials 2021; 271: 120753.
[http://dx.doi.org/10.1016/j.biomaterials.2021.120753] [PMID: 33725585]

[25] Yavvari PS, Verma P, Mustfa SA, *et al.* A nanogel based oral gene delivery system targeting SUMOylation machinery to combat gut inflammation. Nanoscale 2019; 11(11): 4970-86.
[http://dx.doi.org/10.1039/C8NR09599J] [PMID: 30839018]

[26] Laroui H, Theiss AL, Yan Y, *et al.* Functional TNFα gene silencing mediated by polyethyleneimine/TNFα siRNA nanocomplexes in inflamed colon. Biomaterials 2011; 32(4): 1218-28.
[http://dx.doi.org/10.1016/j.biomaterials.2010.09.062] [PMID: 20970849]

[27] Wilson DS, Dalmasso G, Wang L, Sitaraman SV, Merlin D, Murthy N. Orally delivered thioketal nanoparticles loaded with TNF-α–siRNA target inflammation and inhibit gene expression in the intestines. Nat Mater 2010; 9(11): 923-8.
[http://dx.doi.org/10.1038/nmat2859] [PMID: 20935658]

[28] Blanco-García E, Otero-Espinar FJ, Blanco-Méndez J, Leiro-Vidal JM, Luzardo-Álvarez A. Development and characterization of anti-inflammatory activity of curcumin-loaded biodegradable microspheres with potential use in intestinal inflammatory disorders. Int J Pharm 2017; 518(1-2): 86-104.
[http://dx.doi.org/10.1016/j.ijpharm.2016.12.057] [PMID: 28040561]

[29] Duan H, Lü S, Gao C, *et al.* Mucoadhesive microparticulates based on polysaccharide for target dual drug delivery of 5-aminosalicylic acid and curcumin to inflamed colon. Colloids Surf B Biointerfaces 2016; 145: 510-9.
[http://dx.doi.org/10.1016/j.colsurfb.2016.05.038] [PMID: 27239905]

[30] Zhao J, Sun Y, Yang H, *et al.* PLGA-microspheres-carried circGMCL1 protects against Crohn's

colitis through alleviating NLRP3 inflammasome-induced pyroptosis by promoting autophagy. Cell Death Dis 2022; 13(9): 782.
[http://dx.doi.org/10.1038/s41419-022-05226-5] [PMID: 36088391]

[31] Pathak S, Regmi S, Shrestha P, Choi I, Doh KO, Jeong JH. Mesenchymal stem cell capping on ECM-anchored caspase inhibitor–loaded PLGA microspheres for intraperitoneal injection in DSS-induced murine colitis. Small 2019; 15(23): 1901269.
[http://dx.doi.org/10.1002/smll.201901269] [PMID: 31018047]

[32] Wang H, Xing H, Xia Y, *et al.* PLGA microspheres carrying miR-20a-5p improved intestinal epithelial barrier function in patients with Crohn's disease through STAT3-mediated inhibition of Th17 differentiation. Int Immunopharmacol 2022; 110: 109025.
[http://dx.doi.org/10.1016/j.intimp.2022.109025] [PMID: 35853280]

[33] Li J, Qiu H, Gong H, Tong W. Broad-spectrum reactive oxygen species scavenging and activated macrophage-targeting microparticles ameliorate inflammatory bowel disease. Biomacromolecules 2021; 22(7): 3107-18.
[http://dx.doi.org/10.1021/acs.biomac.1c00551] [PMID: 34160209]

[34] Bahram M, Mohseni N, Moghtader M. An introduction to hydrogels and some recent applications. Emerging Concepts in Analysis and Applications of Hydrogels. InTech 2016.
[http://dx.doi.org/10.5772/64301]

[35] Aswathy SH, Narendrakumar U, Manjubala I. Commercial hydrogels for biomedical applications. Heliyon 2020; 6(4): e03719.
[http://dx.doi.org/10.1016/j.heliyon.2020.e03719] [PMID: 32280802]

[36] Ho TC, Chang CC, Chan HP, *et al.* Hydrogels: properties and applications in biomedicine. Molecules 2022; 27(9): 2902.
[http://dx.doi.org/10.3390/molecules27092902] [PMID: 35566251]

[37] Billiet T, Vandenhaute M, Schelfhout J, Van Vlierberghe S, Dubruel P. A review of trends and limitations in hydrogel-rapid prototyping for tissue engineering. Biomaterials 2012; 33(26): 6020-41.
[http://dx.doi.org/10.1016/j.biomaterials.2012.04.050] [PMID: 22681979]

[38] Sudhir Dhote N, Dineshbhai Patel R, Kuwar U, *et al.* Ajazuddin. Application of thermoresponsive smart polymers based *in situ* gel as a novel carrier for tumor targeting. Curr Cancer Drug Targets 2024; 24(4): 375-96.
[http://dx.doi.org/10.2174/1568009623666230803111718] [PMID: 37534485]

[39] Khan I, Saeed K, Khan I. Nanoparticles: Properties, applications and toxicities. Arab J Chem 2019; 12(7): 908-31.
[http://dx.doi.org/10.1016/j.arabjc.2017.05.011]

[40] Joudeh N, Linke D. Nanoparticle classification, physicochemical properties, characterization, and applications: a comprehensive review for biologists. J Nanobiotechnology 2022; 20(1): 262.
[http://dx.doi.org/10.1186/s12951-022-01477-8] [PMID: 35672712]

[41] Yusuf A, Almotairy ARZ, Henidi H, Alshehri OY, Aldughaim MS. Nanoparticles as drug delivery systems: a review of the implication of nanoparticles' physicochemical properties on responses in biological systems. Polymers (Basel) 2023; 15(7): 1596.
[http://dx.doi.org/10.3390/polym15071596] [PMID: 37050210]

[42] Chenthamara D, Subramaniam S, Ramakrishnan SG, *et al.* Therapeutic efficacy of nanoparticles and routes of administration. Biomater Res 2019; 23(1): 20.
[http://dx.doi.org/10.1186/s40824-019-0166-x] [PMID: 31832232]

[43] Mukherjee S, Ray S, Thakur RS. Solid lipid nanoparticles: A modern formulation approach in drug delivery system. Indian J Pharm Sci 2009; 71(4): 349-58.
[http://dx.doi.org/10.4103/0250-474X.57282] [PMID: 20502539]

[44] Xue J, Xie J, Liu W, Xia Y. Electrospun nanofibers: new concepts, materials, and applications. Acc

Chem Res 2017; 50(8): 1976-87.
[http://dx.doi.org/10.1021/acs.accounts.7b00218] [PMID: 28777535]

[45] Torres-Martínez EJ, Cornejo Bravo JM, Serrano Medina A, Pérez González GL, Villarreal Gómez LJ. A summary of electrospun nanofibers as drug delivery system: drugs loaded and biopolymers used as matrices. Curr Drug Deliv 2018; 15(10): 1360-74.
[http://dx.doi.org/10.2174/1567201815666180723114326] [PMID: 30033869]

[46] Al-Tahami K, Singh J. Smart polymer based delivery systems for peptides and proteins. Recent Pat Drug Deliv Formul 2007; 1(1): 65-71.
[http://dx.doi.org/10.2174/187221107779814113] [PMID: 19075875]

[47] Stojanov S, Berlec A. Electrospun nanofibers as carriers of microorganisms, stem cells, proteins, and nucleic acids in therapeutic and other applications. Front Bioeng Biotechnol 2020; 8: 130.
[http://dx.doi.org/10.3389/fbioe.2020.00130] [PMID: 32158751]

[48] Stojanov S, Plavec TV, Kristl J, Zupančič Š, Berlec A. Engineering of vaginal lactobacilli to express fluorescent proteins enables the analysis of their mixture in nanofibers. Int J Mol Sci 2021; 22(24): 13631.
[http://dx.doi.org/10.3390/ijms222413631] [PMID: 34948426]

[49] Al-Malah Kamal I M, Nanomaterials , Metamaterials S, Materials . Nanomaterials, metamaterials, and smart materials: Synthesis and characterization. Bentham Science Publishers 2025.
[http://dx.doi.org/10.2174/97898153242731250101]

[50] Lim EK, Chung BH, Chung SJ. Recent advances in pH-sensitive polymeric nanoparticles for smart drug delivery in cancer therapy. Curr Drug Targets 2018; 19(4): 300-17.
[http://dx.doi.org/10.2174/1389450117666160602202339] [PMID: 27262486]

[51] Rout SR, Gowtham K, Sheikh A, Parvez S, Dandela R, Kesharwani P. Recent advances and future prospective of hybrid drug delivery systems. Hybrid Nanomaterials for Drug Delivery. 2022; pp. 357-74.

[52] Li S, Ge Y, Li H. Smart nanomaterials for sensor application. Bentham Science Publishers. 2012.
[http://dx.doi.org/10.2174/97816080524171120101]

[53] Seth AK, Parmar G, Aundhia C, Shah N, Gohil D. Smart polymer systems: A futuristic approach to enhance therapeutic efficacy. Curr Org Chem 2024; 28(15): 1164-78.
[http://dx.doi.org/10.2174/0113852728305580240429100851]

[54] Abraham BP, Quigley EMM. Probiotics in inflammatory bowel disease. Gastroenterol Clin North Am 2017; 46(4): 769-82.
[http://dx.doi.org/10.1016/j.gtc.2017.08.003] [PMID: 29173520]

[55] Jakubczyk D, Leszczyńska K, Górska S. The effectiveness of probiotics in the treatment of Inflammatory Bowel Disease (IBD)—a critical review. Nutrients 2020; 12(7): 1973.
[http://dx.doi.org/10.3390/nu12071973] [PMID: 32630805]

[56] None N. Western Reserve University Atomic Energy Project: Quarterly Progress Report - April, May, June 1952. Photocrosslinked biodegradable hydrogel United States patent US 9 2017.
[http://dx.doi.org/10.2172/4379873]

[57] Coulter I. Sublimity Therapeutics Ltd, assignee. Oral pharmaceutical composition. United States patent US 10 2019.

[58] Gibson MK, Liu CM, Maltzahn V, Yuan GA, Inventors H. Glycan polymers and related methods thereof. United States patent application US 16/466 2019.

[59] Arzumanyan A, Spector IC, Feitelson MA. Use of short chain fatty acids for the treatment and prevention of diseases and disorders. United States patent application US 18/901. 2025.

[60] Spector IC, Feitelson MA, Arzumanyan A. Temple University of Commonwealth System of Higher Education, assignee. Use of short chain fatty acids for the treatment and prevention of diseases and

disorders. United States patent US 11 2023.

[61] Honda K, Olle B, Atarashi K, *et al.* Compositions containing combinations of bioactive molecules derived from microbiota for treatment of disease United States patent US 10. 2018.

[62] Trachtman IM. Compositions and method for treatment and prophylaxis of inflammatory bowel disease. United States patent US 9. 2015.

[63] Rout SR, Kar B, Pradhan D, *et al.* Chitosan as a potential biomaterial for the management of oral mucositis, a common complication of cancer treatment. Pharm Dev Technol 2023; 28(1): 78-94. [http://dx.doi.org/10.1080/10837450.2022.2162544] [PMID: 36564887]

[64] Haeusler O, Wils D, Siepmann J, Karrout Y, Freres R, SA. Water insoluble polymer: starch-based film coatings for colon targeting. United States patent application US 13/126,212. 2011.

[65] Moon JJ, Yuchen FA, Inventors NJ. Compositions and methods for delivery of polymer/biomacromolecule conjugates. United States patent application US 16/488,031. 2019.

[66] Kulkarni N, Jain P, Shindikar A, Suryawanshi P, Thorat N. Advances in the colon-targeted chitosan based multiunit drug delivery systems for the treatment of inflammatory bowel disease. Carbohydr Polym 2022; 288: 119351. [http://dx.doi.org/10.1016/j.carbpol.2022.119351] [PMID: 35450623]

[67] Duncan R. Polymer conjugates as anticancer nanomedicines. Nat Rev Cancer 2006; 6(9): 688-701. [http://dx.doi.org/10.1038/nrc1958] [PMID: 16900224]

[68] Park JH, Lee S, Kim JH, Park K, Kim K, Kwon IC. Polymeric nanomedicine for cancer therapy. Prog Polym Sci 2008; 33(1): 113-37. [http://dx.doi.org/10.1016/j.progpolymsci.2007.09.003]

[69] Dhal PK, Polomoscanik SC, Avila LZ, Holmes-Farley SR, Miller RJ. Functional polymers as therapeutic agents: Concept to market place. Adv Drug Deliv Rev 2009; 61(13): 1121-30. [http://dx.doi.org/10.1016/j.addr.2009.05.004] [PMID: 19682515]

[70] Cohen RD, Ed. Inflammatory bowel disease: diagnosis and therapeutics. Humana Press 2011. [http://dx.doi.org/10.1007/978-1-60327-433-3]

[71] Liu ZD, Hider RC. Design of clinically useful iron(III)-selective chelators. Med Res Rev 2002; 22(1): 26-64. [http://dx.doi.org/10.1002/med.1027] [PMID: 11746175]

[72] Lloyd AW, Martin GP, Soozandehfar SH. Azopolymers: a means of colon specific drug delivery? Int J Pharm 1994; 106(3): 255-60. [http://dx.doi.org/10.1016/0378-5173(94)90011-6]

[73] Pasut G. Pegylation of biological molecules and potential benefits: pharmacological properties of certolizumab pegol. BioDrugs 2014; 28(S1) (Suppl. 1): 15-23. [http://dx.doi.org/10.1007/s40259-013-0064-z] [PMID: 24687235]

[74] Ramaraju H, Akman RE, Safranski DL, Hollister SJ. Designing biodegradable shape memory polymers for tissue repair. Adv Funct Mater 2020; 30(44): 2002014. [http://dx.doi.org/10.1002/adfm.202002014]

[75] Lima IBC, Moreno LCGAI, Silva-Filho EC, *et al.* Development of nanostructured systems using natural polymers to optimize the treatment of inflammatory bowel diseases: A prospective study. J Drug Deliv Sci Technol 2021; 64: 102590. [http://dx.doi.org/10.1016/j.jddst.2021.102590]

CHAPTER 10

Clinical Applications of Natural Polymers in Inflammatory Bowel Disease: Challenges in Translating Research into Practice

Prashant Tiwari[1,*] and **Sunil Kumar Kadiri**[1]

[1] *Department of Pharmacology, College of Pharmaceutical Sciences, Dayananda Sagar University, Bengaluru 562112, Karnataka, India*

Abstract: Inflammatory Bowel Disease (IBD), including Crohn's disease and ulcerative colitis, is a progressive and disabling disease characterized by relapsing gastrointestinal tract inflammation. However, an age of precision medicine for IBD is still far away, as severe side effects, high relapse rates, and compromised long-term efficacy are still challenging obstacles in conventional therapy. In fact, natural polymers, including alginate, chitosan, pectin, hyaluronic acid, and guar gum, have received considerable attention as novel therapeutic agents and delivery systems in recent years for the treatment of various diseases, which could be attributed to their cell-friendly features (biocompatibility and biodegradability) and their inherent bioactivities, such as anti-inflammatory activity, antioxidant activity, and mucosal healing activity. Several of these polymers have also demonstrated promise in improving drug delivery systems, supporting intestinal repair, and influencing gut microbiota, thereby overcoming certain shortcomings of existing IBD treatments. This chapter discusses natural polymer-based clinical applications in IBD and their functions as advanced drug delivery systems, biomaterials for tissue repair, and prebiotics that maintain gut health. It also discusses the major obstacles that limit the translation of these results into clinical practice, including formulation stability, scalability, patient heterogeneity, and regulatory complexities. Case reports and recent clinical trials are discussed to further illustrate these concepts. In addition, the chapter identifies further research opportunities, in particular, the convergence of polymer engineering, nanotechnology, and personalised medicine in IBD. In doing so, the chapter aims to inspire new approaches to the clinical exploitation of natural polymers to ultimately enhance patient outcomes.

Keywords: Antiinflammation, Biocompatibility, Chitosan, Clinical translation, Drug delivery, Natural polymer.

[*] **Corresponding author Prashant Tiwari:** Department of Pharmacology, College of Pharmaceutical Sciences, Dayananda SagarUniversity, Bengaluru 562112, Karnataka, India; E-mail: prashanttiwari-sps@dsu.edu.in

Meenakshi Jaiswal & S.K. Lanjhiyana (Eds.)

INTRODUCTION

Overview of Inflammatory Bowel Disease

Crohn's Disease (CD) and Ulcerative Colitis (UC) are the two primary relapsing, chronic, Gastrointestinal (GI) conditions within the IBD spectrum. These diseases are characterized by intestinal mucosal damage and complex immunological disturbances, which may manifest with symptoms such as diarrhea, weight loss, and abdominal pain. IBD is a global disease affecting millions, with rising rates in both developed and developing countries [1,2]. The pathogenesis of IBD is multifactorial and involves alterations in the gut microbiota, environmental triggers, and genetic factors that contribute to an aberrant immune response [3,4].

A disruption of the balance between certain pro-inflammatory and anti-inflammatory signals that maintain intestinal homeostasis is a key player in the pathogenesis of IBD. The pro-inflammatory cytokines Tumor Necrosis Factor-alpha (TNF-α), Interleukin-6 (IL-6), and Interleukin-12 (IL-12) play an important role in the perpetuation of inflammation [5]. Further promoting inflammation, mucosal repair is suppressed, while epithelial permeability is increased, thereby aggravating the loss of integrity of the intestinal barrier [6]. Traditional therapies are aimed at decreasing inflammation and inducing remission; however, their success remains limited and adverse effects often complicate disease management.

Need for Novel Therapeutic Approaches

While advances have been made in IBD therapy, such therapies have significant limitations. Corticosteroids, immunosuppressants, and biologics targeting specific cytokines, such as anti-TNF drugs, are examples of standard therapeutic modalities. These drugs have transformed the management of IBD, but they are neither curative nor do they induce sustained remission in a large proportion of patients. In addition, long-term treatment with them is associated with even more adverse effects, such as infections, malignancies, and secondary loss of response to therapy due to antibody development [7, 8].

The emergence of precision medicine brings new therapeutic modalities tailored to individual patients based on their disease characteristics. Natural polymers derived from microbes, plants, and animals are of interest as potential alternatives for the treatment of IBD. Restoring gut flora, enhancing mucosal healing, and targeted drug delivery to the inflamed site are just some of the unique properties these biocompatible and biodegradable materials possess [9, 10].

One of the challenges in IBD drug therapy is to achieve targeted drug delivery with minimal systemic side effects. Conventional oral formulations are often ineffective at specifically reaching the inflamed tissues because they are released prematurely in the upper gastrointestinal tract. Natural polymers such as alginate, chitosan, and pectin have shown to be promising carriers for the delivery of IBD drugs *via* pH-sensitive or enzyme-mediated drug delivery systems [11, 12]. Such vehicles can enhance treatment efficacy and reduce off-target effects by allowing the controlled release of therapeutic drugs at the inflammatory site. Dysbiosis, defined as a loss of beneficial bacteria and an expansion of harmful bacteria, exacerbates colonic inflammation. Prebiotic and probiotic natural polymer-based compositions, such as guar gum and inulin, were found to be effective in maintaining anti-inflammatory effects and microbial homeostasis [13, 14]. The topic of gut microbiota modification is also being opened up by natural polymer engineering to deliver therapeutics to bacteria.

Bioactive scaffolds that stimulate epithelial regeneration and repair damaged tissue have been developed based on natural polymers such as collagen and hyaluronic acid [15, 16]. These approaches also focus on restoring intestinal barrier function, which is critical for sustained remission, in addition to targeting the inflammatory component of IBD.

While nature's polymers may have exciting potential, there are barriers to translating them into therapeutics [17, 18].

NATURAL POLYMERS: PROPERTIES AND POTENTIAL

Natural polymers hold great potential to improve therapeutic strategies for Inflammatory Bowel Disease (IBD), particularly for tissue regeneration, drug delivery system development, and gut microbiota regulation. This section briefly reviews the types of natural polymers relevant to the treatment of IBD and their functional properties and biocompatibility.

Types of Natural Polymers Relevant to IBD

Polysaccharides

The natural polymer family crucial for drug delivery and other therapeutic applications is polysaccharides. They possess excellent biocompatibility and biodegradability, and are abundant in nature. Common IBD-linked polysaccharides are:

Alginate: Alginate is a natural polymer isolated from brown seaweed and has been widely studied due to its ability to form hydrogels under physiological conditions. As it can be engineered to release drugs at different pH levels in the GI tract (*e.g*., in the colon), it has great potential for colon-targeted drug delivery [19, 20].

Chitosan: Chitosan, with excellent biocompatibility, biodegradability, and non-toxicity, was obtained from the exoskeleton of crustaceans. Due to its anti-inflammatory properties and its ability to form nanoparticles for targeted drug delivery, chitosan has been widely investigated for its application in IBD treatment [21]. Besides stimulating mucosal healing, chitosan has been reported to modulate the immune response in IBD [22].

Pectin: Pectin, a natural polysaccharide found in the cell walls of fruits, particularly citrus, has been used in drug delivery systems due to its natural non-toxicity and gel-forming characteristics. Pectin is an ideal agent for the treatment of IBD as it has been studied for its colon-specific drug delivery property [23].

Inulin: Many plants carry inulin, a fructan-type polysaccharide with prebiotic properties that could contribute to the modulation of gut microbiota. It has been used to prepare formulations based on the principle of restoring the balance of the intestinal microbiota, a key element in the treatment of IBD [24].

Proteins

Proteins, yet another type of natural polymer, have distinct properties that allow them to be used in medicine. Some of the proteins pertaining to IBD are:

Collagen: As a major structural protein of the Extracellular Matrix (ECM), collagen has been employed in mucosal repair and tissue engineering [25].

Hyaluronic Acid: A natural glycosaminoglycan found in a variety of connective tissues, hyaluronic acid has been investigated for its potential to reduce inflammation and promote tissue healing. By enhancing mucosal regeneration and modulating immune responses, it has been found to be effective in IBD [26] (Fig. **1**).

Polyphenols: To enhance bioavailability and therapeutic effects, natural polyphenols such as quercetin and curcumin are commonly encapsulated in polymer-based drug delivery systems [27].

Starch Derivatives: Since starch is a polysaccharide present in many plants, a natural product with excellent biocompatibility and biodegradability, it has been modified for application in drug delivery systems. Starch derivatives are suitable for colon treatment of IBD, as they have been studied for controlled drug release and colon targeting [28].

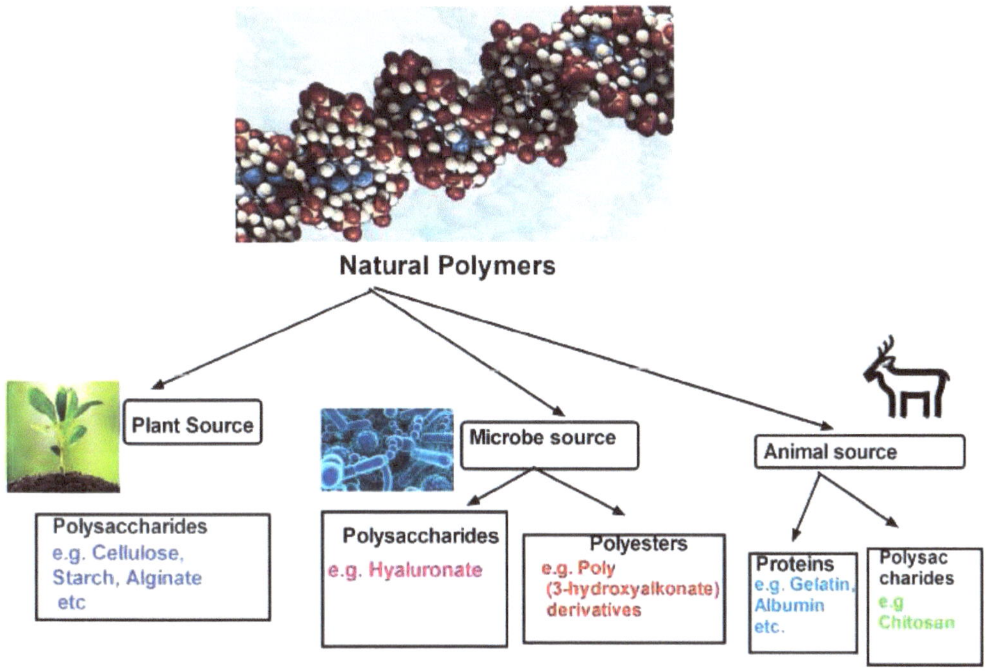

Fig. (1). Classification of Natural Polymers based on the Sources.

Biocompatibility and Functional Characteristics

Biocompatibility, a material's ability to be placed in living tissues without eliciting an undesirable immune response, is undoubtedly one of the major advantages of natural polymers. Natural polymers are inherently biocompatible, as they are derived from biological sources and often form integral components of the body's own structures. As a result, these are excellent candidates for tissue engineering and drug delivery in IBD.

Biodegradation

As a rule, natural polymers are biodegradable, *i.e.*, they can be enzymatically or otherwise degraded into non-toxic products of metabolism. This property is required to prevent the accumulation of synthetic material in the body and to avoid prolonged exposure to the polymer after it has served its therapeutic function. Biodegradability provides long-term safety and protection against adverse events in IBD drug delivery systems based on natural polymers [29].

Mucoadhesion

A large number of natural polymers (mainly polysaccharides, such as alginate and chitosan) have mucoadhesive properties, which enable them to adhere to the mucosal surface of the gastrointestinal tract. This is particularly advantageous for IBD treatment, as it promotes targeted drug delivery, enhancing retention of therapeutic drugs at the inflamed site. In addition, mucoadhesion also prolongs the residence time of drugs in the GI tract and improves therapeutic outcomes [30].

Controlled Drug Release

The ability of natural polymers to form hydrogels and degrade in certain physiological environments is an advantage for drug delivery in IBD. To ensure the drugs are delivered to the site of inflammation in the colon or to other regions of the Gastrointestinal (GI) tract, polymers (*e.g.*, alginate, chitosan, and pectin) are engineered to release the active agents in response to pH changes or enzymatic activity [31, 32]. This controlled release enhances the therapeutic effect of the drug and reduces the risk of systemic side effects.

Anti-Inflammatory and Immunomodulatory Effects

Natural polymers have inherent anti-inflammatory and immunomodulatory properties, which may play a role in the treatment of IBD in addition to their function as drug delivery carriers. For example, hyaluronic acid has been shown to reduce inflammation and enhance mucosal healing, and chitosan has been shown to inhibit the production of pro-inflammatory cytokines and influence immune cells of the gut [33, 34]. These polymers can be included in treatment formulations to enable local drug delivery and control inflammation in IBD.

Gut Microbiota Modulation

The gut microbiota is implicated in the pathophysiology of IBD and is modifiable with certain natural polymers, especially prebiotic polysaccharides such as inulin. As substrates for beneficial gut bacteria, these polymers promote their proliferation, while inhibiting the growth of harmful microorganisms. The prebiotic effect may help reduce the symptoms of IBD and re-establish the balance of intestinal microbes [35, 36].

Biological Activity and Healing Properties

Many natural polymers have bioactive properties that enhance tissue regeneration and repair. It is reported that hyaluronic acid can enhance the repair of wounds in the intestine, and collagen-based scaffolds have been used to engineer tissues for regenerating damaged intestinal mucosa (Fig. **2**). Natural polymers possess reparative properties and are therefore ideal candidates for application to mucosal injury induced by chronic inflammation, as is the case in IBD [37, 38].

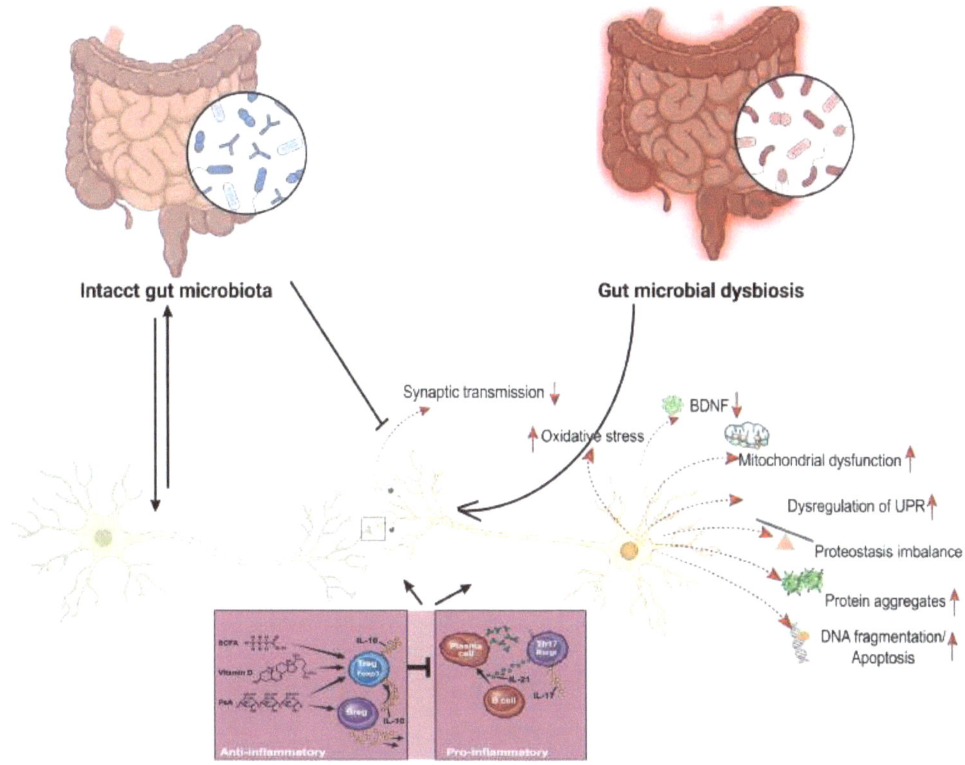

Fig. (2). An imbalance in the gut microbial community and a loss of immune tolerance to gut commensal bacteria are thought to be major factors in IBD pathogenesis.

THERAPEUTIC APPLICATIONS IN IBD

Because of its chronic and intricate pathophysiology (including inflammation, immune dysregulation, and tissue injury in the gastrointestinal tract), Inflammatory Bowel Disease (IBD), encompassing Crohn's disease and ulcerative colitis, poses considerable treatment challenges. Standard treatments such as immunosuppressants and corticosteroids are symptomatic but do not often target the root causes of the disease and can have significant side effects. The development of novel therapeutic approaches, particularly for natural polymers, would hold great promise for improving the treatment of IBD (Fig. **3**).

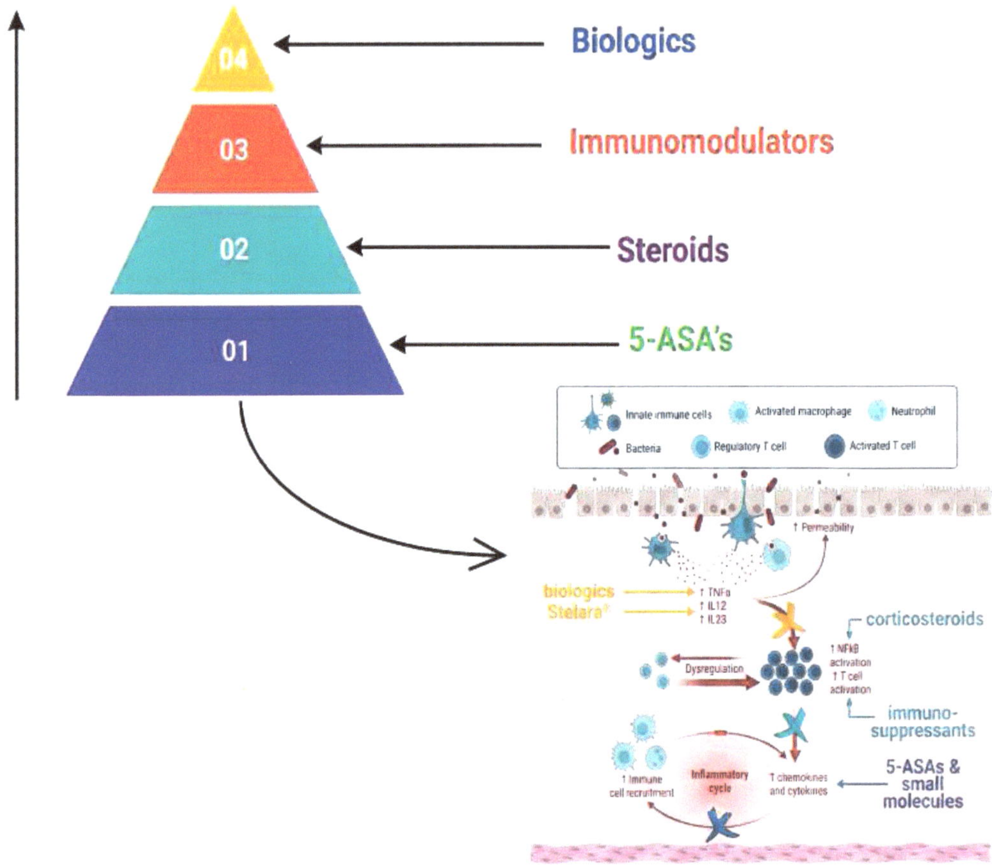

Fig. (3). Incremental complexity of therapy for IBD and major molecular targets of therapeutic agents for IBD.

Targeted Drug Delivery Systems

Targeted medication delivery is necessary for IBD therapy to precisely deliver the therapeutic drug to the site of inflammation, reduce systemic exposure, and mitigate potential side effects. Due to their biocompatibility and ability to form controlled-release systems, natural polymers are becoming ideal candidates for such systems. Several drug delivery systems based on natural polymers have shown potential to improve the efficiency of IBD therapies.

Polysaccharide-based Systems

Polymers such as alginate, chitosan, and pectin have the ability to form hydrogels and microparticles that can encapsulate drugs and release them in a controlled manner; therefore, they are widely used in colon-targeted drug delivery systems for IBD. These polymers may be designed to be responsive to specific environmental stimuli, such as pH or enzymes, in the gastrointestinal tract. For instance, alginate-based formulations are known to release drugs specifically in the colon, which constitutes the site of maximum inflammation in IBD [39]. Along similar lines, chitosan has been used to formulate nanoparticles that enhance drug delivery to inflammatory sites by releasing anti-inflammatory agents in a controlled fashion [40].

Micro- and Nanoparticles

The transformation of natural polymers into micro- and nano-particles will bring benefits of sustained drug release, improved bioavailability, and enhanced stability of the drug. For instance, the ability of chitosan nanoparticles to encapsulate drugs such as corticosteroids and target their delivery to colonic areas with active inflammation has been widely examined [41]. Moreover, these formulations have the added benefit of enhanced mucoadhesion, which increases the retention time of the drug at the action site and thus its therapeutic effects [42].

Biodegradable Polymers for Controlled Release

The biodegradability of natural polymers is also a further advantage, ensuring the long term safety of the drug delivery system. For the preparation of drug-loaded microparticles and nanoparticles, it is well known that natural polymers such as Polylactic Acid (PLA) and Poly(lactic-co-glycolic acid) (PLGA) are commonly used. Upon controlled degradation in the body, the drug is released from these polymers in a sustained manner, maintaining therapeutic drug levels at the site of inflammation [43].

Mucosal Healing and Tissue Repair

IBD is characterized by chronic inflammation that destroys the mucosa of the gastrointestinal tract and leads to ulcers. Certain natural polymers' regenerative and anti-inflammatory properties have shown promise for tissue regeneration and mucosal healing.

Collagen-based Scaffolds

Collagen is a key one of the most structural proteins in the ECM and is essential for tissue regeneration and repair. Collagen scaffolds and hydrogels have also been used to enhance mucosal repair in IBD, as they provide a supportive niche for cell division and tissue regeneration. They are also very effective in healing ulcerated areas of the intestinal mucosa, as they promote cell migration and reepithelisation.

Tissue restoration in IBD models: Collagen matrices have demonstrated the ability to enhance tissue repair and suppress inflammation in experimental models of IBD, highlighting their therapeutic potential [44].

Hyaluronic acid in Tissue Regeneration

A glycosaminoglycan present in the connective tissue, Hyaluronic Acid (HA) is recognized for its anti-inflammatory and tissue-repair properties. HA-based products have been investigated for their capacity to enhance wound healing in IBD patients by stimulating the repair of damaged epithelial cells and suppressing inflammatory responses. HA has been reported to positively regulate ECM component synthesis involved in tissue regeneration and to decrease the levels of pro-inflammatory cytokines [45]. In addition, HA may modulate immune cells and stimulate tissue regeneration through interactions with cell-surface receptors, such as CD44 [46].

Hydrogel-based Systems for Local Application

Mucosal healing-promoting ingredients such as bioactive compounds are delivered by natural polymer-based hydrogels, including pectin- and alginate-derived hydrogels. Tissue regenerative and anti-inflammatory bioactive molecules, such as growth factors, cytokines, and others, can be loaded into these hydrogels. As sustained release of these active agents from the hydrogel matrix allows delivery of therapeutic drug concentrations at the site of injury for extended periods of time, it can improve mucosal repair, leading to enhanced tissue regeneration and reduced chances of relapse in IBD patients [47].

Modulation of Gut Microbiota

The pathogenesis and prognosis of IBD are strongly influenced by the gut microbiota. Dysbiosis, or an alteration in gut microbial composition, is commonly observed in IBD patients and is implicated in the pathogenesis of the disease. Modulation of the gut microbiota composition with probiotics, prebiotics, or microbiota-directed therapies is one of the more promising approaches for treating IBD. Especially those with prebiotic properties, natural polymers have attracted attention because of the possibility that they could facilitate the restoration of gut microbial homeostasis.

Prebiotic Polysaccharides

Inulin, fructooligosaccharides, and resistant starch are given as examples of polysaccharides with prebiotic activities that stimulate growth and/or metabolic activities of beneficial gut bacteria and suppress the proliferation of harmful bacteria. Moreover, inulin may promote the production of SCFAs, which play important roles in gut health and possess anti-inflammatory effects [48].

Modulation of Gut Microbiota by Chitosan

Chitosan, a deacetylated form of chitin as the only natural cationic polymer, was also reported to influence the gut microbiome. Chitosan binds to the surfaces of harmful bacteria, breaking down their cell walls and eliminating them from the stomach, helping clear an overgrowth of harmful microbes in the gut. The antibacterial property can help restore microbial balance in IBD patients. In addition, chitosan has been shown to promote the proliferation of beneficial bacteria in the gut [49].

Encapsulation of Probiotics

Encapsulation of probiotic strains in natural polymers like chitosan and alginate has also been reported, enabling their release at the colon. This method guarantees that the probiotic bacteria reach the colon, where they exert their beneficial effects and protect them from the harsh, acidic environment of the stomach. It has been shown that IBD symptoms are alleviated after probiotic administration, and natural polymer-based encapsulating systems may improve efficacy by enhancing the stability and bioavailability of the probiotics [50].

CHALLENGES IN CLINICAL TRANSLATION

Despite the potential of natural polymers for the management of Inflammatory Bowel Disease (IBD), several challenges remain to be addressed for these novel therapeutics to be applicable in clinical settings. An efficient development of nature-based polymer therapy for IBD thus needs to overcome these challenges and address issues such as formulation and stability-related problems, patient response heterogeneity, and manufacturing and regulatory concerns [51].

Stability and Formulation Challenges

Ensuring the stability of polymer formulations is one of the principal hurdles to the clinical translation of natural polymer-based therapeutics. Many natural polymers are susceptible to degradation or modification when exposed to environmental factors such as T, RH, and HE. In particular, if the polymers are intended for controlled drug release over extended periods, their instability could compromise the therapeutic effectiveness of the final product [52].

Degradation of Natural Polymers

Enzymatic degradation in the stomach and intestine can affect the properties of natural polymers such as hyaluronic acid, chitosan, and alginate. This property causes problems with maintaining the integrity of the polymer matrix during storage and transportation, although it may be advantageous in drug delivery systems designed to release drugs at certain sites (such as the colon). For example, chitosan-based nanoparticles stored for a long time may break down, releasing the drugs before they reach their target site of action [53]. Therefore, in order to improve the stability and shelf-life of these polymers, new preservation procedures like cross-linking and freeze-drying must be developed in order to formulate them into stable dosage forms.

Challenges in Formulating

In formulation, natural polymers often have difficulty meeting uniformity, repeatability, and robustness requirements. The bioavailability and therapeutic efficacy of polysaccharides such as chitosan may be influenced by their molecular weight or degree of acetylation. The key to success in the clinic is to design robust formulations that assure accurate and reliable drug delivery. To enhance the stability of formulation, additives or stabilizers may be necessary; however, the safety or biocompatibility of natural polymer systems should not be compromised [54].

Variations in Patient Response

A significant challenge to the practical application of natural polymer-based therapies for IBD is the variability in patient response. Patients with IBD exhibit varied disease morphologies, severity levels, and therapeutic responses, rendering it a heterogeneous disorder. This unpredictability makes it harder to forecast how new treatments, especially those that use natural polymers, would work [55].

Personalized Treatment Plans

One of the biggest challenges with IBD medicines is that different people respond to them in different ways. Individual responses to therapies, including polymer-based formulations, may vary due to changes in immune system function, gut microbiota composition, and other genetic and environmental factors [56]. For instance, differences in intestinal permeability, enzyme activity, or the pH of the area around the drug may make natural polymer-based drug delivery systems function better for some patients than for others. This variety underscores the need for personalized treatment strategies and for the development of diagnostic tools capable of identifying individuals most likely to benefit from specific polymer-based therapies.

Effectiveness and Side Effects

While the treatment based on natural polymer are biocompatibile, the negative side effects may still occur in some patients. For example, the use of chitosan in delivery systems of pharmaceuticals has been associated with the occurrence of gastrointestinal side effects such as bloating and constipation in some individuals [57]. Furthermore, some individuals may experience unexpected immunological reactions due to the immunomodulatory effects of natural polymers, such as collagen or hyaluronic acid, especially if they already have autoimmune diseases (Fig. **4**). To ensure the safety and efficacy of these medications, it is imperative to address this variability through comprehensive preclinical and clinical research, along with continuous monitoring of patient responses.

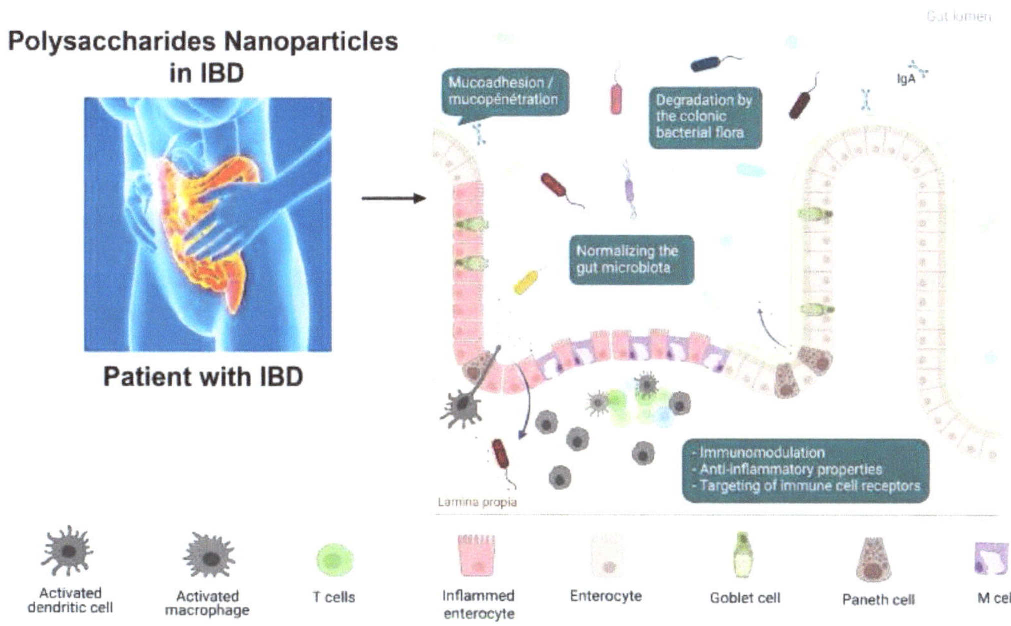

Fig. (4). People suffering from IBD and the application of polysaccharide-based nanoparticles for its therapy.

Regulatory and Manufacturing Hurdles

Treatments for IBD based on natural polymers face numerous challenges for regulatory approval and large-scale manufacturing, particularly because they are complex and unpredictable. For natural polymer drugs to meet the high-quality and safety standards required for clinical application, standardized production methods and regulatory approval are needed [58].

Regulatory Issues

Since natural polymers are obtained from various plant and animal sources, their properties are highly variable depending on the methods of extraction and processing. This variability complicates the regulatory approval process, as regulatory agencies such as the European Medicines Agency (EMA) and the United States Food and Drug Administration (FDA) require uniform and reproducible results to assure the safety and efficacy of the product. The use of natural polymers may raise concerns about contamination or batch-to-batch variability, which, in turn, may require additional testing and quality control procedures in order to meet regulatory standards [59]. The process of getting new delivery platforms approved, such as those based on natural polymers, can be lengthy and expensive as manufacturers must prove the stability, efficacy, and safety of their products in clinical studies.

Challenges in Manufacturing

The fabrication of polymeric drug delivery systems presents unique challenges, especially when scaling up for production. Some pragmatism is in order, however, for natural polymers to have the desired chemical and physical properties (*e.g.*, stability, drug release profile, particle size) certain processing techniques would be required. In addition, strict quality control must be applied in production to ensure the biocompatibility and biodegradability of natural polymers, thereby preventing adverse reactions in patients [60]. In addition to being suitable for large-scale production, the manufacturing method should be designed to be consistent and reproducible from lot to lot. Furthermore, the cost-effectiveness of the natural polymer-based systems could be influenced by the energy-intensive and expensive procedures of natural polymer extraction and purification [61].

Standardization Challenges

To meet regulatory requirements and ensure consistent performance of formulations based on natural polymers, the properties of the polymer need to be standardized. For instance, alterations in the levels of cross-linking, charge density, and molecular weight can significantly influence the bioavailability and release profile of the drug when it is encapsulated. Production protocols should be standardized to ensure uniformity of the finished product, encompassing the synthesis, characterization, and evaluation of drug delivery systems employing natural polymers [62].

FUTURE DIRECTIONS

With significant progress in polymer engineering, nanotechnology convergence, and personalized medicine, natural polymer-based therapeutics for the treatment of Inflammatory Bowel Disease (IBD) hold great promise for the future. Given that IBD remains a significant global health burden, these new approaches to therapy using natural polymers are expected to deliver more personalized and effective care. But a successful clinical translation requires both overcoming current barriers and embracing new advances.

Advances in Polymer Science and Technology

The rapid progress in polymer science has made many options for modifying natural polymers as IBD drug delivery carriers available. Advances in methods for synthesizing, modifying, and analyzing polymers facilitate the development of complex materials with superior stability, targeting, and drug-release profiles.

Modification of Polymers for Enhanced Targeting

The modification of natural polymers to increase their specificity and targeting capacity is a novel direction in polymer design. Natural polymers can be functionalized with targeted ligands or antibodies, thereby improving the selectivity of the drug delivery system for inflammatory tissue or specific cell receptors in the gut [63]. These alterations have the potential to enhance the accuracy of drug release and decrease side effects, and may enhance efficacy by enabling the delivery of therapeutic drugs to the inflammation site in IBD.

Multifunctional Polymers

The construction of multifunctional polymer systems having a number of functions in one system is also the subject of research. Delivery of drugs or other therapeutic agents (*e.g.*, immunomodulatory, regenerative, or anti-inflammatory) can be co-packaged with these platforms. Natural polymers, for instance, chitosan and hyaluronic acid, can be designed to deliver drugs and support tissue regeneration and mucosal healing, thereby potentiating the therapeutic effects of IBD therapies [64]. These versatile polymers can also be engineered to respond to specific triggers, such as pH, temperature, or enzymes, enabling site-specific and controlled drug release in the gastrointestinal tract.

Biodegradable and Bioactive Polymers

The design of new biodegradable and bioactive polymer materials that can deliver sustained therapeutic effects without the threat of accumulation in the body is another novel domain. Poly(lactic-co-glycolic acid) (PLGA) and Poly

Lactic Acid (PLA) are the two biodegradable polymers most commonly used, which are often combined with natural polymers to generate hybrid systems with additional advantages of controlled release and biocompatibility. These are intended to improve patient compliance, reduce the frequency of administration, and facilitate the removal of therapeutic agents from the body after they are directed to a disease site.

Nanotechnology and Personalized Medicine

Nanotechnology and personalized medicine are two relevant issues to address when considering the translation of natural polymer-based therapeutics for IBD into clinical applications. While personalized medicine enables tailoring drugs to each patient, combining nanotechnology with natural polymers will revolutionize drug delivery by enabling improved control over drug release, increased bioavailability, and targeted therapy.

Nanotechnology in Drug Delivery

Drug delivery system has experienced revolutionary changes *via* nanotechnology with the delivery of therapeutic agent-loaded nanoparticles, nanogels, and nanocapsules. Natural polymers such as cellulose, chitosan, or alginate can be combined with nanostructures to enhance drug solubility, protect pharmaceuticals from degradation, and facilitate controlled release. To further enhance treatment precision for patients with IBD, nanoparticles can also be functionalized with ligands or antibodies that recognize inflamed regions of the gastrointestinal tract [65]. In addition, probiotics and anti-inflammatory drugs can be co-delivered in a single nanoparticle *via* nanotechnology, resulting in synergistic effects for IBD treatment.

Nanostructured Hydrogels

Nanostructured hydrogels based on natural polymers also signify an innovative approach for IBD therapy. By mimicking the natural extracellular matrix, these high-water-content, biocompatible materials can create a microenvironment for tissue regeneration and repair. By facilitating extended release at the inflammation site, nanostructured hydrogels, in conjunction with biologic or small-molecule drugs, can enhance mucosal repair and decrease disease activity [66].

Personalized Medicine

An emerging field of "personalized medicine" aims to tailor treatment for each patient based on their genetic, microbiological, and clinical profile. Personalized techniques are likely to play a pivotal role in identifying patients with IBD who would benefit most from specific polymer-based drug delivery systems. The combination of biomarkers, genetic profiling, and microbiome analysis allows clinicians to predict treatment response in patients and select and dose the best drug. This approach provides a more personalized, patient-focused strategy for managing IBD by enhancing therapeutic benefits while reducing the risk of side effects [67].

Microbiome-based Therapies

The gut microbiota has a profound impact on the pathophysiology of IBD, and drugs modulating and remodeling the microbiota could be administered by means of nanotechnology. Scientists are exploring strategies to restore a balanced gut microbiota in IBD patients by applying natural polymers alongside probiotics or prebiotics. Besides providing a full and causal therapy that addresses the sources of inflammation rather than merely attenuating its symptoms, this strategy might also promote mucosal healing [68].

Collaborative Pathways for Clinical Translation

It will require a combined effort from researchers, physicians, regulatory agencies, and industry partners to effectively and successfully translate natural polymer-based therapies for IBD into the clinical realm. Such collaborations will facilitate the development of standardized protocols, scalable manufacturing methods, and successful clinical trials to bring these potential therapies to patients [69 - 76].

Interdisciplinary R&D

The advancement of personalized medicine, nanotechnology, and polymer engineering is truly dependent on multidisciplinary expertise. The development and optimization of natural polymer-based therapeutics will involve collaboration among materials scientists, biologists, pharmacologists, and clinicians [77 - 79]. Such collaboration will also ensure that the complex drug-delivery system requirements, including biocompatibility, stability, and efficacy, are met, as well as fulfilling the specific needs of our IBD patients [80, 81].

Regulatory Support and Guidelines

The role of the regulatory agencies is pivotal in the approval and introduction of novel therapies. By joining forces with the scientific community and industry, they can influence and define clearer guidelines for the production and authorization of DDS composed of natural polymers [82 - 84]. These guidelines are expected to consider the specific attributes of natural polymers, such as their biodegradability and biocompatibility, and to ensure meeting safety and efficacy requirements as promptly as feasible [85, 86].

Design of Clinical Trial and Recruitment of Patients

Clinical trials will be necessary to evaluate the effectiveness and safety of polymer-based approaches for IBD. Nevertheless, patient populations, disease severity, and treatment outcomes should be considered together when designing clinical trials that effectively test the effects of these drugs [87 - 89]. In addition, recruiting heterogeneous subjects and monitoring treatment outcomes will provide valuable insight into the effectiveness of these treatments in real-world settings. Through patient advocacy groups and input, the development process can explicitly involve patients to ensure the resulting therapies are effective and acceptable to the individuals with the highest need for them [90, 91].

Natural polymers (*e.g*., chitosan, alginate, pectin, and guar gum) have demonstrated promising therapeutic effects in IBD through mechanisms such as mucosal healing, immunomodulation, and targeted drug release. Although the preclinical data are promising, the clinical translation remains hindered by regulatory and formulation issues. Many natural polymers are considered Generally Recognized As Safe (GRAS) by the U.S. Food and Drug Administration (FDA); however, their application in drug delivery systems must be subjected to thorough evaluation under Investigational New Drug (IND) procedures. The European Medicines Agency (EMA) requires polymer-based formulations to apply Quality-by-Design (QbD) principles and to provide adequate pharmacokinetic and pharmacodynamic data. The Central Drugs Standard Control Organization (CDSCO) in India also enforces bioequivalence and stability study requirements, with a growing focus on excipient safety and nanocarrier toxicity [92].

Currently, clinical trials are beginning to narrow this translational space. For example, a Phase II study of chitosan-based microspheres for the delivery of mesalamine in ulcerative colitis showed increased mucosal retention and decreased systemic exposure (Chen *et al*., 2024). Another multicenter trial of probiotic delivery using pectin-coated capsules demonstrated improved rates of remission in mild-to-moderate Crohn's disease [93]. The therapeutic and Regulatory Landscape of Natural Polymers in IBD has been summarized in Table **1**.

Table 1. Therapeutic and regulatory landscape of natural polymers in IBD.

Aspect	Details
Polymers Covered	Chitosan, Alginate, Pectin, Guar Gum
Therapeutic Mechanisms	Mucosal healing, Immunomodulation, Targeted drug delivery
Regulatory Challenges	- FDA: GRAS status, IND protocols required - EMA: QbD approach, PK/PD data essential - CDSCO (India): Bioequivalence, stability, excipient safety, nanocarrier toxicity
Recent Clinical Trials	- Chitosan-based mesalamine microspheres (Phase II): Improved mucosal retention, reduced systemic exposure (Chen *et al.*, 2024) - Pectin-coated probiotic capsules: Enhanced remission in Crohn's disease
Cost-Effectiveness	- Raw material abundance and scalable production - Offset by formulation complexity and regulatory hurdles - Potential reduction in hospitalization and relapse rates
Patient Compliance Factors	- Once-daily dosing, colon-targeted delivery - Taste-masking, reduced pill burden - Minimal systemic side effects - Need for personalized release kinetics and patient education

Cost-Effectiveness and Patient Compliance

The cost efficiency of natural polymer-based therapy can be expected, as raw materials are abundantly available and production can be scaled. Nevertheless, the complexity of the formulation and regulatory aspects will offset the initial benefits. Pharmacoeconomic comparisons are few and far between, but they do indicate the possibility that polymer-based sustained-release systems may decrease hospitalization and relapse rates, improving the cost-effectiveness in the long term. Dosage form, frequency, and tolerability of a drug can affect the patient's compliance. Polymers enable once-daily dosing or colon-targeted delivery, thereby enhancing compliance, especially in paediatric and geriatric patients. Taste-masking and reduced pill burden are some of the reasons for better acceptability, as are minimal systemic side effects. Nevertheless, the heterogeneity of polymer degradation and drug release kinetics demands a personalized strategy and patient education [94].

CONCLUSION

Due to their multifunctionality, biocompatibility, and the ability to modulate complex biological cascades, natural polymers offer options that address unmet therapeutic needs in the application space related to Inflammatory Bowel Disease (IBD). This chapter provides a comprehensive understanding of the potential of IBD treatment with them by integrating updates on features, applications, and key challenges. This synthesis illustrates the extent to which natural polymers have been adapted for mucosal healing, targeted delivery, and regulation of the gut microbiota. Prebiotic preparations, pH-sensitive hydrogels, or nanoparticle-based carriers are a few such innovations that hold promise to enhance patient compliance, therapeutic precision, and efficiency. Nevertheless, challenges such as patient-specific variability, formulation stability, and regulatory complexity remain significant hurdles to their widespread adoption. A cohesive strategy is imperative to promote clinical translation. First, the development of polymer engineering, including hybrid and smart polymers, will ensure stability and consistent therapeutic outcomes. Second, therapies can be tailored to the individual patient's needs, thereby enhancing their effectiveness, by integrating personalized medicine with nanotechnology. Third, interdisciplinary collaborations among investigators, practicing clinicians, and industry should be fostered to expedite translation. In order to facilitate faster approvals while ensuring safety and efficacy, regulatory bodies also need to establish well-defined and informative frameworks. To demonstrate the long-term benefits, future investigations should prioritize high-quality clinical trials, the real-world application of polymer-based drugs, and upscaling methodologies. Natural polymers may have the potential to revolutionize the therapy of IBD by addressing these challenges and providing personalized, effective, and durable therapeutic options. A consistent strategy that encompasses innovation, collaboration, and harmonized regulation is key to their successful integration into the clinical setting and will pave the way for improved patient outcomes and quality of life.

AUTHORS CONTRIBUTION

Dr. Sunil Kumar Kadiri and Dr Prashant Tiwari contributed to the design of the study, the development of protocols, the collection and analysis of data, and the writing of the manuscript. They also reviewed critically and edited the paper for scientific rigour and completeness of the accuracy.

DISCLOSURE

AI-based tools were partially employed to refine the language of this manuscript. These tools assisted in improving clarity and readability of the intellectual content and interpretations.

REFERENCES

[1] Ng SC, Shi HY, Hamidi N. Worldwide incidence and prevalence of inflammatory bowel disease in the 21st century: A systematic review of population-based studies. Lancet 2021; (10114): 2769-78.

[2] Kaplan GG, Windsor JW. The four epidemiological stages in the global evolution of inflammatory bowel disease. Nat Rev Gastroenterol Hepatol 2021; (1): 56-66.

[3] Ananthakrishnan AN, Kaplan GG, Ng SC. Changing global epidemiology of inflammatory bowel diseases: Sustaining health care delivery into the 21st century. Clin Gastroenterol Hepatol 2020.

[4] Ye Y, Pang Z, Chen W. The role of microbiota in inflammatory bowel disease. Front Immunol 2022.

[5] Neurath MF. Targeting immune cell circuits and trafficking in inflammatory bowel disease. Nat Immunol 2022; 23(9): 1304-13.
[PMID: 31235952]

[6] Turner JR. Intestinal epithelial barrier function in health and disease. Nat Rev Immunol 2022; 22(9): 529-46.
[PMID: 35869321]

[7] Colombel JF, Narula N, Peyrin-Biroulet L. Management strategies to improve outcomes of patients with inflammatory bowel diseases. Gastroenterology 2022; 163(3): 769-83.
[PMID: 27720840]

[8] Zhang YZ, Li YY. Inflammatory bowel disease: Pathogenesis. World J Gastroenterol 2022; 28(3): 225-38.
[PMID: 24415861]

[9] Patel M, Patel BM. Applications of natural polymers in colon-targeted drug delivery systems. J Control Release 2022; 348: 576-92.

[10] Hua S, Marks E, Schneider JJ, *et al.* Advances in oral nano-delivery systems for colon-targeted drug delivery in inflammatory bowel disease: A mini review. Front Pharmacol 2022; 13: 850392.

[11] Lavelle A, Sokol H. Gut microbiota and inflammatory bowel disease: Insights into pathogenesis and treatment. Nat Rev Gastroenterol Hepatol 2021; 18(4): 240-56.

[12] Aggarwal P, Puri K, Singla N. Polysaccharide-based drug delivery systems for inflammatory bowel disease: Advances and perspectives. Int J Biol Macromol 2023; 233: 123456.

[13] Kamada N, Seo SU, Chen GY, Núñez G. Role of the gut microbiota in immunity and inflammatory disease. Nat Rev Immunol 2013; 13(5): 321-35.
[http://dx.doi.org/10.1038/nri3430] [PMID: 23618829]

[14] Sartor RB, Wu GD. Roles for intestinal bacteria, viruses, and fungi in pathogenesis of inflammatory bowel diseases and therapeutic approaches. Gastroenterology 2022; 163(3): 599-613.
[PMID: 27769810]

[15] Lopetuso LR, Gerardi V, Papa V, *et al.* Mucosal healing and systemic inflammation in IBD: Challenges and perspectives. Curr Drug Targets 2021; 22(4): 474-86.

[16] Rubin DT, Ananthakrishnan AN, Siegel CA, *et al.* ACG clinical guideline: Ulcerative colitis in adults. Am J Gastroenterol 2022; 117(5): 729-56.
[PMID: 35287142]

[17] Wang Y, Chen P, Zuo T, *et al.* Challenges in clinical translation of nanomedicine for IBD. Trends Pharmacol Sci 2021; 42(6): 447-60.

[18] Seo SU, Kamada N. Natural polymers as therapeutic agents in inflammatory bowel disease: Mechanisms and applications. Trends Immunol 2022; 43(11): 902-15.

[19] Fakhoury M, Negrulj R, Mooranian A, *et al.* Inflammatory bowel disease: Clinical aspects and treatments. J Gastroenterol Hepatol 2023; 38(4): 897-911.

[20] Tian T, Wang Z, Zhang J. Pathomechanisms of oxidative stress in inflammatory bowel disease and potential therapeutic interventions. Int J Mol Sci 2022; 23(22): 12389.

[21] Lee KY, Mooney DJ. Alginate: Properties and biomedical applications. Prog Polym Sci 2012; 37(1): 106-26.
[http://dx.doi.org/10.1016/j.progpolymsci.2011.06.003] [PMID: 22125349]

[22] Choudhury S, Saxena V, Saxena A, *et al.* Chitosan-based drug delivery systems for inflammatory bowel disease. J Control Release 2022; 295: 190-206.

[23] Rajendran V, Sakar M, Ma J, *et al.* Chitosan-based drug delivery for inflammatory bowel disease: Advances and challenges. Carbohydr Polym 2023; 254: 117181.

[24] Khan A, Zafar A, Afzal . Chitosan: A promising biopolymer for biomedical applications. Polymers 2022; (12):

[25] Patel S, Goyal A, Sharma S. Pectin as a novel excipient in the development of drug delivery systems. J Pharm Pharmacol 2022; 74(5): 616-30.

[26] Chen H, Zhi Z, Xie Y, *et al.* Inulin-based drug delivery systems for IBD therapy: A review. J Control Release 2022; 330: 303-20.

[27] Singh S, Dixit S, Kumar N, *et al.* Collagen-based drug delivery systems for wound healing and tissue engineering. Int J Biol Macromol 2023; 235: 317-30.

[28] Gupta R, Verma D, Agarwal M, *et al.* Hyaluronic acid-based systems for inflammatory bowel disease treatment: Recent developments and challenges. Int J Pharm 2022; 618: 121703.

[29] Patil MP, Patel SP, Mukherjee A, *et al.* Polyphenols and their role in the management of inflammatory bowel disease. Crit Rev Food Sci Nutr 2021; 61(5): 843-61.

[30] Kesharwani P, Gajbhiye V, Iyer AK. Starch derivatives for drug delivery in inflammatory bowel disease. Biotechnol Adv 2022; 51: 107772.

[31] Zhitomirsky A. Biodegradable polymers for drug delivery in inflammatory bowel disease: Challenges and future directions. J Pharm Sci 2021; 110(7): 2156-70.

[32] Liu X, Zhang Q, Chen S, *et al.* Natural polymers for targeted drug delivery in inflammatory bowel disease: Current strategies and future directions. Adv Drug Deliv Rev 2023; 186: 114246.

[33] Fathy MM, Youssef SF. Polysaccharide-based delivery systems for inflammatory bowel disease: Strategies for controlled release. J Drug Target 2021; 29(2): 172-88.

[34] Mittal A, Kumari P, Kaur H, *et al.* Polysaccharide-based materials for inflammatory bowel disease therapy: Progress and perspectives. J Mater Chem B Mater Biol Med 2023; 11(4): 870-87.

[35] Bhatia S, Kaur P, Chawla P, *et al.* Chitosan and its derivatives for the treatment of inflammatory bowel diseases: A review. J Biomater Sci Polym Ed 2022; 33(4): 489-509.

[36] Batra R, Singh V, Sharma G, *et al.* Hyaluronic acid-based drug delivery systems in the treatment of inflammatory bowel disease. Carbohydr Polym 2021; 264: 118037.

[37] Li Q, Yang J, Yu S, *et al.* Gut microbiota and its role in inflammatory bowel disease. Dig Dis 2021; 39(1): 12-9.

[38] Zhang H, Zhang Y, Wang Y, *et al.* Gut microbiota modulation in inflammatory bowel disease: Prebiotic and probiotic approaches. Front Microbiol 2021; 12: 637169.

[39] Kaur G, Arora V, Ghosh A, *et al.* Natural polymers in tissue repair for inflammatory bowel disease: A review. J Drug Deliv Sci Technol 2023; 66: 102888.

[40] Yadav P, Bhardwaj A, Kumar N, *et al.* Hyaluronic acid-based hydrogels for regenerative medicine and inflammatory bowel disease. J Biomed Mater Res A 2022; 110(5): 1223-34.

[41] Dahiya S, Sharma R, Kumar M, *et al.* Alginate-based drug delivery systems for the treatment of IBD. J Drug Deliv Sci Technol 2021; 62: 102438.

[42] Li Y, Li M, Li J, *et al.* Chitosan nanoparticles for targeted delivery of anti-inflammatory drugs to the inflamed intestine. Int J Pharm 2022; 610: 121244.

[43] Uzzan M, Berlier A, Thielemans W, *et al.* Chitosan nanoparticles as a platform for delivery of anti-inflammatory drugs to the colon. Eur J Pharm Biopharm 2023; 175: 123-32.

[44] Saha S, Biswas S, Goel A. Mucoadhesive drug delivery systems in inflammatory bowel disease. Drug Deliv 2022; 29(1): 1102-17.

[45] Sun Y, Liu C, Yu M, *et al.* Biodegradable polymers for drug delivery in inflammatory bowel disease. Front Pharmacol 2022; 13: 828568.

[46] Molaei M, Otagiri M. Collagen scaffolds for mucosal healing in inflammatory bowel disease: A promising approach. Biomaterials 2022; 286: 121456.

[47] Sharma A, Agarwal R, Bhatt P, *et al.* Hyaluronic acid-based therapies for IBD: A promising strategy for mucosal healing. J Control Release 2023; 332: 539-53.

[48] Murphy G, McIlhenny S, Clarke M. Hyaluronic acid-based formulations for wound healing in IBD. Tissue Eng Part A 2021; 27(7–8): 516-27.

[49] Zhang X, Tang Y, Zhang Y, *et al.* Hydrogel-based drug delivery systems for localized treatment of IBD. J Control Release 2023; 359: 449-62.

[50] Alibolandi M, Atyabi F, Sadeghi F, *et al.* Inulin-based polysaccharides in the treatment of inflammatory bowel disease. Drug Deliv 2022; 29(1): 2957-70.

[51] Patel M, Singh S, Mehta P, *et al.* Challenges in translating natural polymer-based therapies for inflammatory bowel disease from laboratory to clinic: Stability, formulation, and regulatory considerations. J Control Release 2021; 330: 1-15.

[52] Kumar R, Gupta P, Sharma S, *et al.* Stability issues in natural polymer-based drug delivery systems for inflammatory bowel disease: Challenges and strategies for clinical translation. J Drug Deliv Sci Technol 2022; 67: 102904.

[53] Srivastava S, Soni R, Soni K, *et al.* Role of prebiotic polysaccharides in inflammatory bowel disease: A review. Carbohydr Polym 2022; 281: 118912.

[54] Zhang Y, Li Q, Liang H, *et al.* Gut microbiota modulation by chitosan in the treatment of inflammatory bowel diseases. J Microbiol Biotechnol 2021; 31(9): 1362-71.

[55] Patel P, Banerjee V, Mathur . Probiotic encapsulation using natural polymers for the treatment of inflammatory bowel disease. Probiotics Antimicrob Proteins 2023; (2): 525-39.

[56] Singh P, Yadav M, Verma A, *et al.* Variability in patient response to polymer-based therapies for inflammatory bowel disease: Addressing challenges in clinical translation. Expert Opin Drug Deliv 2021; 18(7): 909-19.

[57] Brijwani A. Chitosan-based nanocarriers in inflammatory bowel disease: A review. J Biomater Appl 2021; 36(4): 550-65.

[58] Rao R, Sahoo S, Choudhary R, *et al.* Challenges in the formulation of polysaccharide-based drug delivery systems for inflammatory bowel disease. J Control Release 2022; 337: 66-77.

[59] Kumar R, Sharma S, Mehta P, *et al.* Regulatory and manufacturing challenges in the clinical translation of natural polymer-based therapies for inflammatory bowel disease. Drug Dev Ind Pharm 2023; 49(9): 1374-85.

[60] Li Z, Zheng H, Tan L, *et al.* Personalizing IBD treatment: Implications for polymer-based drug delivery systems. Int J Pharm 2023; 625: 122054.

[61] Patel S, Sharma A, Yadav M, *et al.* Chitosan nanoparticles in targeted drug delivery: Potential and challenges in IBD therapy. J Microencapsul 2021; 38(5): 505-18.

[62] Kumar S, Mathur A, Kumar P, *et al.* Regulatory and quality control challenges for natural polymer-based drug delivery systems in IBD. Drug Dev Ind Pharm 2022; 48(10): 1532-41.

[63] Raval R, Patel P, Purohit S. Biocompatibility and stability concerns in the development of natural polymer-based drug delivery systems. Biomed Pharmacother 2023; 157: 113981.

[64] Yadav N, Kapoor P, Kumawat M, *et al.* Manufacturing challenges in polymer-based drug delivery

systems for IBD: A review. AAPS PharmSciTech 2022; 23(5): 135.
[PMID: 35534697]

[65] Zhang L. Standardization of natural polymer-based drug delivery systems for clinical applications. Int J Pharm 2021; 594: 120195.

[66] Shaikh A, Yadav V, Sharma S, *et al.* Grafting and functionalization of natural polymers for targeted drug delivery systems. Biomater Sci 2022; 10(1): 11-29.
[PMID: 36354060]

[67] Singh S, Roy S, Verma A, *et al.* Multifunctional natural polymer systems in inflammatory bowel disease therapy: Recent advancements. J Drug Target 2021; 29(3): 215-29.

[68] Zhang X, Li Y, Li . Nanotechnology in IBD therapy: Natural polymer-based nanoparticles for targeted drug delivery. Drug Dev Ind Pharm 2023; (7): 890-901.

[69] Pathak S, Yadav M, Sharma P, *et al.* Nanostructured hydrogels for tissue repair in IBD: Natural polymer-based strategies. Nanomaterials (Basel) 2023; 13(6): 1019.
[PMID: 36985914]

[70] Liu Z, Wang Y, Zhang N. Micelle-like nanoassemblies based on polymer–drug conjugates as an emerging platform for drug delivery. Expert Opinion on Drug Delivery 2022; (7): 805-22.
[http://dx.doi.org/10.1517/17425247.2012.689284]

[71] Wang Y, Li X, Yang X, *et al.* Microbiome-based therapies and natural polymers in IBD: A promising synergy. World J Gastroenterol 2024; 30(1): 45-58.
[http://dx.doi.org/10.3748/wjg.v4.i1.45] [PMID: 38293326]

[72] Gupta P. Collaborative efforts in the clinical translation of polymer-based drug delivery systems for inflammatory bowel disease: Challenges and opportunities. J Control Release 2022; 341: 42-57.

[73] Patel S, Sharma P, Singh . Interdisciplinary collaboration in polymer-based therapies for inflammatory bowel disease: Bridging research and clinical applications. Drug Dev Ind Pharm 2023; (1): 11-9.

[74] Kim YH, Lee HJ, Lee JW, *et al.* Regulatory considerations and industry partnerships in the clinical translation of natural polymers for IBD therapies. Eur J Pharm Sci 2021; 161: 105769.

[75] Zhang Y, Wang J, Li J, *et al.* Advancements in polymer engineering for targeted therapies in IBD: A collaborative approach. Biomaterials 2024; 273: 120768.

[76] Kumar S, Verma P, Malik . Standardization and clinical translation of natural polymer-based drug delivery systems for inflammatory bowel disease: Collaborative pathways for success. AAPS PharmSciTech 2022; (4):

[77] Singh P, Kumar M, Sharma . Advancements in nanotechnology: Revolutionizing drug delivery systems for precision targeted cancer therapy. Journal of Scientific Advances 2023; (1): 23-33.
[http://dx.doi.org/10.63665/jsa.v1i1.01]

[78] Patel P, Sharma S, Kumar R, *et al.* The role of interdisciplinary research in advancing personalized polymer-based therapies for inflammatory bowel disease. J Control Release 2022; 337: 219-32.

[79] Zhang Y, Wu X, Li J, *et al.* Collaborative efforts in nanotechnology and polymer engineering for optimizing IBD therapies: Addressing challenges in drug delivery systems. Nanomedicine (Lond) 2021; 16(8): 1059-74.

[80] Lee HJ, Park S, Kang YJ, *et al.* Interdisciplinary strategies in the development of natural polymer-based drug delivery systems for inflammatory bowel disease. Drug Dev Ind Pharm 2022; 48(6): 909-17.

[81] Yadav V, Kumar S, Verma A, *et al.* Collaborative pathways for optimizing polymer-based drug delivery systems in personalized medicine for IBD treatment. AAPS PharmSciTech 2024; 25(1): 28.

[82] Singh P, Yadav M, Verma A, *et al.* Regulatory guidelines for the approval of natural polymer-based drug delivery systems: Ensuring safety and efficacy in IBD therapy. Drug Deliv Transl Res 2023;

13(4): 815-28.

[83] Kumar S. The role of regulatory agencies in the commercialization of natural polymer-based drug delivery systems for inflammatory bowel disease. J Control Release 2021; 337: 208-21.

[84] Zhang Y, Lee S, Kim H, *et al.* Regulatory challenges in the approval of biodegradable and biocompatible natural polymers for drug delivery. Eur J Pharm Biopharm 2022; 175: 33-45.

[85] Patel P, Kumar S, Gupta P, *et al.* Establishing clear regulatory pathways for natural polymer-based drug delivery systems in inflammatory bowel disease. AAPS J 2024; 26(1): 15-28. [PMID: 38267593]

[86] Chen L, Yang X, Liu J, *et al.* Regulatory perspectives on natural polymer-based therapies for inflammatory bowel disease: Addressing biodegradability and biocompatibility. Biomater Sci 2021; 9(7): 2564-76.

[87] Liu Y, Zhang Y, Li X, *et al.* Clinical trial design for evaluating polymer-based therapies in inflammatory bowel disease: Key considerations for patient populations and treatment outcomes. J Clin Pharmacol 2022; 62(4): 541-51. [PMID: 34657303]

[88] Gupta P, Kumar R, Sharma M, *et al.* Designing clinical trials for polymer-based drug delivery systems in IBD: Addressing patient heterogeneity and treatment efficacy. J Drug Target 2023; 31(2): 132-45.

[89] Singh P, Patel V, Yadav . Patient-centered clinical trial design in inflammatory bowel disease: Ensuring effective and acceptable polymerbased therapies. AAPS J 2021; (3).

[90] Lee HJ, Park J, Kim H, *et al.* The role of patient cohorts and real-world data in the clinical evaluation of natural polymer-based drug delivery systems for IBD. Clin Transl Sci 2023; 16(5): 1256-64.

[91] Zhang L, Li J, Wang Y, *et al.* Involving patients in the clinical development of polymer-based therapies for inflammatory bowel disease: Insights from advocacy groups and feedback mechanisms. Patient Educ Couns 2022; 105(9): 2145-53.

[92] Gonciarz W, Balcerczak E, Brzeziński M, *et al.* Chitosan-based formulations for therapeutic applications. A recent overview. J Biomed Sci 2025; 32(1): 62. [http://dx.doi.org/10.1186/s12929-025-01161-7] [PMID: 40629425]

[93] Martău GA, Mihai M, Vodnar DC. The use of chitosan, alginate, and pectin in the biomedical and food sector iocompatibility, bioadhesiveness, and biodegradability. Polymers (Basel) 2019; 11(11): 1837. [http://dx.doi.org/10.3390/polym11111837] [PMID: 31717269]

[94] Jangra N, Singla A, Puri V, *et al.* Herbal bioactive-loaded biopolymeric formulations for wound healing applications. RSC Advances 2025; 15(16): 12402-42. [http://dx.doi.org/10.1039/D4RA08604J] [PMID: 40248229]

SUBJECT INDEX

A

Accumulation 23, 119, 180, 182, 204, 214
Acidic conditions 19, 55, 98, 99, 105, 147
Active targeting strategies 27
Adalimumab 10, 165, 166
Adhesion 56, 121
Administration 80, 106, 147, 215
Algae 42, 50, 51, 123
Alterations 8, 22, 31, 126, 201, 209, 213, 214
Amino acids 45, 53, 123, 182
Animal 95, 97, 98, 107, 108, 133, 145, 178
  models 145, 178
  derived polymers 95, 97, 98, 107, 108, 133
Anti-inflammatory drugs 118, 123, 133, 176, 178, 186, 215
Antibiotics 12, 166, 167, 174, 190
Antibodies 150, 188, 214, 215
Antigen-presenting cells (APCs) 7, 161 `
Antigens 7, 55, 174
Antimicrobial properties 48, 55, 57
Antioxidant 55, 63, 103, 107, 143

B

Bacteria 2, 3, 5, 6, 21, 22, 50, 51, 76, 77, 82, 83, 164, 165, 202
Bacteroidetes 21, 127, 128
Barriers 21, 74, 194, 202, 214
Bifidobacterium 100, 132, 165
Biocompatible materials 89, 215
Biodegradable polymers (BDPs) 58, 143, 151, 153, 183, 194, 208, 215
Biological origins 121, 122
Biologics 8, 10, 12, 95, 98, 104, 160, 163, 164, 165, 166, 167
Biomarkers 53, 162, 216
Biopolymers 50, 60, 62, 80, 97, 108, 119, 122, 123, 133, 149
Biosynthesis 47, 48, 49, 51, 165, 182
Blood vessels 50, 53, 101, 106
Budesonide 27, 30, 84, 103, 105, 184, 186

C

Cancer treatment 55, 145, 183
Carbohydrates 41, 43, 44, 45, 54, 55, 146, 175
Carboxymethyl chitosan 128, 150
Carriers 20, 32, 83, 90, 144, 183, 188
Cartilage 47, 48, 53, 64, 101, 106
Cases 2, 5, 48, 50, 58, 96, 166, 167, 187, 200
CD4+ 161
CD44 receptors 103, 106
Cell 48, 49, 51, 55, 56, 61, 81, 82, 87, 203, 210
  encapsulation 51, 55, 61
  growth 48, 49, 55, 56, 87
  walls 55, 81, 82, 203, 210
Cellular uptake 19, 149, 184
Chemical modifications 42, 46, 88, 121, 129
Chitin 41, 44, 48, 50, 51, 98
Chondroitin sulfate (CS) 48, 51, 86, 95, 106, 107, 108, 148
Chronic inflammation 7, 18, 21, 22, 31, 74, 160, 206, 208
Ciprofloxacin 146, 166, 167, 174
Clinical 18, 62, 63, 121, 153, 163, 165, 180, 213, 215, 216, 217
  applications 18, 62, 63, 121, 153, 165, 180, 213, 215
  trials 163, 216, 217
Collagen-based scaffolds 133, 205, 208
Colonic bacteria 99, 105, 120, 184
Compounds 78, 80, 177, 189

Connective tissues 44, 47, 48, 53, 63, 103, 203, 209
Controlled 45, 48, 49, 55, 56, 59, 61, 63, 88, 97, 146, 164, 165, 166, 185, 186, 215
drug release 45, 88
release 48, 49, 55, 56, 59, 61, 63, 97, 146, 164, 165, 166, 185, 186, 215
Corticosteroids 8, 9, 104, 117, 133, 173, 174, 194, 201, 206, 208
Crohn's disease (CD) 1, 2, 4, 5, 6, 7, 12, 18, 20, 22, 74, 75, 84, 85, 95, 96, 117, 149, 161, 166, 174, 191, 200, 201, 206
Cross-linking 48, 51, 57, 85, 211, 213
Curcumin 30, 101, 128, 177, 203
Cyclodextrins 74, 78, 79, 82, 84, 88, 89, 90, 143, 145, 153
Cytotoxicity 148, 149, 180

D

Dextran sodium sulfate (DSS) 23, 24, 84, 86, 100, 126, 131, 132, 185
Diagnosis 75, 161, 162, 173
Diagnostic tools 26, 32, 52, 212
Differentiation 51, 53, 54, 60, 161, 183
Disease severity 20, 26, 107, 217
Drug 18, 31, 32, 45, 52, 55, 76, 88, 134, 143, 148, 149, 153, 178, 183, 215
accumulation 148, 149
carriers 32, 52, 55, 76, 134, 143, 178
release kinetics 18
solubility 31, 45, 88, 153, 183, 215
Dysbiosis 3, 12, 18, 19, 21, 26, 31, 166, 202, 209

E

Elasticity 53, 54, 55, 56, 60
Enzymatic 99, 103, 106, 129, 130, 178, 183, 211
breakdown 103
degradation 99, 106, 129, 130, 178, 183, 211
Epithelial cells 21, 24, 28, 32, 118, 133, 176
European Medicines Agency (EMA) 108, 163, 176, 213, 217, 218
Exopolysaccharides 118, 123, 129

F

Fabrication 50, 144, 146, 147, 183, 213
Factors 1, 3, 4, 12, 49, 58, 62, 63, 132, 163
Fibrosis 18, 21, 22, 31
Films 41, 50, 52, 55, 133
Functional groups 43, 58, 79, 127
Fungi 2, 50, 63, 117, 119, 128

G

Gastrointestinal tract 12, 23, 96, 120, 125, 162, 178, 180, 184, 193, 202
Gelatin nanoparticles 100, 101
Gelling agents 45, 88
Gels 52, 55, 59, 133, 165
Genetic variables 4, 201
Glucose units 49, 51, 145
Glycosaminoglycans 47, 48, 103, 106, 127, 209
Glycosidic bonds 48, 49, 52, 77
Growth factors 48, 55, 56, 61, 118, 209
Gut 6, 88, 89, 174, 175, 205, 210
bacteria 6, 88, 89, 174, 205, 210
barrier 175

H

Histological examination 102, 104
Homeostasis 1, 126, 189

I

IL-1a 21, 89, 100, 101, 102, 104, 126, 128, 129
IL-4 128, 129
IL-10 8, 100, 128, 129, 177
IL-17 21, 128, 129
Immune 19, 20, 22, 23, 24, 31, 117, 206
cell infiltration 22, 23, 24
dysregulation 19, 20, 31, 117, 206

Immunomodulatory effects 54, 74, 123, 205, 212
Immunosuppressants 9, 11, 117, 118, 166, 194, 201, 206
In-vitro dissolution studies 130
Infections 12, 21, 49, 51, 55, 57, 165, 173, 201
Infliximab 10, 125, 150, 165, 166
Intestinal 21, 84, 89, 118, 211
  epithelium cells 118
  permeability 21, 84, 89, 211

J

Junction proteins 100, 102, 126, 127

L

Ligands 27, 32, 121, 183, 186, 215
Limitations 40, 51, 88, 89, 160, 165, 167, 180, 183, 193, 201
Liposomes 28, 30, 48

M

Macrophages 2, 8, 20, 23, 24, 30, 32, 89, 126, 179
Manufacturing techniques 43, 153
Mechanisms 1, 4, 8, 25, 118, 125, 133, 151, 152, 153, 163
Medication delivery methods 176
Mesalamine 87, 102, 133, 217
Metronidazole 130, 166, 167, 174
Microencapsulation 59, 62
Microenvironment 18, 20, 60, 83, 215
Microorganisms 1, 3, 41, 57, 78, 119, 185
Microparticles 85, 97, 125, 177, 179, 185, 207
Modifications 43, 55, 59, 82, 85, 149, 179, 210, 214
Molecular weight (MW) 54, 58, 78, 82, 118, 119, 175, 177, 180, 182, 184, 211, 213
Monoclonal antibodies 10, 117, 174, 178, 185
Monomers 41, 48, 49, 59, 179
Mucosa 173, 208
Mucosal healing 20, 95, 161, 162, 203, 205, 208, 214, 216, 217, 219
Multifunctional nanocarriers 20, 32

N

Nano-carriers 19, 95, 98
Nanogels 106, 107, 215
Nanotechnology 18, 19, 20, 23, 26, 31, 32, 184, 187, 194, 215, 216, 219
Natural polymers 41, 56, 59, 63, 88, 153, 164, 214, 216
Negative charges 48, 76, 88, 103, 105, 122, 184
Neutrophils 2, 20, 23, 24
Nucleic acids 41, 50, 51, 184, 186, 192

O

Oligosaccharides 78, 126, 145
Organs 50, 52, 59, 60, 61
Outcomes 5, 146, 148, 149, 175
Oxidative stress 19, 23, 29, 132, 133, 179

P

Packaging 44, 46, 47, 52, 63
Particle size 88, 120, 213
Patent 66, 67, 152, 153, 188, 189, 190, 191, 192
Pathogenesis 1, 3, 209
Pathophysiology 3, 11, 21, 132, 160, 163, 205, 206, 216
Patient compliance 117, 215, 218, 219
Peptides 55, 102, 147, 192
Permeability 89, 124, 143
Pharmacokinetics 59, 147, 167, 183, 217
Polyacrylates 175, 177, 179
Polyesters 41, 122, 123, 175, 180
Polyethylene glycol (PEG) 57, 145, 175, 178, 183
Polyglutamic acid (PGA) 122, 123, 130, 131, 183
Polyhydroxyalkanoates 57, 182
Polyisoprenes 41, 55
Polymer chains 43, 49, 57, 185
Polymeric 183, 184, 186
  drug conjugates 183
  nanoparticles 184, 186
Polyphenols 104, 175, 177, 178, 184,

203
Polysaccharides 41, 42, 47, 48, 49, 50, 51, 61, 62, 63, 76, 122, 127, 128, 202
Porosity 183, 185
Prebiotics 76, 82, 88, 200, 202, 209, 216
Prednisolone 9, 104, 107, 186
Pro-inflammatory cytokines 8, 10, 18, 21, 84, 89, 118, 128, 178, 205, 209
Probiotics 11, 84, 87, 130, 132, 160, 164, 165, 166, 167, 187, 209, 210, 215, 216
Production 9, 11, 44, 49, 55, 78, 82, 89, 126, 127, 213, 216, 218
Proliferation 51, 53, 54, 55, 61, 84, 126, 183, 205, 210
Proteases 22, 29, 105
Proteobacteria 6, 21

R

Reactive oxygen species (ROS) 18, 19, 23, 25, 28, 32, 86, 104, 105, 126, 127, 128, 132, 174, 177, 180, 185, 186, 187
Receptors 24, 27, 86, 161, 214
Regeneration 47, 59, 183
Remission 7, 174, 217
Renewable resources 41, 67
Reproducibility 26, 58, 153, 182, 183
Retention time 143, 208

S

Safety profiles 108, 166
Scaffolds 48, 51, 53, 55, 56, 59, 61, 85, 98, 103, 183
Scalability 26, 133, 153, 182, 200
Signaling pathways 47, 179
Smoking 3, 5, 6, 7
Sodium alginate 123, 126, 130
Soft tissues 47, 52, 61, 62, 65
Solubility 43, 74, 80, 85, 98, 117, 145, 151, 184
Stability 45, 46, 88, 89, 90, 97, 119, 120, 129, 130, 178, 184, 210, 211, 213
Starch derivatives 46, 203
Stem cells 48, 60, 186
Structure 45, 48, 49, 52, 53, 54, 55, 56, 58, 60, 64, 175, 182
Substrates 48, 49, 75, 182, 205
Sulfated polysaccharides 81, 119, 132
Synthetic polymers 43, 44, 46, 49, 50, 119, 175, 176, 180, 181, 182
Systemic 18, 105, 166, 173, 207
  exposure 166, 173, 207
  toxicity 18, 105, 173

T

Targeted drug delivery 25, 66, 74, 80, 95, 97, 201, 202, 203, 205
Techniques 88, 184, 191, 192
Technologies 62, 65, 143, 146, 150, 214
Temperature 48, 62, 101, 129, 151, 152, 183, 186, 214
Textiles 41, 44, 51, 67, 81, 145, 147
Therapeutic 12, 18, 30, 76, 88, 95, 99, 100, 103, 105, 106, 107, 108, 119, 125, 129, 147, 151, 153, 163, 164, 165, 167, 177, 180, 184, 188, 193, 205, 207, 211, 214, 215
  agents 76, 95, 163, 184, 193, 207, 214, 215
  choices 12
  effectiveness 88, 95, 108, 125, 129, 147, 177, 188, 211
  efficacy 99, 100, 103, 105, 106, 107, 119, 151, 153, 164, 165, 180, 184
  outcomes 18, 30, 167, 205
Therapies 10, 53, 62, 200, 201, 207, 211, 212, 214, 217, 219
Tissue engineering 47, 49, 51, 53, 54, 55, 63
Tissues 21, 31, 47, 50, 51, 53, 55, 56, 57, 59, 60, 61, 82, 183, 185
Tofacitinib 11, 106, 164, 166
Toxicity 59, 151, 163, 176, 180
Transcription factors 118, 161

U

Ulcerative colitis (UC) 1, 2, 4, 6, 7, 11, 12, 75, 95, 96, 102, 106, 107, 131, 161, 162, 165, 166, 174, 201

V

Variability 20, 42, 211, 212, 213, 219
Variations 31, 97, 162, 211
Vedolizumab 165, 166
Viscosity 49, 54, 85, 97, 147, 182

W

Weight management 88
Wound 44, 48, 49, 50, 51, 52, 53, 54, 55, 60, 61, 62, 65, 67, 133
  dressings 44, 49, 50, 51, 52, 53, 55, 60, 61, 65
  healing 48, 51, 52, 53, 54, 55, 60, 62, 65, 67, 133

X

Xanthan gum 42, 117, 119, 129, 130, 133, 164

www.ingramcontent.com/pod-product-compliance
Lightning Source LLC
LaVergne TN
LVHW070949210926
848482LV00002B/157